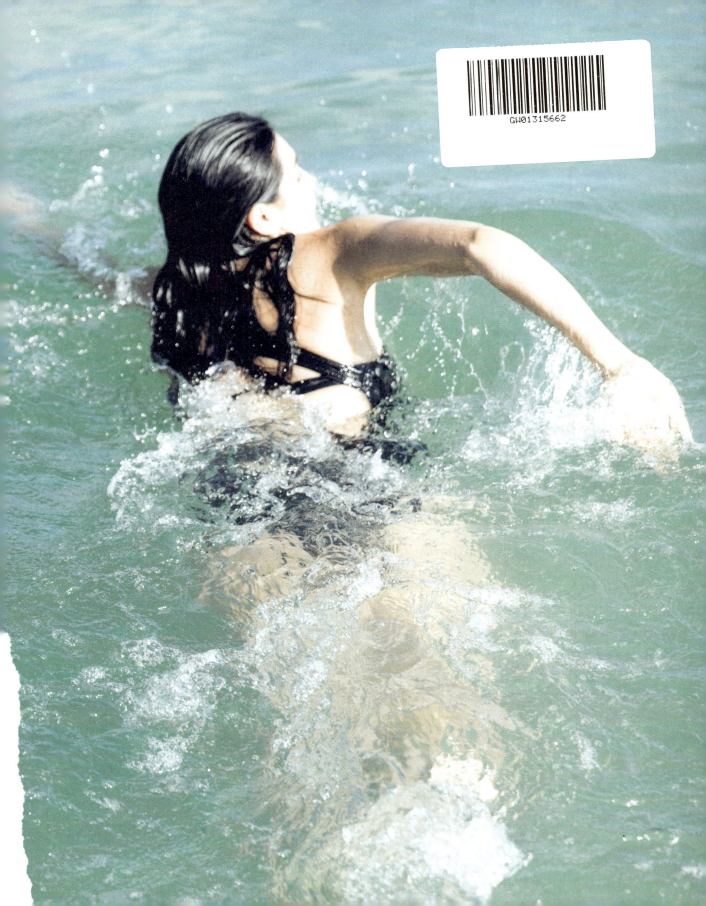

NADIA LIM'S
FRESH START COOKBOOK

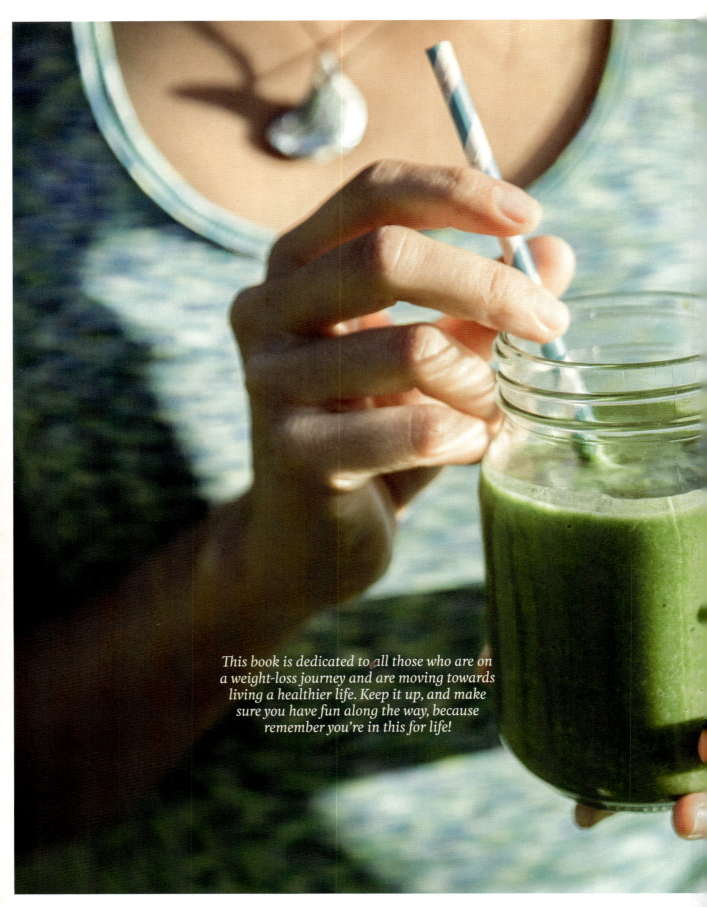

This book is dedicated to all those who are on a weight-loss journey and are moving towards living a healthier life. Keep it up, and make sure you have fun along the way, because remember you're in this for life!

NADIA LIM'S
FRESH START
COOKBOOK

Over 100 delicious everyday recipes for lasting good health and weight loss

Photography by Tam West

RANDOM HOUSE
NEW ZEALAND

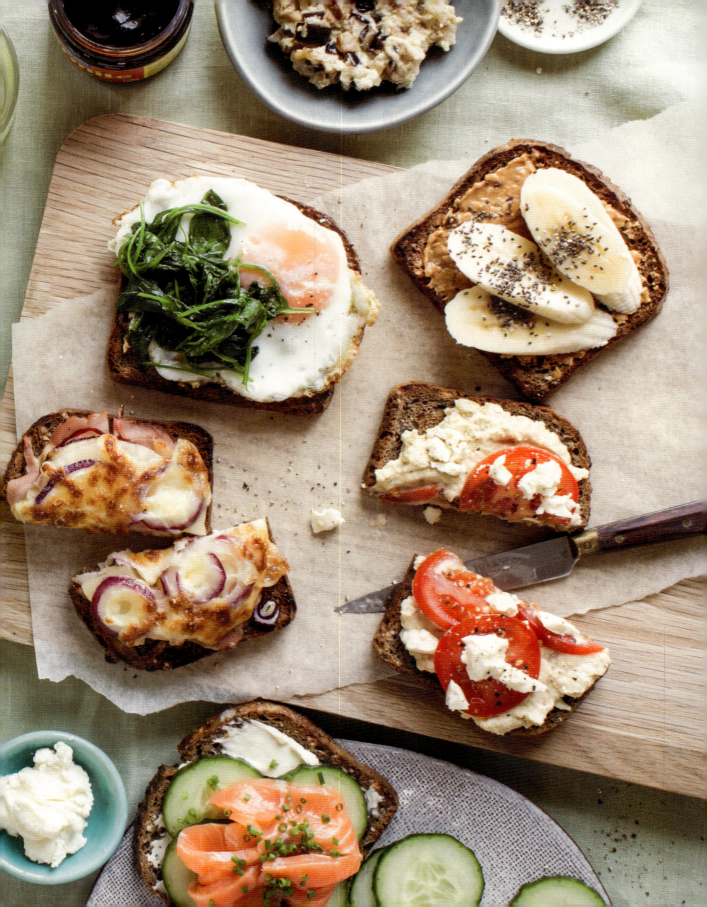

7	**A FRESH START**
11	**HOW TO USE THIS BOOK**
18	**YOUR NEW HEALTH RULES**
29	**BREAKFAST**
69	**LUNCH**
111	**DINNER**
112	VEGETARIAN
133	MEAT
166	CHICKEN
194	FISH + SEAFOOD
217	**DESSERTS + TREATS**
253	**HEALTHY SNACKS**
276	**ESSENTIALS**
281	**TIME TO GET MOVING**
307	**FIT TIPS**
313	**ACKNOWLEDGEMENTS**
314	**RECIPE INDEX**

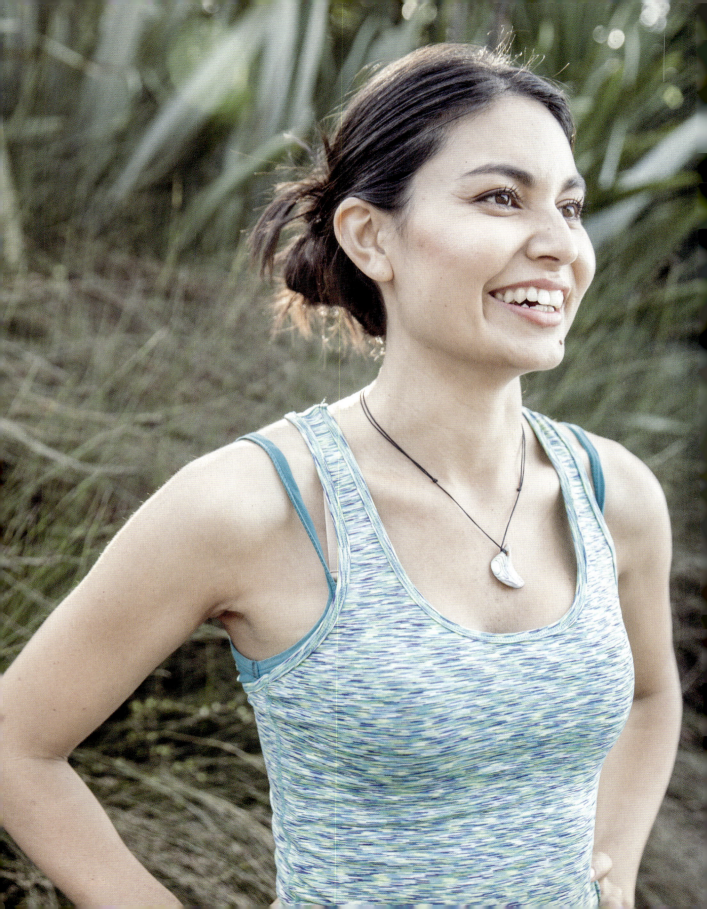

A FRESH START

This is not a diet book. Although I'm a qualified dietitian, I don't believe in diets. What I do believe in, though, is eating real food that nourishes you and in keeping active in a way that is easy and enjoyable so that it becomes a long-lasting, sustainable practice.

I felt compelled to write this book because it's clear that there is still a lot of confusion around what it means to be healthy and how to lose weight. I receive countless requests from people asking for recipes, meal plans and dietary advice. There's a lot of nonsense health and weight-loss information out there that simply isn't necessary, sustainable or good for your body (and mind). We're constantly bombarded with the latest diets and studies, but isn't it ironic that the more nutrition information becomes available, the unhealthier we become? I want to set the record straight, get back to basics and show you what it really means to be and feel healthy, and lose weight (if you need to) in a simple, enjoyable and sustainable way that will last forever.

I came up with the idea of Nude Food when I was just 12 years old, and it has been my mantra ever since. I wasn't referring to cooking or eating in the nude, in case that's what you were thinking! Rather, Nude Food simply signifies food that is free from being dressed up in fancy packages, marketing and additives. You don't have to shop at fancy stores for special 'health' ingredients, be a label-reading expert, rack up a big grocery bill, or be a whizz in the kitchen to eat nutritious, delicious food every day.

Being a Nude Foodie is all about focusing on what you should eat and add to your life, not take out. It's about leading a positive lifestyle, not obsessing over inflexible food rules or sticking to a stringent gym routine. In this age of confusing information overload, we seem to have forgotten the basics of living a gratifying, healthy life. What if we stripped away the ongoing distractions — food fads, latest science and media hype — and began listening to our bodies? When it comes to wellbeing, one size does not fit all (we're far too genetically varied!). For something to work long-term, it has to fit in with your lifestyle, your genetics and your taste buds.

So I'm not going to prescribe you a strict diet or set of food rules to follow. My focus has always been on making healthy eating as simple, easy and delicious as possible for everyday, busy people like me. I like flexibility, so I've created over 100 delicious, easy recipes, covering every meal, that you can choose from to create your own tailored everyday healthy eating plan. All you have to do is flick through the pages and choose what delicious breakfast, lunch, dinner, snacks (and sometimes dessert!) you want to eat. I've done all the work to make sure they fit the bill in terms of nutrition and calorie count. If you're looking to lose weight, I suggest following this eating and exercise plan for 12 weeks. The great thing about this plan is its flexibility — you can chop and change the meals as you like!

Nutrition comes first and foremost; you can only lose weight if you're properly nourished; an undernourished body will crave more food in an attempt to get the nutrients it needs. For that reason I don't like to highlight calorie counting, as you won't learn how to fuel your body properly if you focus on numbers instead of nutrients. So while I've ensured that all of these recipes meet a certain calorie criteria (around 350 calories for breakfast, 450 calories for lunch, 550 calories for dinner and 100 calories per snack), I want you to pay more attention to your food groups and portion sizes, and this book will show you exactly how to do that.

Now to the other important part of the equation — exercise! I'm no gym bunny, but with the help of fitness expert Michael McCormack (aka 'Coach Dingo') I've found a way to fit exercise into my hectic life and make it fun. With Michael's help I've created an exercise plan to get you on track to being the healthiest, fittest, most energetic version of yourself, and to lose weight, if you need to, in a safe, realistic way.

Michael's put together some great exercises that will get results, no matter what your current fitness level is. No special equipment is needed — the exercises are designed to do in the comfort of your own home or outdoors — so you can easily incorporate them anywhere, anytime.

So, are you ready to refresh the way you live, and find your fittest, healthiest, happiest self? Add a little zest and inspiration and become a Nude Foodie! Flick the page and let's make a fresh start!

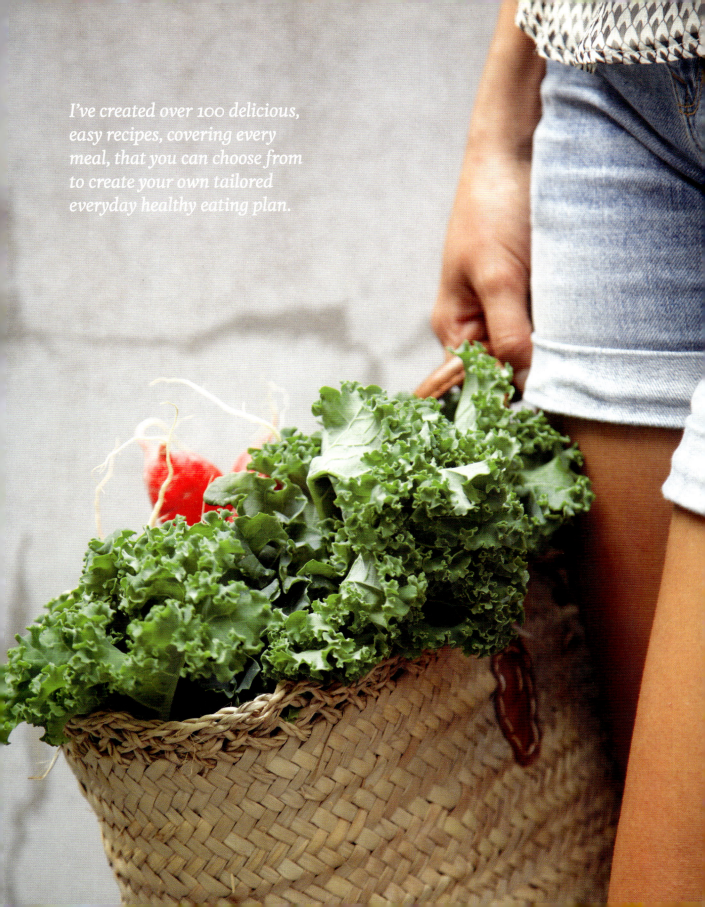

I've created over 100 delicious, easy recipes, covering every meal, that you can choose from to create your own tailored everyday healthy eating plan.

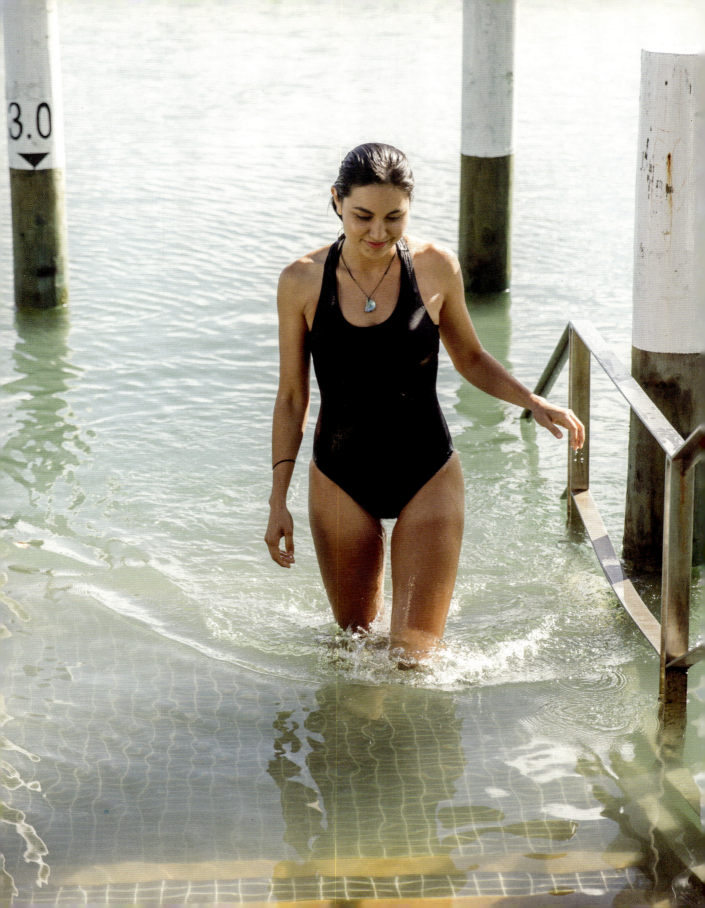

HOW TO USE THIS BOOK

The recipes in this book are designed to fit into three levels of eating plans providing all the nutrition you need from protein, vegetables, unprocessed carbohydrates and healthy fats.

Women who want to lose weight should go on Plan 1. To maintain weight, Plan 2 or Plan 3 is right for most women. Most men who want to lose weight should go on Plan 3, or add in an extra serve of protein at lunch and dinner for weight maintenance (see pages 16-17 for informatin on food groups).

The best rate of weight loss to aim for is 0.5-1kg per week (unless you are substantially overweight, in which case you may lose more). Any more than this is too fast as you will be losing muscle and water. Muscle mass increases your metabolism, helping you to burn calories faster. Keep in mind that weight loss is only one measure, and not always the best measure of progress. Equally important is your body shape and muscle tone — if you are not substantially overweight you may find that your weight does not change much, but that your muscle mass and tone increases and your body shape changes.

On the following pages is an example of a menu for one week. You can substitute any of the meals for any of the other recipes in the book. Because all the recipes are nutrition and calorie controlled, you can choose any breakfast, lunch, dinner, snack and dessert to make up your daily plan throughout the entire 12 weeks that I suggest you do this for, to see results and make sure good habits are well and truly formed.

In addition, to help you get moving, fitness expert Michael McCormack has developed three exercise plans (see pages 281-309), based on whether you are at a beginner, intermediate or more advanced level of fitness. These are practical and able to be done by anyone, in any environment, so you don't need a gym membership or any special equipment (other than a Swiss ball and a skipping rope).

PLAN 1 (approx. 1500cal/day)

Breakfast
Lunch
Dinner
Snacks (2 per day including 1 fruit)
Dessert (1 per week)
Extras (up to 2 per week)

PLAN 2 (approx. 1600cal/day)

Breakfast
Lunch
Dinner
Snacks (2-3 per day including 1 fruit)
Dessert (2 per week)
Extras (up to 3 per week)

PLAN 3 (approx. 1700cal/day)

Breakfast
Lunch
Dinner
Snacks (3 per day including 1 fruit)
Dessert (2 per week)
Extras (up to 4 per week)

SAMPLE MENU

Here is a sample menu plan for a week on the Plan 1 programme (see page 11). If you're following a Plan 2 or Plan 3 programme, simply add in a dessert, snack or extra as specified on page 11.

You can follow this menu exactly, or change up the meals as you like, substituting any recipe from this book. On some days you might even like to make up your own meal, as long as you substitute an equal quantity of each food group, e.g. 150g steak for 150g chicken, or ½ cup cooked pasta for ½ cup couscous. See pages 16-17 for what constitutes a portion size for each food group. You can tailor your meals to suit your taste buds and lifestyle, just as long as you tick off all the food groups and stick to the recommended quantities you need each day (see pages 15-17).

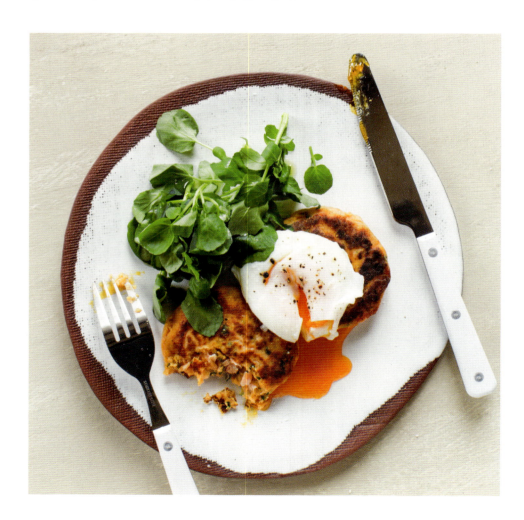

DAY	BREAKFAST	LUNCH	DINNER	SNACKS	DESSERTS + EXTRAS
1	Cherry + coconut granola (p.40) made on the weekend	French tuna, egg + caper pan bagnat (p.97)	Lamb baharat with braised parsnips, carrots + barley (p.136)	Avocado, tomato, olive + basil Ryvita (p.267) Piece of fruit	
2	Green colada (p.32) Scrambled eggs	Lamb with Moroccan chickpeas (p.90) using leftover lamb from dinner	Mediterranean baked fish (p.204)	Hummus with vegetable sticks (p.270) Piece of fruit	
3	Instant cinnamon, apple + almond bircher bowl (p.34)	Maple-roasted pumpkin + onion soup (p.75) from the freezer	Oriental poached chicken noodle bowl (p.181)	Oaty apple + sultana muffin (p.257) from the freezer Piece of fruit	
4	Swedish breakfast smörgås (p.47)	Vietnamese chicken noodle box (p.84) using leftover chicken from dinner	Asian steak tacos (p.155)	Hummus with vegetable sticks (p.270) Piece of fruit	
5	Cherry + coconut granola (p.40) made on the weekend	Maple-roasted pumpkin + onion soup (p.75) from the freezer	Turkish lamb kofte (p.133)	Oaty apple + sultana muffin (p.257) from the freezer Piece of fruit	Apple, blackberry + date nut crumble (p.240)
6	Smoked salmon cakes (p.39)	Steak open sandwich (p.97)	Cauliflower-crust pizza (p.112)	Kale chips (p.274) Piece of fruit	2 x 130ml glasses of wine
7	The works (p.43)	Sweet chilli prawn noodle box (p.87)	Tandoori roast chicken + vegetables (p.176)	2 biscotti (p.264) with a coffee Piece of fruit	

HOW TO USE THIS BOOK

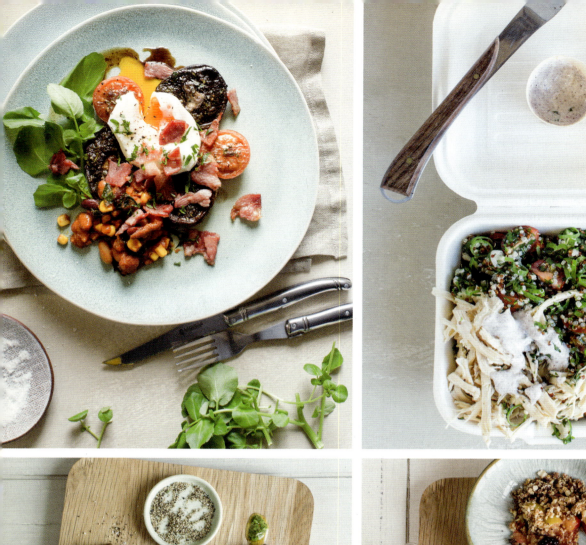
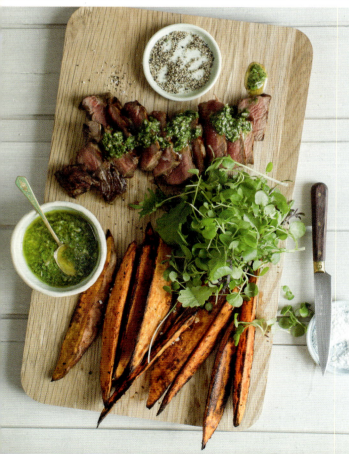
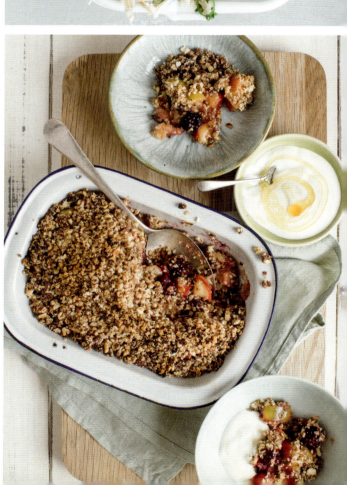

THE RIGHT BALANCE

I don't believe in calorie counting, as you won't learn how to fuel your body properly if you focus on numbers instead of nutrients. So while I have developed all these recipes to meet certain calorie and nutrition requirements, instead of counting calories I want you to get used to knowing your food groups and portion sizes (see pages 16-17). If there's anything you should be counting, it should be nutrients!

Every day you should be having: 3 portions unprocessed carbohydrates, at least 4-5 portions of (non-starchy) vegetables, 2 portions fruit, 2 portions protein, 3 portions healthy fats and 1-2 portions dairy (or dairy substitutes). This will ensure you're getting a healthy balance of fat, protein and carbohydrates, as well as vitamins and minerals. Then you can have a few little extras on top of this for pleasure! This sample menu from Plan 1 shows how easy it is to cover all your food groups by choosing meals from this book. Remember to make sure you are drinking enough fluid every day.

	RECIPE	FOOD GROUPS
Breakfast	Cherry + coconut granola with banana and milk (p.40)	1 unprocessed carbohydrate 1 dairy (or dairy substitute) 1 fruit
Lunch	Chicken quinoa tabouleh with yoghurt dressing + a piece of fruit (p.99)	1 unprocessed carbohydrate 1 protein 2½ vegetables 1½ healthy fats 1 fruit
Dinner	Steak, smoky kumara fries + salsa verde (p.141)	1 unprocessed carbohydrate 1 protein 2 vegetables 1 healthy fat
Snacks	2 prune, cocoa + coconut bliss balls (p.261)	1 snack (also provides 1 healthy fat)
Dessert **(1 per week)**	Apple, blackberry + date nut crumble (p.240)	1 dessert (also provides 1 healthy fat and 1 fruit)
Extras **(up to 2 per week)**	1 x 130ml glass of wine	1 extra
Drinks	6 glasses water 3 herbal teas	9 cups fluid

KNOW YOUR FOOD GROUPS

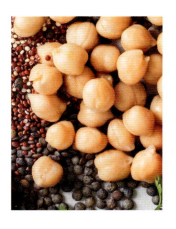

VEGETABLES (at least 4–5 per day)

1 portion is equal to:

- 1 cup cooked or raw vegetables
- 1 cup leafy green salad leaves

* Non-starchy vegetables are the one food group that you can eat as much as you like!

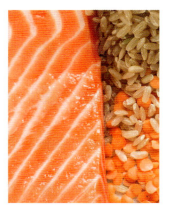

UNPROCESSED CARBOHYDRATES (about 3 per day)

1 portion is equal to:

- 1 medium potato (approximately 150g)
- 150g sweet potato or kumara
- ½ cup cooked brown rice
- ½ cup cooked pasta or noodles
- ½ cup cooked quinoa or barley
- ¾ cup cooked legumes, e.g. beans, chickpeas, lentils
- 2 crispbreads, e.g. Ryvita
- ⅓ cup muesli, cereal or oats
- 1 thin slice wholegrain bread

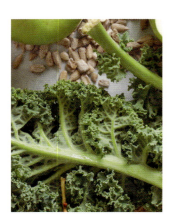

FRUIT (about 2 per day)

1 portion is equal to:

- roughly what fits in the palm of your hand for fresh fruit, e.g. 2 small apricots, 1 small apple, 1 orange, 1 small or ½ large banana, 1 pear, ½ cup diced mango
- ½ cup frozen fruit, e.g. berries
- ½ cup tinned fruit, e.g. tinned peaches

LEAN PROTEIN (about 2 per day)

1 portion is equal to:

- 125–150g raw meat or chicken
- 100g cooked meat or chicken
- 150g raw fish
- 100g smoked or cooked fish
- 2 eggs
- 100g tofu
- 1 cup beans, lentils or chickpeas
- 80g haloumi

DAIRY PRODUCTS OR SUBSTITUTES (about 2 per day)

1 portion is equal to:

- 1 cup milk of any kind, e.g. almond, cow's, soy, oat, rice milk
- ½ cup yoghurt
- 20-25g full-fat cheese, e.g. parmesan or cheddar
- 50-60g lower fat cheese, e.g. haloumi, feta or mozzarella

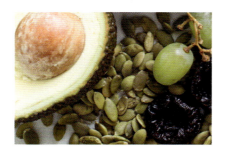

HEALTHY FATS (about 3 per day)

1 portion is equal to:

- ¼ avocado
- 20g (1½-2 tablespoons) nuts and seeds
- 1 tablespoon oil, butter or substitute
- 2 tablespoons nut butter (e.g. peanut butter)

DRINKS (at least 8 per day)

- You can drink water and herbal teas freely
- Have a small coffee no more than once per day
- Alcohol comes under 'extras'

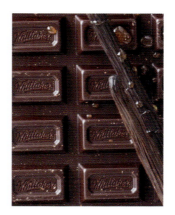

EXTRAS (up to 2-4 per week)

1 portion is equal to any extra food that equates to approximately 100kcal (420kJ), such as:

- 1 x 130ml glass of wine
- 250ml beer
- 1 small 200ml hot chocolate or Milo
- 20g chocolate

YOUR NEW HEALTH RULES

Great health is more than just eating well and exercising. Stress, sleep, caffeine, alcohol, breathing and digestive health are all equally important factors.

Once you get these areas of your life sorted, it makes the eating and exercising part easier too. These are your new health rules — they'll not only make you fitter and healthier, but give you energy, vitality, clearer thinking and a sense of purpose.

1. **CHANGE YOUR MINDSET TO THE GLASS IS HALF FULL**
Think about what foods you need to *add* for health instead of subtract. Diets make you feel guilty about indulging in something you 'shouldn't' have. That's a negative approach, and negative thoughts lead to negative outcomes, hence diets simply aren't sustainable. Turn the traditional diet mentality on its head and focus on what you *should* be having every day, rather than what you're 'not allowed'. When you take this positive approach to include all the things your body needs to be nourished, it leaves very little room for the less healthy things. Take a few seconds before you choose a food to ask yourself whether it's useful to you, i.e. does it provide lots of useful nutrients?

2. **LOVE REAL FOOD**
Real food is food that comes from the ground, sea and sky, not the highly processed stuff in packets. Real food goes off if it's not refrigerated, and has a limited shelf life — think of all your fresh produce. These foods are nutrient-dense, providing the most 'bang for buck' in terms of the nutrients they contain for their number of calories. Instead of trying to decipher food labels and being fooled by health claims, buy less processed, packaged foods, which are often stripped of nutrients and laden with fat, salt, sugar and preservatives during processing to prolong their shelf life. They provide nothing but empty calories, leaving your body hungry for more food in an attempt to gain the nutrition it needs.

3. **STOP COUNTING NUMBERS**
This applies to calories, grams of fat, carbohydrates and the number on the bathroom scales. If you want to count something, count the nutrients you're getting by making sure you're ticking off all the food groups you need every day (see page pages 16-17). I strongly recommend that you don't weigh yourself any more than once a month. It's important to turn your attention towards focusing on nutrition rather than weight, as it's only once you're in a relaxed, happy (and healthy body) state that you will start to lose weight. Your food choices should be based on whether they provide useful nutrients to you, not on their number of calories.

    Set a new goal every week (e.g. this week I will have a green smoothie

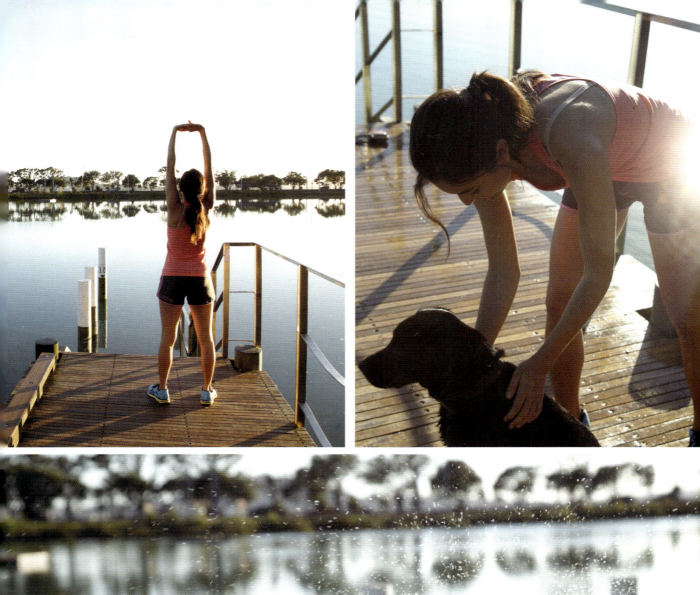
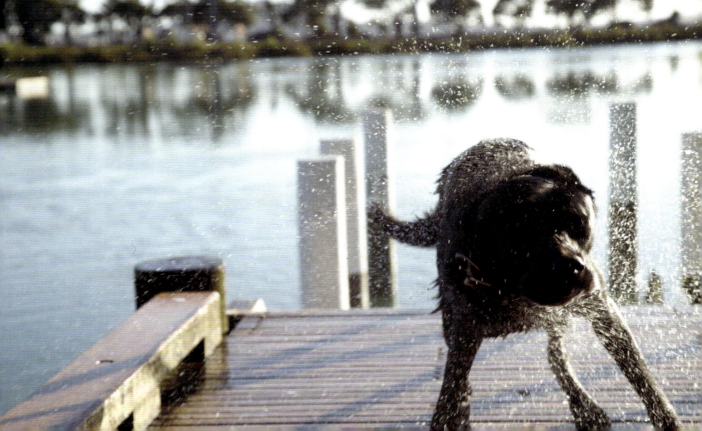

every day as a snack to boost my leafy green intake); measure your success by what healthy eating and exercise behaviours or goals have now formed into habits. You will find that weight loss will be a by-product of these habits later down the track. The number on the scales can sabotage your efforts and motivation, and is completely irrelevant to begin with. Fluctuations in body weight often naturally occur as your body adjusts, and if you are gaining muscle and losing fat it is possible your weight may not change much to begin with (as muscle weighs more than fat), so it is much better to go by how you feel and how your clothes fit. In fact, I suggest you throw your scales away (I haven't owned any for more than five years) and only get weighed every month — you can just drop in to your doctor's and do this for free. What is most important is how you feel — the positive reinforcement of feeling good is what will see you ultimately succeed in the long run.

4 HYDRATION

Keeping well hydrated is essential for a healthy digestive system, properly functioning kidneys, hydrating your skin and other organs, and keeping your brain alert. Thirst is often mistaken for hunger, so if you're not drinking enough you can tend to overeat. Dehydration is also one of the most common causes of constipation and feeling 'fuzzy'. You should drink little else other than water and herbal teas (other than smoothies, which are more like a small meal blended up). At least eight cups of water a day is a good guide, but it will depend on how much you sweat as well (from the weather or exercise). The best guide is to look at the colour of your pee: it should be a very pale straw colour, not at all dark or yellow. Eventually, your natural thirst mechanism will kick in and let you know when and how much you need to drink.

5 ORGANISATION

Spending some time and effort getting organised will make things ten times easier throughout the week, and the easier things are, the more likely you will do them. Plan your meals for the week and cook at least two meals a week that you can freeze. For example: a batch of soup that you can freeze in portions in ziplock bags, ready to take to work for a 'heat and eat' lunch, and something for dinner that you can simply heat up and eat at the end of the day. You should always have lunch, dinner and snack options in the freezer for those days when you can't be bothered. You'll most certainly come across times like these, and you don't want this to be a road block that ruins all your good efforts!

Schedule in your exercise times in advance, so that you don't risk filling up your diary and leaving no time for it. Instead of catching up with friends for coffee, try meeting up for a walk or some yoga or stretching in the park. Or, if you've got to have that weekend coffee, pick a place that's a 30-minute walk from your house — that way you do your exercise and get your reward!

Have healthy habit triggers ready and waiting — for example, I always have my smoothie ingredients out on the bench by the blender, ready for me when I wake up in the morning. And on my exercise days I have my gear all laid out ready to go when I wake up or when I get home from work.

6   TAKE A BREAK FROM CAFFEINE AND ALCOHOL

If you drink coffee, limit it to one cup per day, and never have it after midday. Caffeine is a stimulant and has a very long half-life — it can still be in your system six hours after consumption, so if you have one in the afternoon it can severely interfere with your ability to sleep. Drink green tea, other herbal teas and hot water with lemon or ginger instead.

Alcohol is not only very high in calories and devoid of nutrients, but it is also a stimulant. While you might think it helps you to nod off, it decreases the quality of your sleep, and you won't feel as energised in the morning. Because it is metabolised by the liver, it also impedes many other important functions the liver has, such as breaking down glycogen into glucose for energy and detoxifying substances. I recommend being alcohol-free throughout the week and only drinking in moderation (i.e. not more than 2–3 drinks) on the weekend. In this eating plan, alcohol comes under 'extras'.

7   THE POWER OF SLEEP

Get at least eight hours' sleep a night, with ideally two hours before midnight (every hour before midnight is worth two after). Good-quality sleep is a strong factor linked to weight loss and maintenance. For good sleep, don't drink alcohol during the week, and limit caffeine to one small cup before midday. You need to have a cool room (around 18°C) and no screens at least 30 minutes before bedtime (i.e. no TV, computers, laptops or mobile phones). Turn your electronic devices onto flight mode so you don't get woken up and don't have any bright lights present, e.g. from your alarm clock. Sleep-train yourself by getting into a regular routine throughout the week — if you reinforce a rhythm, it will start to produce melatonin around the right time to make you feel sleepy, and release serotonin at the right time to help you wake up. Even if occasionally you aren't able to get to bed on time, still try to wake up at your routine wake-up time.

8   INCREASE INCIDENTAL MOVEMENT AND BUILD MUSCLE MASS

It's easy to build more exercise into your daily routine without slogging it out at the gym three hours a day. Here are some simple tips:

- Get up and move at least once every hour. For example, walk to the kitchen for a drink every hour.
- Build little bouts of activity into your everyday life. You should be stoked that you have stairs to take to get to your office — what a great opportunity to get a little butt workout in (this is what I think every time I have to climb four flights of stairs to get to my apartment!).
- Build muscle mass with resistance exercises to increase your metabolism,

Measure your success by what healthy eating and exercise behaviours or goals have now formed into habits. You will find that weight loss will be a by-product of these habits later down the track.

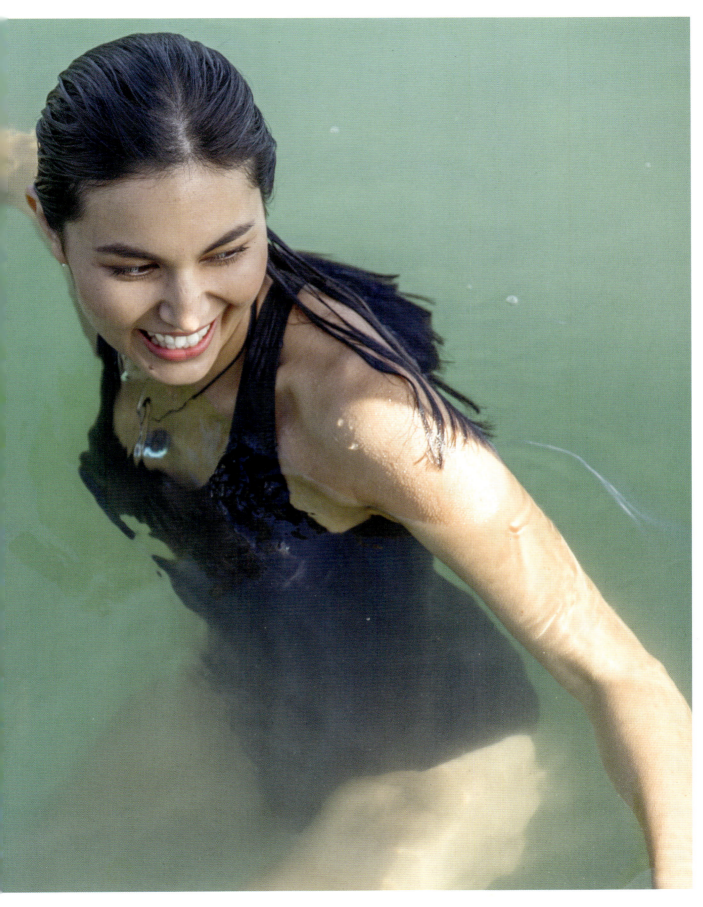

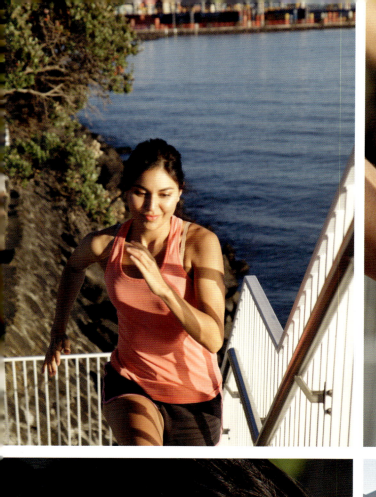
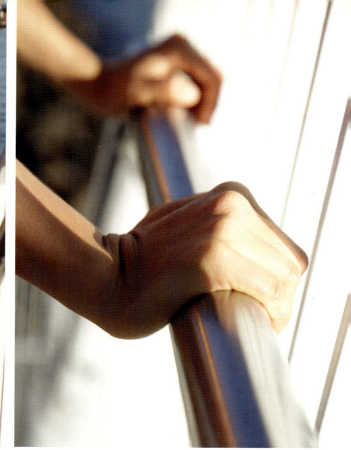
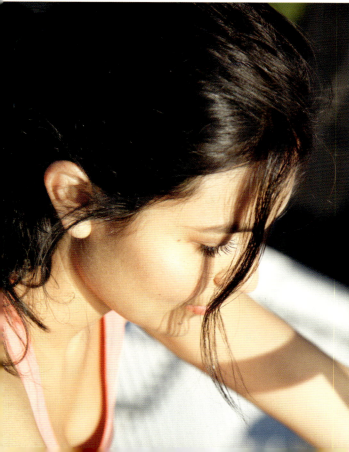
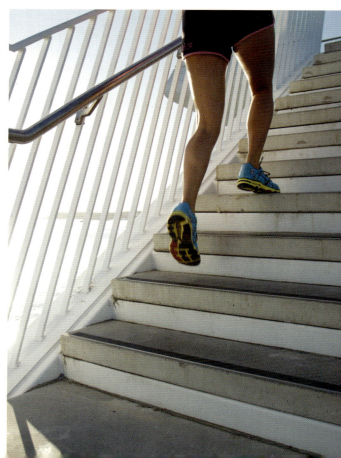

- Try interval training — short bursts of high intensity exercise mixed with relaxed walking burns more calories. For example, a fast 5-minute run followed by a 10-minute walk, repeated. This mix will help burn more calories!

9 DIGESTION AND GUT FUNCTION

I can't emphasise enough how vital it is to have a well-functioning gut that breaks down your food (avoiding any digestion problems) and eliminates toxic waste in a timely manner. Sorry to be blunt, but when your bowels aren't working properly and you're not doing your number twos regularly and easily enough, you feel awful, and are often lethargic and unsettled.

As mentioned, a common cause of gut problems is dehydration. Consistent fluid intake gets things moving. So does movement — moving around stimulates peristalsis (the involuntary wave-like movement of your intestines to push things through). That's why you're often constipated after sitting on a plane for hours. So, if you're at a desk job you should get up at least every hour for a quick walk. We all know that fibre intake is important, but high-fibre foods alone won't work — you need to eat lots of hydrating (high-water content) foods, too (e.g. fruit and vegetables!). The combination of water and fibre in these foods is far more effective than the two components separately.

Good digestion starts with chewing your food well, and eating slowly over at least 15–20 minutes. This allows enough time to stimulate your digestive system to release the stomach acid and enzymes needed to break down food in your gut, so it can move along and be absorbed more easily. You can also imagine how chewing your food well and breaking it up into smaller pieces will be kinder on your digestive system by putting less strain on it. If you're a fast eater, I suggest you simply practise putting your knife and fork down between each bite and chewing at least 20 times before swallowing (yes, count until you get used to how mashed up your food should be). Another important reason for eating more slowly is that it takes approximately 20 minutes for the hormone leptin to signal to your brain that you are full, so by eating fast you will over-eat. Apple cider vinegar and lemon juice can help your digestion by stimulating stomach acid production, so try having a tablespoon in a small glass of water before eating. You should never continue eating until you are completely full (and slightly uncomfortable); stop when you are 80 percent full, when you are no longer hungry.

10 RELAX

Being calm and relaxed is immensely important for good health in more ways than most people realise. Stress, nowadays caused by being so busy and the pressures of work, social and family life, results in adrenaline and cortisol production. Cortisol is a fat storage hormone, while adrenaline stimulates a rise in blood glucose levels, which is counteracted by a surge of insulin (another fat storage hormone). The best thing you can do every day to keep your body in a relaxed state (even if things get a little crazy), is to breathe deeply through your diaphragm, not take short breaths through your chest. Take at least 5 minutes every day (perhaps after work) to just lie on your back and concentrate on your breathing.

Take regular breaks. At work, take a quick 3-5-minute break ever hour: get up and walk to get a drink or go to the bathroom. Take a complete break from technology for at least a few hours every week (no phones, TV or computers) — it may seem weird at first, but you'll discover a new sense of freedom and relaxation. If you can, I also suggest taking a break away every 90 days or so — it doesn't have to be a full-on holiday, it could just be camping for the weekend. It's amazing how this can restore motivation as I have more recently discovered.

Get rid of negative thoughts. Negative thoughts or feelings of guilt result in stress, and stress results in not sleeping well. Not sleeping well results in relying on caffeine and making poor food choices, which results in more negative feelings and stress hormone production, leading to more sleeping problems. It becomes a never-ending downward spiral. Turn the cycle around. Positive thoughts have the power to change the course of your life.

A relaxed attitude to food is key to having a healthy relationship with it, which means having treats every now and again — whether it's a glass of wine with friends, buttered popcorn at the movies, fish and chips on the beach, or a few squares of your favourite chocolate. It's good to have things that give you pleasure and not feel guilty about it — be happy and proud that you can live a little and not be uptight about it! Remember, it's what you do most of the time that counts, not what you do on the odd occasion. Eat in a relaxed manner, at the table, with no distractions.

11 CREATE AN ENCOURAGING ENVIRONMENT

Fill your kitchen with nutritious food so that it's easily and readily available to snack on or turn into a meal. Make sure 'super foods' such as dark leafy greens, berries, avocados and eggs are on your shopping list every week, and that you always have some lean protein in the fridge or freezer so you've always got ingredients on hand to make a healthy meal, removing the risk of having to resort to takeaways. Enlist a friend or your partner to exercise with, or join an exercise group — having others in the same boat will encourage you more. Even having an energising environment at home with upbeat music and essential oils or candles will make you feel more motivated.

12 LISTEN TO YOUR BODY AND EAT MINDFULLY

You need to work with your body, not force it, as it knows best what it needs. This means you need to eat when you are hungry (i.e. don't starve yourself), sleep when you are tired, and stop an exercise if it hurts. It's good to push yourself out of your comfort zone, but only in ways that are kind to your body and rejuvenate it to make you feel energised.

Mindless eating is often where excess calories can stack up without you even realising. Picking at a few chips, nuts or biscuits here and there throughout the day can easily add up to a full meal. Always put a portion out on a plate (even if it's just one cookie), then put the leftovers or packet away. This way your mind consciously registers what it is eating. Never eat straight from the pot or packet. Mindful eating means consciously stopping for a few seconds to think if you really need this snack or second helping, before you automatically put it in your mouth.

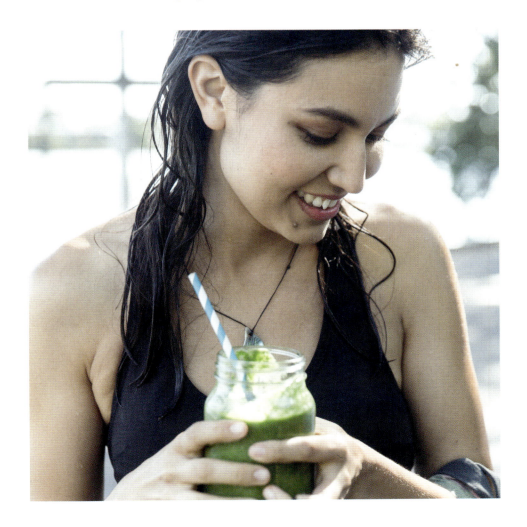

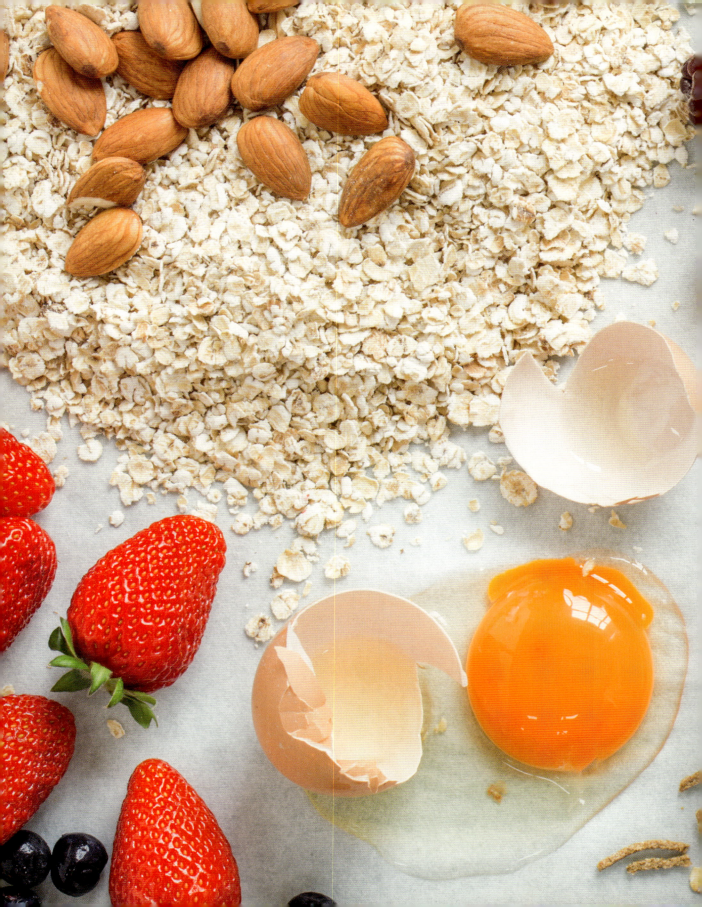

Recipes approx. 350 calories per serve

BREAKFAST

+ Eat within one hour of waking — a big mistake people often make is leaving breakfast too late. The longer you leave breakfast, often the hungrier you become, making it harder to be satisfied.

+ The morning rush can quickly sabotage your healthy eating plans. If you don't have time to eat at home, take your breakfast with you to eat on your commute or at work. You can even leave your muesli, milk and fruit at work to have when you get in.

+ Have some protein, fat and fibre at breakfast, whether from eggs, milk, yoghurt, avocado or nut butter. Foods high in protein, fat and fibre have a low glycaemic index, helping to keep you fuller for longer.

+ Unless you prefer them, there's no need to have low-fat dairy products if you're only eating 1–2 serves a day. Low-fat dairy products often contain more additives and can contain more sugar.

+ If you don't feel hungry first-thing, have a smoothie and something else an hour later.

SMOOTHIES

Breakfast in a glass can be a very convenient way to start the day. You can always take your smoothie in a jar with you. Adding avocado or nuts to your smoothie makes it creamy and filling, and adds a great boost of healthy fats.

Chocolate oat

Per serve
Energy (kJ) 1321 (311 kcal)
Protein (g) 16.1
Total fat (g) 2.3
Saturated fat (g) 0.8
Carbohydrate (g) 58.5
Sugars (g) 24.04

Creamy mint, mango + kiwifruit

Per serve
Energy (kJ) 1314 (310 kcal)
Protein (g) 2.7
Total fat (g) 21.7
Saturated fat (g) 3.3
Carbohydrate (g) 26.4
Sugars (g) 25.39

Creamy cashew, banana + cinnamon

Per serve
Energy (kJ) 1303 (307 kcal)
Protein (g) 6.2
Total fat (g) 14.4
Saturated fat (g) 2.3
Carbohydrate (g) 39.6
Sugars (g) 13.28

Raspberry, apple, avocado + yoghurt

Per serve
Energy (kJ) 825 (194 kcal)
Protein (g) 6.3
Total fat (g) 11.4
Saturated fat (g) 1.9
Carbohydrate (g) 17.3
Sugars (g) 16.83

TIP Creamier smoothies can be a meal on their own. However, if you're having one of the lighter smoothies, you might want to have 2 scrambled eggs for breakfast, too, to keep you going until lunch. If you're only making a smoothie for one person, just halve the recipe.

Beetroot, apple + berry
Per serve
Energy (kJ) 516 (121 kcal)
Protein (g) 2.9
Total fat (g) 1.1
Saturated fat (g) 0.1
Carbohydrate (g) 25.6
Sugars (g) 25.18

Tamarillo, berry, vanilla + almond milk
Per serve
Energy (kJ) 595 (140 kcal)
Protein (g) 3.2
Total fat (g) 1.8
Saturated fat (g) 0.2
Carbohydrate (g) 27.4
Sugars (g) 15.40

Banana coconut caramel
Per serve
Energy (kJ) 1316 (310 kcal)
Protein (g) 16.6
Total fat (g) 6.7
Saturated fat (g) 1.3
Carbohydrate (g) 47.7
Sugars (g) 26.13

Green colada
Per serve
Energy (kJ) 631 (149 kcal)
Protein (g) 2.2
Total fat (g) 0.7
Saturated fat (g) 0.2
Carbohydrate (g) 34.2
Sugars (g) 23.71

GREEN COLADA

SERVES: 2   PREP TIME: 5 MINUTES

Place 1½ cups **baby spinach** or **chopped spinach leaves**, 1½ cups **chopped frozen, fresh or canned pineapple**, 1 ripe **banana**, juice of 1 **lime**, ⅓ cup **coconut milk** (optional), 1-2 teaspoons **liquid honey** and ⅓ cup **water** in a blender and blend until smooth. Add a little more liquid if needed. Pour into glasses and serve.

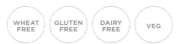

CREAMY MINT, MANGO + KIWIFRUIT

SERVES: 2   PREP TIME: 5 MINUTES

Place flesh of 1 ripe **mango**, 2 ripe **green kiwifruit**, 1 ripe **avocado**, 1½ cups **water**, 5-6 **ice cubes**, ¼ cup **mint leaves** and 1-2 teaspoons **liquid honey** to taste in a blender and blend until smooth. Add a little more liquid if needed in order to achieve desired consistency. Pour into glasses and serve.

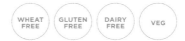

BEETROOT, APPLE + BERRY

SERVES: 2   PREP TIME: 5 MINUTES

Place 1½ cups **frozen berries** (e.g. raspberries, boysenberries, blackberries, blueberries), 1 cup grated fresh **beetroot**, 1 ripe **peach** or **nectarine**, 1 grated **apple**, 2-3 teaspoons **liquid honey** to taste, ¾ cup **water** and 5-6 ice cubes in a blender and blend until smooth. Add a little more liquid if needed in order to achieve desired consistency. Pour into glasses and serve.

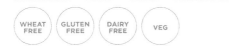

CREAMY CASHEW, BANANA + CINNAMON

SERVES: 2   PREP TIME: 5 MINUTES

Place ⅓ cup soaked **raw natural cashew nuts***, 2 ripe **bananas**, 1½ cups **milk** (e.g. almond, cow's, rice, oat), ¼ teaspoon **ground cinnamon**, 1-2 teaspoons **liquid honey** to taste, and 5-6 **ice cubes** in a blender and blend until smooth. Add a little more liquid if needed in order to achieve desired consistency. Pour into glasses and serve.

* Soak cashew nuts in cold water for at least 8 hours, or boil in water for 15 minutes, then drain. This softens the cashews, giving them a creamy texture when blended.

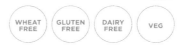

Use dairy-free milk

RASPBERRY, APPLE, AVOCADO + YOGHURT

SERVES: 2   **PREP TIME:** 5 MINUTES

Place 1½ cups **frozen raspberries**, 1 grated **apple**, ½ ripe **avocado**, ¾ cup **natural yoghurt** (a runnier yoghurt is better in this case), 1-2 teaspoons **liquid honey** to taste and ¾ cup **water** in a blender and blend until smooth. Add a little more liquid if needed in order to achieve desired consistency. Pour into glasses and serve.

* If you only have really thick yoghurt in the fridge, thin it out with a little water.

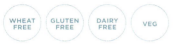

Dairy-free with coconut yoghurt

CHOCOLATE OAT

SERVES: 2   **PREP TIME:** 5 MINUTES

Place 2 ripe **bananas**, 1 tablespoon **good-quality dark cocoa powder** or **raw cacao powder**, ½ cup **fine rolled oats**, 1 cup **milk** (e.g. cow's, almond, rice, oat), 1-2 tablespoons **liquid honey**, **pure maple syrup** or **agave nectar** to taste, and 5-6 **ice cubes** in a blender and blend until smooth. Add a little more liquid if needed in order to achieve desired consistency. Pour into glasses and serve.

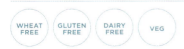

Use dairy-free milk

TAMARILLO, BERRY, VANILLA + ALMOND MILK

SERVES: 2   **PREP TIME:** 5 MINUTES

Place ¾ cup **frozen raspberries**, flesh of 3 ripe **tamarillos**, ¾ cup **almond milk**, 1 large ripe **banana**, 2 teaspoons **liquid honey** and ½ teaspoon **vanilla extract** or **essence** in a blender and blend until smooth. Add a little more liquid if needed in order to achieve desired consistency. Pour into glasses and serve.

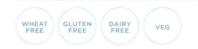

BANANA COCONUT CARAMEL

SERVES: 2   **PREP TIME:** 5 MINUTES

Place 2 ripe **bananas**, 3 **pitted medjool dates**, ¼ cup **coconut milk**, 2 tablespoons **peanut butter**, 1 cup **milk** (e.g. cow's, almond, rice, oat) and 5-6 **ice cubes** in a blender and blend until smooth. Add a little more liquid if needed in order to achieve desired consistency. Pour into glasses and serve.

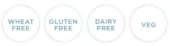

Use dairy-free milk

BREAKFAST

INSTANT CINNAMON, APPLE + ALMOND BIRCHER BOWL

Bircher muesli is the spring or summer version of porridge. Each mouthful is full of creamy goodness, with a refreshing fruity twist. Most bircher mueslis need overnight to soak, but this one is instant, as it uses fine rolled oats which soak up liquid very fast.

1. Mix grated apple with oats, milk, yoghurt, vanilla, lemon juice, cinnamon and honey in a bowl. Leave in fridge for about 5 minutes (while you get ready!).

2. Stir through half of the almonds. Divide between bowls and top with remaining almonds.

SERVES: 2

PREP TIME: 5 MINUTES

apple (e.g. Granny Smith or Braeburn) 1 large, coarsely grated
fine rolled oats ¾ cup
milk ½ cup
natural unsweetened yoghurt ¼ cup
vanilla bean paste or **vanilla extract** or **essence** 1 teaspoon
lemon juice of ½
ground cinnamon ½ teaspoon
liquid honey or **pure maple syrup** or **apple syrup** 1-2 tablespoons to taste
roasted almonds ¼ cup, finely chopped

Use dairy-free milk + coconut yoghurt

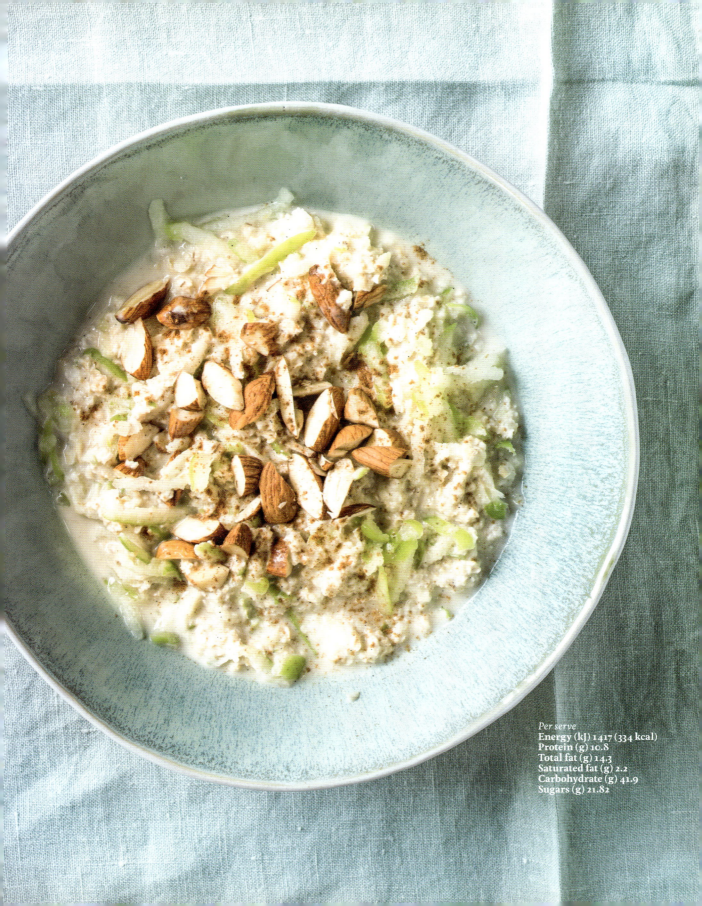

Per serve
Energy (kJ) 1417 (334 kcal)
Protein (g) 10.8
Total fat (g) 14.3
Saturated fat (g) 2.2
Carbohydrate (g) 41.9
Sugars (g) 21.82

ONE-PAN TURKISH EGGS + CHICKPEAS IN SMOKY TOMATO SAUCE

In this dish, the eggs are cooked in the sauce, infusing them with smoky tomato flavour (and saving on dishes!). Chickpeas are full of fibre, vitamins and minerals, and have a low glycaemic index — they make a delicious, healthy change to having bread.

SERVES: 4

PREP TIME: 10 MINUTES

COOK TIME: 15 MINUTES

olive oil 1 tablespoon
onion 1, diced
garlic 2 cloves, finely chopped
ground cumin 1 teaspoon
smoked paprika 2 teaspoons
tomato paste 3 tablespoons
chilli flakes ½–1 teaspoon (optional)
crushed tomatoes 1 x 400g can
water ¼ cup
chickpeas 1 x 390g can, rinsed, drained
salt
freshly ground black pepper
free-range eggs 4
feta 30g, crumbled
coriander or **flat-leaf parsley** ¼ cup chopped

1. Heat oil in a frying pan over medium heat. Cook onion and garlic until soft, 3–4 minutes. Add cumin and smoked paprika and cook for 1 minute. Stir in tomato paste, chilli flakes, if using, crushed tomatoes, water and chickpeas. Simmer for 4–5 minutes until sauce has thickened. Season to taste with salt and pepper.

2. Use a wooden spoon to create four 'pockets' in the sauce and carefully crack one egg into each pocket. Cover frying pan with a lid and steam over low heat for 7–10 minutes until whites are just set but yolks are still runny (or cook a little longer if you prefer a firmer yolk).

3. To serve, spoon some smoky tomato sauce, chickpeas and an egg onto each plate. Crumble over feta and garnish with coriander or parsley.

TIP The chickpea sauce freezes well, so you can simply heat it up and add the eggs to it for a quick meal.

WHEAT FREE · GLUTEN FREE · DAIRY FREE · VEG

Dairy-free without feta

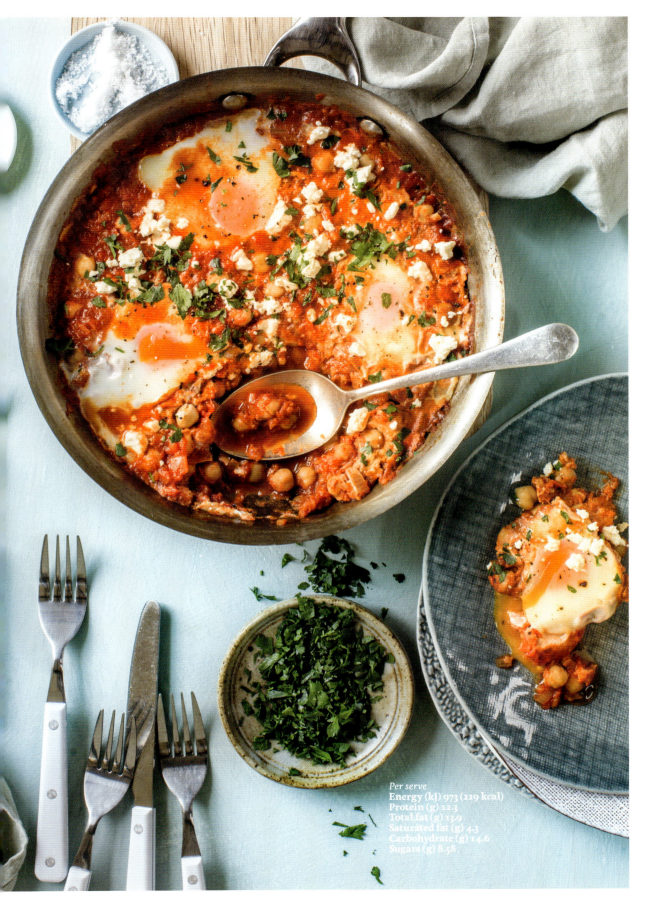

Per serve
Energy (kJ) 973 (229 kcal)
Protein (g) 12.3
Total fat (g) 13.9
Saturated fat (g) 4.3
Carbohydrate (g) 14.6
Sugars (g) 8.58

BREAKFAST

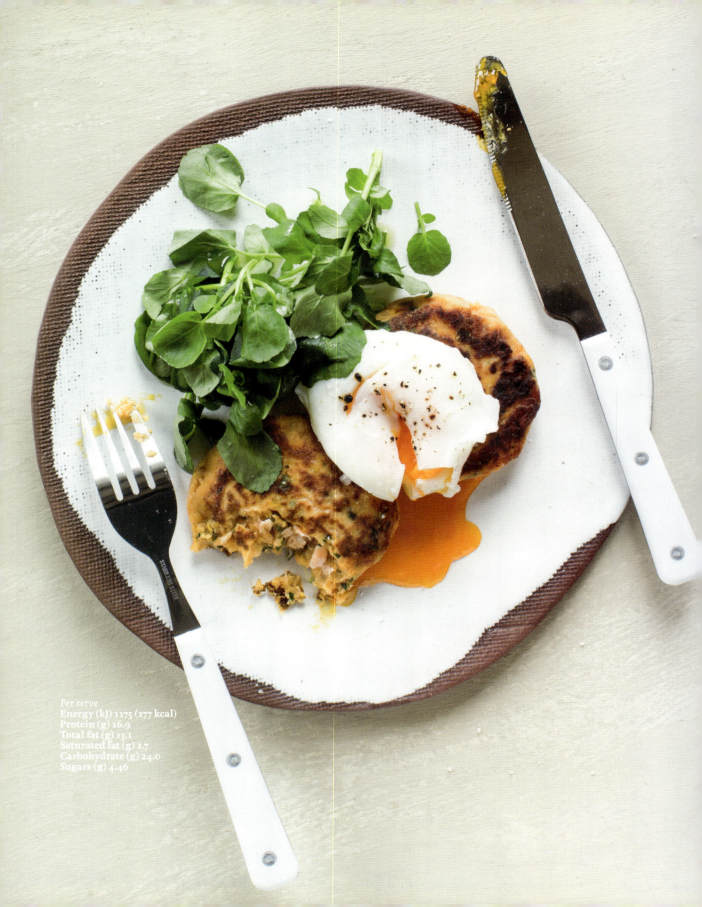

Per serve
Energy (kJ) 1175 (277 kcal)
Protein (g) 16.9
Total fat (g) 13.1
Saturated fat (g) 2.7
Carbohydrate (g) 24.0
Sugars (g) 4.46

SMOKED SALMON CAKES

This makes a delicious brunch. You can use any other smoked fish instead of salmon if you prefer.

1. Preheat oven to 50°C. Cook kumara or sweet potato in a saucepan of boiling salted water until soft, 12–15 minutes. Drain well, return to the pan and place back onto low heat for a few minutes — this will help the kumara dry out a bit. Mash kumara, then mix with salmon, spring onion, parsley, egg, lemon zest, and salt and pepper.

2. Scoop out ⅓ cup portions of fishcake mixture and shape into patties. The mixture will be quite soft. Carefully dust each patty in flour.

3. Heat 1 tablespoon oil in a large non-stick frying pan over medium heat. Cook fishcakes in batches for about 3 minutes each side until golden brown. Wipe the pan clean with a paper towel in between batches and add a little more oil as needed. Keep fishcakes warm in the oven as you cook them.

4. Bring a saucepan of water to a gentle simmer to poach the eggs. Carefully crack eggs into simmering water and poach for 1–2 minutes until whites are just set, but yolks are still runny.

5. To serve, place two fishcakes on each plate and top with a poached egg. Garnish with parsley and serve with watercress or rocket on the side. Squeeze over lemon juice just before eating.

TIP Don't skip the step of drying the kumara out over a low heat — this will ensure the mixture is not too wet. Once you've cooked the fishcakes, you can freeze them (they will keep for a couple of months). Then just defrost and reheat in the oven until hot through for a convenient meal.

SERVES: 6

PREP TIME: 15 MINUTES

COOK TIME: 25 MINUTES

- **kumara** (red kumara works best but you can use any sweet potato) 500g, peeled, chopped
- **hot smoked salmon** (or other smoked fish) 200g, flaked
- **spring onions** 2–3, finely sliced
- **flat-leaf parsley** 3–4 tablespoons finely chopped
- **free-range egg** 1
- **lemon** zest of 1
- **salt** ½ teaspoon
- **freshly ground black pepper** ½ teaspoon
- **flour** (e.g. plain, rice, buckwheat) 2–3 tablespoons
- **oil** 2 tablespoons

TO SERVE

- **free-range eggs** 6
- **flat-leaf parsley** ¼ cup chopped
- **watercress** or **baby rocket** 4 small handfuls
- **lemon** 1, cut into wedges

WHEAT FREE • GLUTEN FREE • DAIRY FREE • FREEZES WELL

Use gluten-free flour

BREAKFAST

CHERRY + COCONUT GRANOLA

Making your own golden, crunchy granola is easier than you think, and it saves your dollars and your waistline.

1. Preheat oven to 150°C. Line an oven tray with baking paper. Melt honey, butter or coconut oil, vanilla and cinnamon together in a medium-sized saucepan. Stir in oats, ensuring they are well coated.

2. Spread oats out on prepared oven tray. Bake for 15 minutes, then add coconut and dried fruit and bake for a further 3-5 minutes until coconut is very lightly toasted.

3. Allow to cool completely before storing in an airtight container. Serve with milk or yoghurt and fruit of your choice.

TIP This muesli will keep, stored in an airtight container, for a couple of months. You can substitute the dried cherries for any other dried fruit, e.g. apricots, if you like.

MAKES: 7 x ½ CUP SERVINGS
PREP TIME: 5 MINUTES
COOK TIME: 20 MINUTES

honey ¼ cup
butter or **coconut oil** 2 tablespoons
vanilla extract or essence 1 teaspoon
ground cinnamon 1 teaspoon
large jumbo rolled oats 2 cups
thread coconut ¼ cup
dried cherries, berries or cranberries (or other dried fruit) ½ cup, chopped

TO SERVE

milk or **yoghurt** ¼ cup per serving
fresh or canned fruit ½ cup per serving

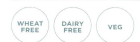

Dairy-free with coconut oil
+ serve with dairy-free milk
+ coconut yoghurt

Per serve
Energy (kJ) 1144 (270 kcal)
Protein (g) 7.0
Total fat (g) 10.8
Saturated fat (g) 7.3
Carbohydrate (g) 36.5
Sugars (g) 21.38

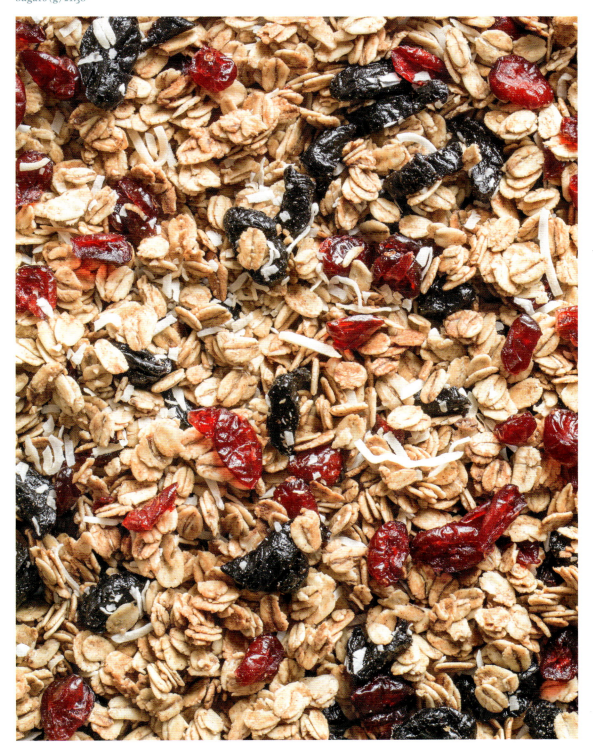

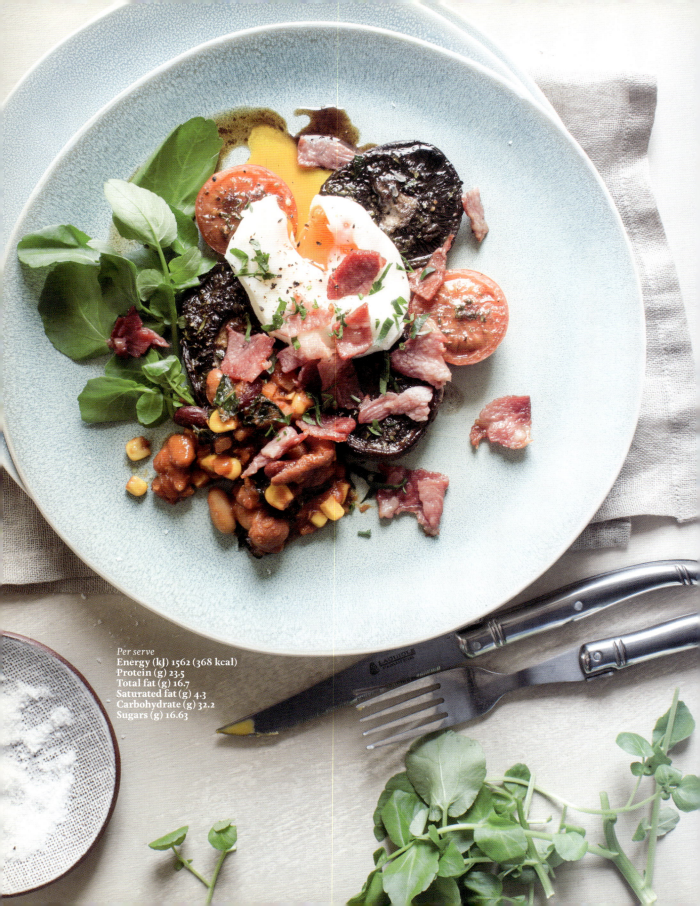

Per serve
Energy (kJ) 1562 (368 kcal)
Protein (g) 23.5
Total fat (g) 16.7
Saturated fat (g) 4.3
Carbohydrate (g) 32.2
Sugars (g) 16.63

THE WORKS
BALSAMIC-GRILLED MUSHROOMS, TOMATO, BACON, BEANS + EGGS

Here's my lighter but equally delicious version of the weekend brunch classic that will put you in a good mood for the weekend.

1. Preheat oven grill to 200°C. Line an oven tray with baking paper. Place mushrooms, gill side up, and tomatoes, cut side up, on oven tray. Mix balsamic vinegar, olive oil, thyme, garlic and honey together and spoon over mushrooms and tomatoes. Season with salt and pepper.

2. Scatter bacon next to mushrooms and tomatoes on prepared tray. Grill mushrooms, tomatoes and bacon together until the bacon is crispy and mushrooms are soft, 12–15 minutes.

3. Meanwhile, bring a small saucepan of water to a gentle simmer to poach the eggs. Warm up beans on the stovetop or in the microwave.

4. Carefully crack eggs into the simmering water and poach for 1–2 minutes or until whites are just set, but yolks are still runny. Remove with a slotted spoon.

5. To serve, arrange three mushrooms and two tomato halves on each plate, a couple of spoonfuls of beans and place a poached egg on top. Scatter crispy bacon over the top, and garnish with watercress or spinach, and parsley.

TIP You can use canned chilli beans or baked beans if you haven't prepared any bean chilli.

SERVES: 2

PREP TIME: 10 MINUTES

COOK TIME: 15 MINUTES

portobello mushrooms 6 large, stems removed
vine-ripened tomatoes 2 small, halved
balsamic vinegar 1 tablespoon
olive oil 1 tablespoon
thyme leaves 1 teaspoon chopped
garlic 2 cloves, minced
liquid honey 1½ teaspoons
salt
freshly ground black pepper
lean shoulder bacon 80g (about 2 rashers), chopped

TO SERVE
free-range eggs 2
bean, corn + kale chilli (see page 122) or **canned chilli beans** 1 cup
watercress or **baby spinach** handful, chopped
flat-leaf parsley 2–3 tablespoons chopped

WHEAT FREE   GLUTEN FREE   DAIRY FREE

BREAKFAST

GRILLED STONE FRUIT + VANILLA LEMON RICOTTA

Grilling fruit softens it and brings out its natural sweetness and juiciness. It's delicious when served with creamy ricotta or yoghurt — it's like having dessert at breakfast.

1. Preheat oven grill to medium-high heat. Pour water into a baking dish and arrange stone fruit, cut side up, in the dish. Drizzle 1-2 tablespoons honey over the fruit and grill until soft and caramelised on top, 12-15 minutes. Watch the fruit doesn't burn.

2. Beat ricotta or yoghurt until smooth, then add 1 tablespoon honey, vanilla and lemon zest.

3. To serve, divide grilled fruit and ricotta or yoghurt between breakfast bowls and drizzle with a little extra honey.

TIP Make sure you use soft, ripe fruit that is not too firm. If stone fruit is not in season you can use other fruit like pears, apples or feijoas.

SERVES: 4

PREP TIME: 5 MINUTES

COOK TIME: 12-15 MINUTES

water ½ cup
peaches 2 large ripe, halved and stoned
apricots 4 ripe, halved
nectarines 2 large ripe, halved
cherries 12
liquid honey 2-3 tablespoons + a little extra to serve
soft ricotta or **thick natural yoghurt** 1½ cups
vanilla bean paste or **vanilla extract** or **essence** ¾ teaspoon
lemon zest of 1

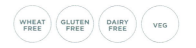

Dairy-free with coconut yoghurt

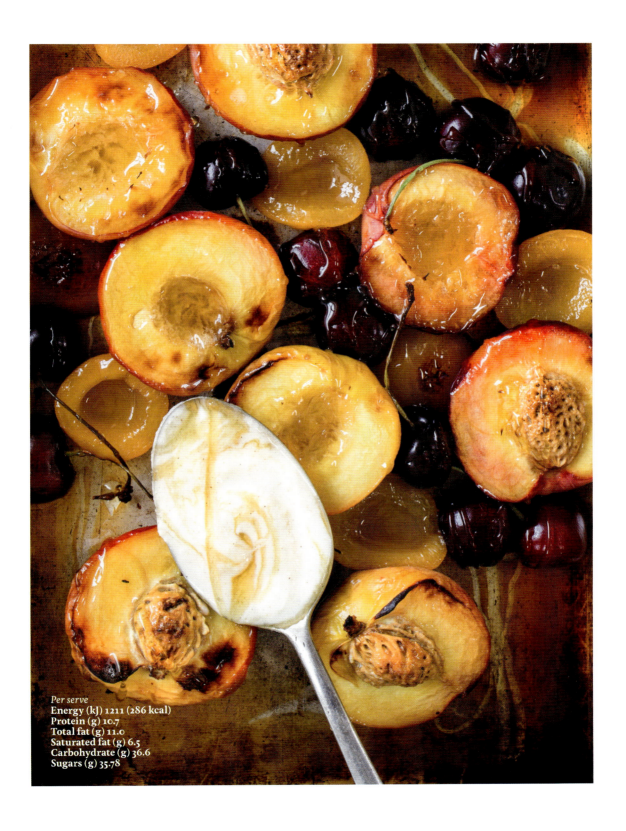

Per serve
Energy (kJ) 1211 (286 kcal)
Protein (g) 10.7
Total fat (g) 11.0
Saturated fat (g) 6.5
Carbohydrate (g) 36.6
Sugars (g) 35.78

BREAKFAST

Per serve
Energy (kJ) 1486 (350 kcal)
Protein (g) 20.5
Total fat (g) 24.4
Saturated fat (g) 7.5
Carbohydrate (g) 13.2
Sugars (g) 5.93

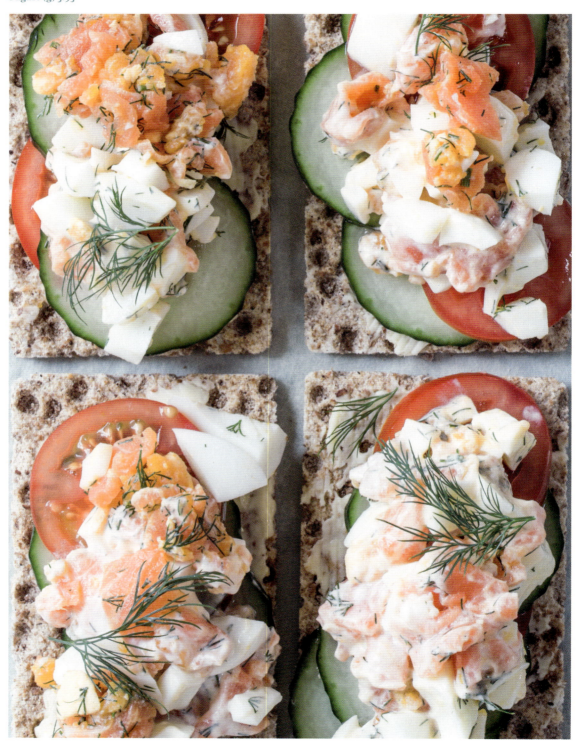

SWEDISH BREAKFAST SMÖRGÅS

Breakfast in Sweden is usually based around smörgås (an open-faced sandwich), often using crispbread. I love this smoked salmon, egg, cucumber and tomato combination — it's fresh, light, tasty and quick! Hardboil your egg the night before to speed up breakfast in the morning.

1. Roughly chop hardboiled egg and smoked salmon and mix with dill and crème fraîche or mayonnaise. Season to taste with a little salt and pepper.

2. To serve, butter the crispbreads and top with tomato, cucumber and egg, salmon and dill mixture. Squeeze over a little lemon juice just before eating.

TIP You could substitute ham for the salmon if you prefer.

SERVES: 1

PREP TIME: 5 MINUTES

hardboiled free-range egg 1, shelled
cold smoked salmon 2 slices (about 30–40g)
dill 1 teaspoon finely chopped
crème fraîche or **good-quality mayonnaise** 1 tablespoon
salt
freshly ground black pepper

TO SERVE
butter 1 teaspoon
rye crispbreads 2
tomato 1 small, sliced
cucumber 6–8 slices
lemon wedge 1

Dairy-free without butter

BREAKFAST

47

BACON, PEA + EGG BREAKFAST FRIED RICE

Fried rice for breakfast might sound odd, but it's really just another way of having some carbohydrate and protein at breakfast. It's very tasty and a great way to use up leftover rice.

1. Combine fried rice sauce ingredients and set aside.

2. Heat 1 teaspoon oil in a wok or large non-stick frying pan over high heat. Cook bacon for about 2 minutes until it starts to crisp up, then add rice and stir-fry for another 2 minutes, tossing to combine. Add peas, spring onion and fried rice sauce, and toss for 1–2 more minutes to mix and heat through, then set fried rice aside on a serving plate.

3. Add remaining teaspoon oil to the hot pan and add beaten eggs. Cook quickly for about 1 minute, using a wooden spoon or fish slice to scramble the eggs slightly and break them up. When they are just beginning to set as an omelette, roughly chop or cut up in the pan.

4. To serve, top fried rice with omelette and some fresh chilli, if using.

TIP 1–2-day-old chilled cooked rice makes the best fried rice because it has had time to dry out, so you get a fluffy fried rice. Once you have cooled cooked rice, you can freeze it.

SERVES: 2

PREP TIME: 5 MINUTES

COOK TIME: 10 MINUTES

FRIED RICE SAUCE

soy sauce 1½–2 teaspoons
sesame oil 1 teaspoon
ginger 1 teaspoon minced
garlic 1 clove, minced

FRIED RICE

oil 2 teaspoons
lean shoulder bacon 80g (about 2 rashers), diced
leftover cooked rice 1½ cups (from 1–2 days earlier is best)
frozen peas ¾ cup, defrosted
spring onions 1–2, finely sliced
free-range eggs 2, beaten with a good pinch of **salt**

TO SERVE

red chilli ½, finely chopped (optional)

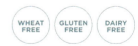

Use wheat-free tamari soy sauce

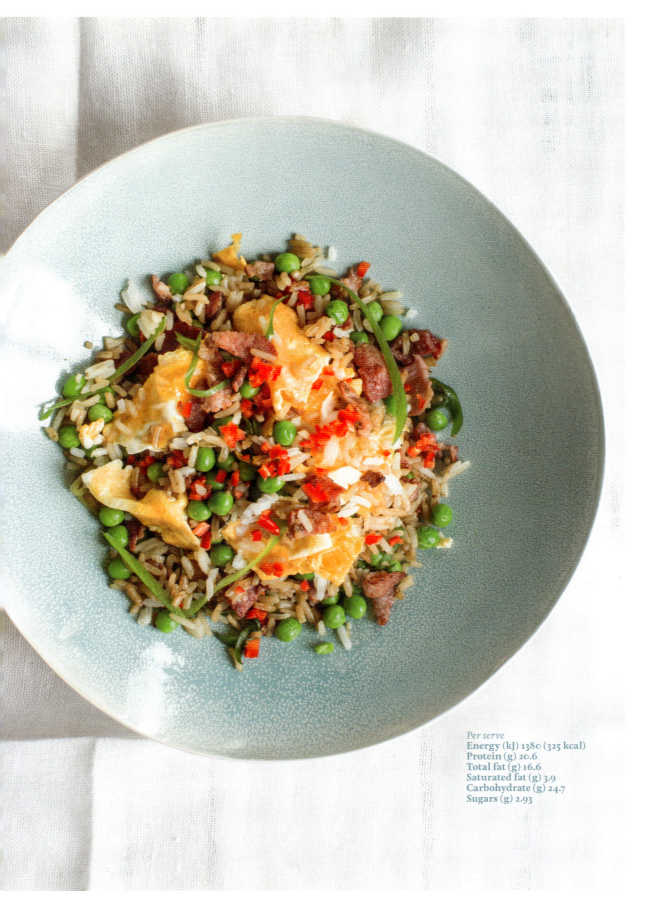

Per serve
Energy (kJ) 1380 (325 kcal)
Protein (g) 20.6
Total fat (g) 16.6
Saturated fat (g) 3.9
Carbohydrate (g) 24.7
Sugars (g) 2.93

BREAKFAST

EVERYDAY BANANA PANCAKES

Pancakes are usually a weekend treat, but these ones are healthy and quick enough to make every day! They're made pretty much out of nothing but banana and egg, so are healthy, light and fluffy (and very 'bananary').

1. Place bananas in a mixing bowl and use a potato masher or fork to mash well until smooth and lump-free — you should end up with about ¾ cup mashed banana. Whisk in eggs, baking powder, flour, salt and cinnamon until well combined.

2. Melt butter or coconut oil in a large non-stick frying pan over medium heat. Spoon half ladlefuls of pancake mixture into the frying pan and cook for 1-2 minutes until set, then flip over and cook on the other side for about 1 minute until golden.

3. To serve, divide pancakes between plates, top with fruit and drizzle over syrup or honey.

SERVES: 2

PREP TIME: 5 MINUTES

COOK TIME: 5-10 MINUTES

bananas 1-2 ripe
free-range eggs 2
baking powder ¼ teaspoon
flour (e.g. buckwheat, coconut, plain wheat) 1 tablespoon
salt good pinch of
ground cinnamon ½ teaspoon
butter or **coconut oil** 2 teaspoons

TO SERVE

fresh or canned fruit or **frozen or fresh berries** ½ cup per serving
pure maple syrup, apple syrup, liquid honey or **agave nectar** 1 tablespoon per serving

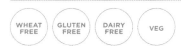

Wheat-free with buckwheat or coconut flour + dairy-free with coconut oil

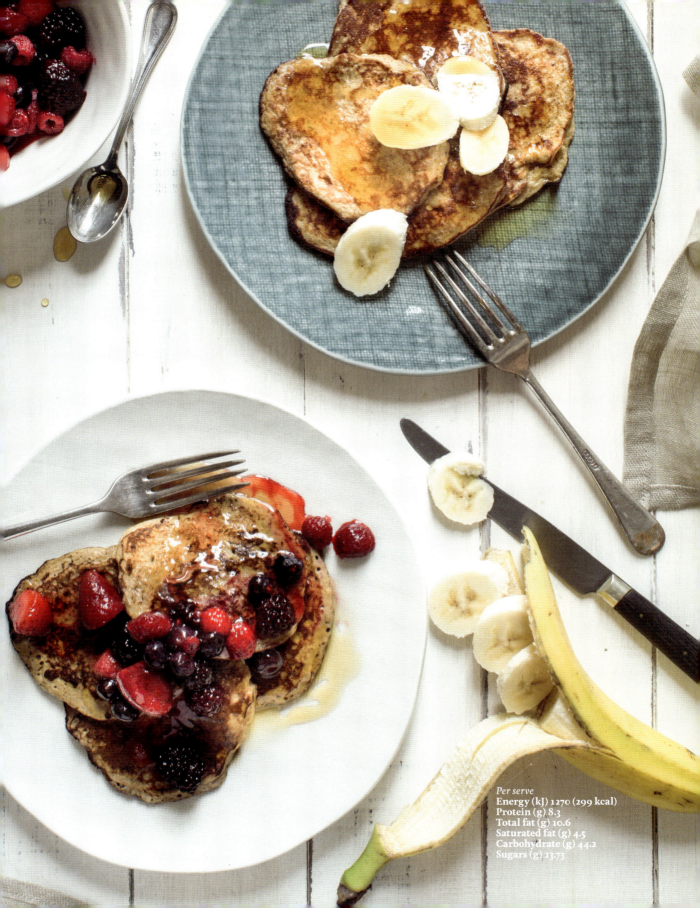

Per serve
Energy (kJ) 1270 (299 kcal)
Protein (g) 8.3
Total fat (g) 10.6
Saturated fat (g) 4.5
Carbohydrate (g) 44.2
Sugars (g) 23.73

JAZZED-UP SCRAMBLED EGGS

Eggs are truly an amazing food — they contain an array of vitamins and minerals, and protein: everything needed to create new life! I love eggs for breakfast — they're yummy, nourishing and sustaining. Here are some great ways to flavour them to take them up another notch.

SMOKED SALMON + CHIVES SCRAMBLED EGGS

SERVES: 1 **PREP TIME:** 5 MINUTES

In a small bowl, whisk 2 **free-range eggs** and a pinch of **salt** and tiny grind of **black pepper** together. Heat 1 teaspoon **butter** in a non-stick frying pan on low heat. When it starts to bubble, pour eggs into the pan and, using a wooden spoon or rubber spatula, stir eggs over low heat for about 1 minute to create soft, creamy curds. Turn off the heat (it's best to take them off the heat when they are still slightly underdone as they will continue cooking off the heat). Sprinkle over 50g chopped **smoked salmon** and 2 teaspoons chopped **chives** or **flat-leaf parsley**.

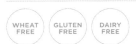

Use olive oil instead of buter

Per serve
Energy (kJ) 916 (216 kcal)
Protein (g) 22.7
Fat (g) 14.1
Saturated fat (g) 5.7
Carbohydrate (g) 0.4
Sugar (g) 0.1

SPINACH + PARMESAN SCRAMBLED EGGS

SERVES: 1 **PREP TIME:** 5 MINUTES

In a small bowl, whisk 2 **free-range eggs** and a pinch of **salt** and tiny grind of **black pepper** together. Heat 1 teaspoon **butter** in a non-stick frying pan on low heat. When it starts to bubble, pour eggs into the pan and, using a wooden spoon or rubber spatula, stir eggs over low heat for about 1 minute to create soft, creamy curds. Sprinkle over 1 tablespoon of grated **parmesan** cheese. Spoon eggs onto serving plate, and keep pan on the heat (it's best to take them off the heat when they are still slightly underdone as they will continue cooking off the heat). Add a tiny drizzle of **olive oil** to pan and 1 handful **baby or chopped spinach**, and cook for about 1 minute or until just wilted. Serve on top of scrambled eggs.

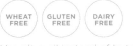

Use olive oil instead of buter

Per serve
Energy (kJ) 784 (185 kcal)
Protein (g) 14.7
Fat (g) 14.1
Saturated (g) fat 6.7
Carbohydrate (g) 0.4
Sugar (g) 0.1

CURRIED SCRAMBLED EGGS WITH TOMATO + CORIANDER

SERVES: 1   **PREP TIME:** 5 MINUTES

In a small bowl, whisk 2 **free-range eggs** and a pinch of **salt** and tiny grind of **black pepper** together. Heat 1 teaspoon **butter** in a non-stick frying pan on low heat. When it starts to bubble, add ¼–½ teaspoon **curry powder** and sizzle for 30 seconds, then pour eggs into the pan and, using a wooden spoon or rubber spatula, stir eggs over low heat for about 1 minute to create soft, creamy curds. Turn off the heat (it's best to take them off the heat when they are still slightly underdone as they will continue cooking off the heat). Serve topped with 1 diced **tomato** and 1 tablespoon chopped **coriander**, and a few slices of **green chilli** (if desired).

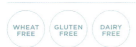

Use olive oil instead of buter

Per serve
693 kJ (163 kcal)
6.7g protein
12.3g fat
5.2g saturated fat
5.6g carbs
1.7g sugar

KALE + PROSCIUTTO SCRAMBLED EGGS

SERVES: 1   **PREP TIME:** 5 MINUTES

In a small bowl, whisk 2 **free-range eggs** and a pinch of **salt** and tiny grind of **black pepper** together. Heat 1 teaspoon **butter** in a non-stick frying pan on low heat. When it starts to bubble, pour eggs into the pan and, using a wooden spoon or rubber spatula, stir eggs over low heat for about 1 minute to create soft, creamy curds. Turn off the heat (it's best to take them off the heat when they are still slightly underdone as they will continue cooking off the heat). Spoon eggs onto serving plate, and keep pan on the heat. Add a tiny drizzle of **olive oil** to the pan and 1 handful finely sliced **kale**, and cook for about 2 minutes or until just wilted. Serve on top of scrambled eggs, with 1 slice **prosciutto**, torn.

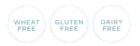

Use olive oil instead of buter

Per serve
Energy (kJ) 852 (201 kcal)
Protein (g) 13.2
Fat (g) 16.4
Saturated fat (g) 7
Carbohydrate (g) 0.9
Sugar (g) 0.1

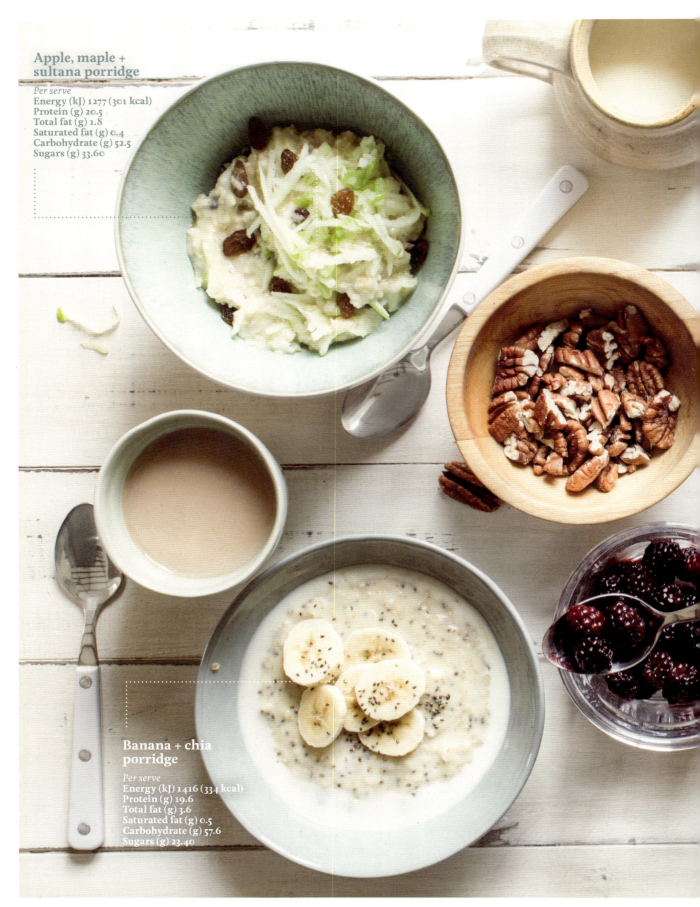

Apple, maple + sultana porridge

Per serve
Energy (kJ) 1277 (301 kcal)
Protein (g) 20.5
Total fat (g) 1.8
Saturated fat (g) 0.4
Carbohydrate (g) 52.5
Sugars (g) 33.60

Banana + chia porridge

Per serve
Energy (kJ) 1416 (334 kcal)
Protein (g) 19.6
Total fat (g) 3.6
Saturated fat (g) 0.5
Carbohydrate (g) 57.6
Sugars (g) 23.40

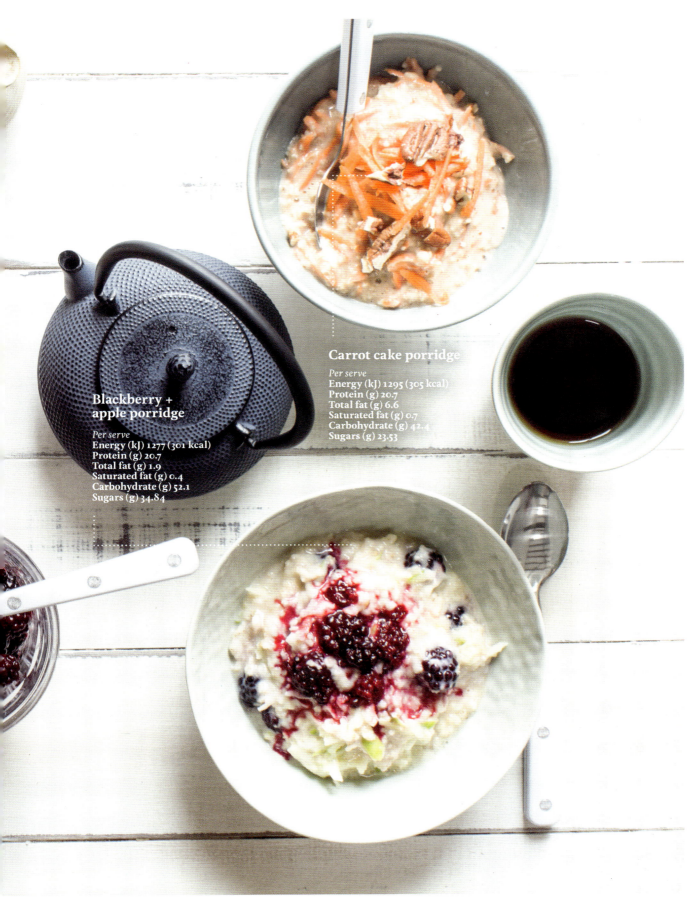

Carrot cake porridge
Per serve
Energy (kJ) 1295 (305 kcal)
Protein (g) 20.7
Total fat (g) 6.6
Saturated fat (g) 0.7
Carbohydrate (g) 42.4
Sugars (g) 23.53

Blackberry + apple porridge
Per serve
Energy (kJ) 1277 (301 kcal)
Protein (g) 20.7
Total fat (g) 1.9
Saturated fat (g) 0.4
Carbohydrate (g) 52.1
Sugars (g) 34.84

JAZZED-UP PORRIDGE

To make basic porridge, combine ⅔ cup fine rolled oats, 1 cup milk, ½ cup water and a good pinch of salt in a saucepan, and simmer for a few minutes over medium heat, stirring until thickened.

APPLE, MAPLE + SULTANA

SERVES: 2   **PREP TIME:** 3 MINUTES

Coarsely grate 1 **Granny Smith apple** and add to the basic porridge ingredients, along with 2 tablespoons **pure maple syrup** and 2 tablespoons **sultanas** or **raisins**. Serve with ¼ cup **milk** or **yoghurt** per serving.

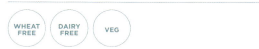

Use dairy-free milk or yoghurt

BLACKBERRY + APPLE

SERVES: 2   **PREP TIME:** 3 MINUTES

Coarsely grate 1 **apple** and add to the basic porridge ingredients, along with 2 tablespoons **liquid honey**. Gently fold through ½ cup **canned or frozen blackberries** just before serving. Serve with ¼ cup **milk** or **yoghurt** per serving.

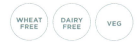

Use dairy-free milk or yoghurt

CARROT CAKE

SERVES: 2   **PREP TIME:** 3 MINUTES

Coarsely grate 1 peeled **carrot** and add to the basic porridge ingredients, along with ½ teaspoon **ground cinnamon** and 2 tablespoons **pure maple syrup**. Serve with ¼ cup **milk** or **yoghurt** and 1 tablespoon chopped toasted **pecan nuts** per serving.

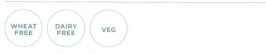

Use dairy-free milk or yoghurt

BANANA + CHIA

SERVES: 2   **PREP TIME:** 3 MINUTES

Add 2 teaspoons **chia seeds**, 1 mashed ripe **banana**, and an extra ¼ cup **milk** to the basic porridge ingredients. Sweeten with 1-2 tablespoons **honey, pure maple syrup** or **agave nectar**. Top with a few extra slices of **banana**.

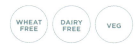

Use dairy-free milk

BREAKFAST FRUIT PARFAITS

Breakfast parfaits are quick and easy to assemble, and so yummy it's almost like you're having dessert for breakfast. Get creative with the fruit and flavours you use.

STRAWBERRY, MINT + LIME

SERVES: 2   **PREP TIME:** 5 MINUTES

Combine 1 punnet **fresh strawberries**, quartered, 1 teaspoon finely chopped **mint** or **basil**, finely grated zest and juice of 1 **lime** and 1 teaspoon **liquid honey** in a small bowl. In a separate bowl, mix 1 cup **natural unsweetened yoghurt** or **coconut yoghurt** with 2 teaspoons honey. To serve, layer strawberry mixture with yoghurt and ½ cup **granola** (see page 40) or **muesli** in two parfait glasses.

WHEAT FREE · DAIRY FREE · VEG

Dairy-free with coconut yoghurt

MANDARIN, PEACH + GINGER

SERVES: 2   **PREP TIME:** 5 MINUTES

Combine 2 large or 3 small **mandarins**, chopped, 1 cup **canned or fresh peaches**, drained and chopped, ½ teaspoon finely grated **ginger** and 1 teaspoon **liquid honey** in a small bowl. Mix 1 cup **natural unsweetened yoghurt** or **coconut yoghurt** with 2 teaspoons honey. To serve, layer fruit mixture with yoghurt and ½ cup **granola** (see page 40) or **muesli** in two parfait glasses.

WHEAT FREE · DAIRY FREE · VEG

Dairy-free with coconut yoghurt

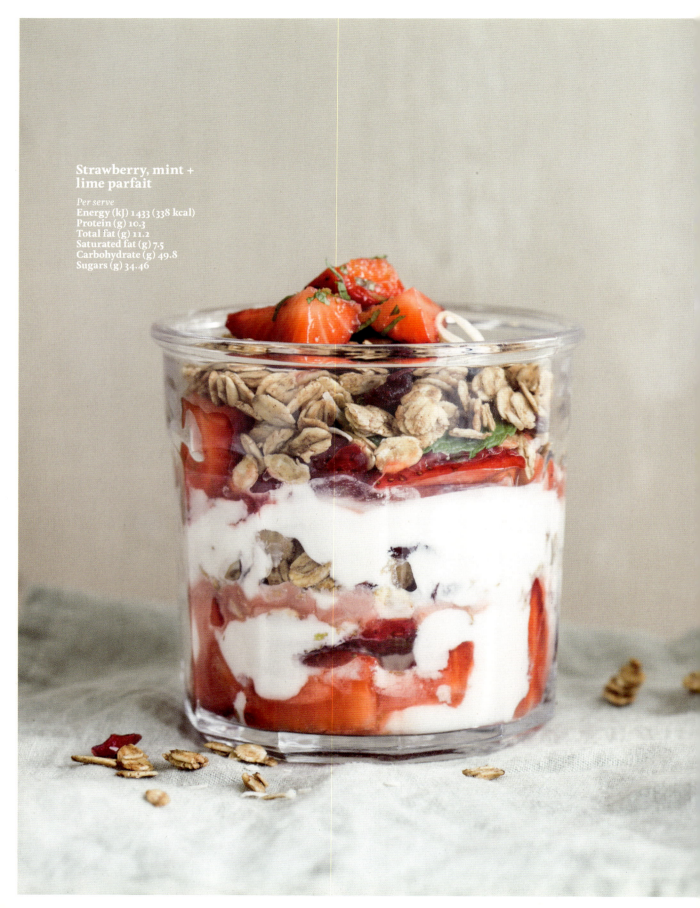

Strawberry, mint + lime parfait

Per serve
Energy (kJ) 1433 (338 kcal)
Protein (g) 10.3
Total fat (g) 11.2
Saturated fat (g) 7.5
Carbohydrate (g) 49.8
Sugars (g) 34.46

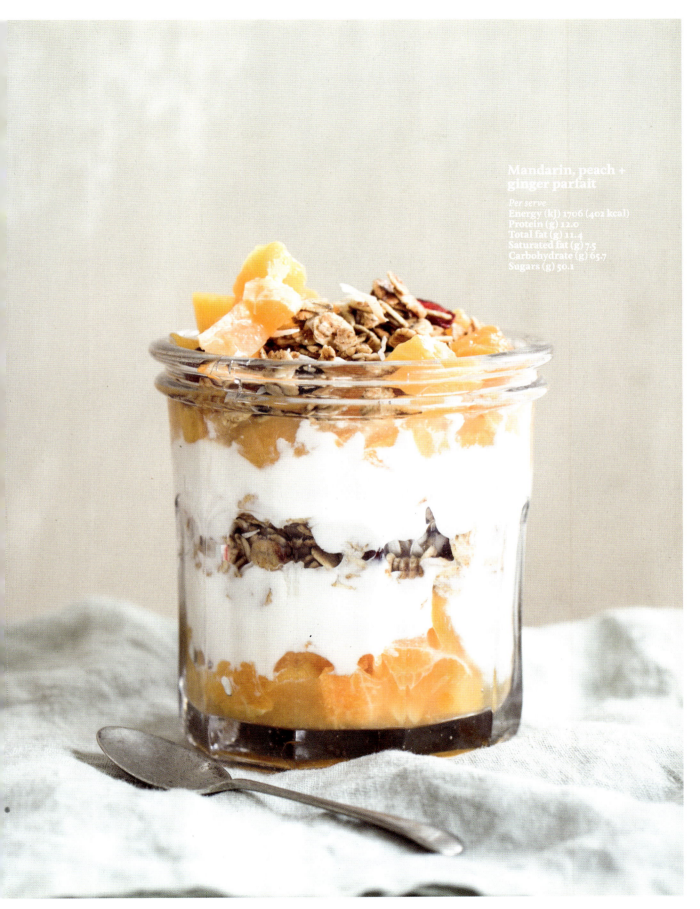

Mandarin, peach + ginger parfait

Per serve
Energy (kJ) 1706 (402 kcal)
Protein (g) 12.0
Total fat (g) 11.4
Saturated fat (g) 7.5
Carbohydrate (g) 65.7
Sugars (g) 50.1

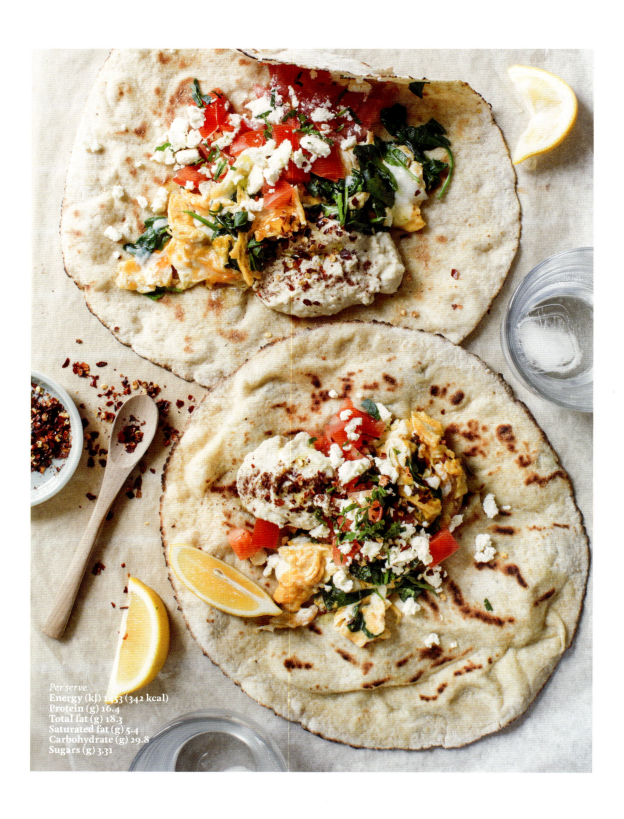

Per serve
Energy (kJ) 1,453 (342 kcal)
Protein (g) 16.4
Total fat (g) 18.3
Saturated fat (g) 5.4
Carbohydrate (g) 29.8
Sugars (g) 3.31

LEBANESE BREAKFAST WRAP WITH HUMMUS, TOMATO, SPINACH + FETA

This is a quick, simple 'Middle Eastern inspired' alternative way of having scrambled eggs — with spinach, hummus, feta and tomato, in a wrap.

1. Heat olive oil in a non-stick frying pan over medium heat. Add beaten eggs, parsley and spinach and leave to cook for about 1 minute. Lightly stir with a wooden spoon or spatula to scramble the eggs and cook for 1 more minute, or until the eggs are cooked to your liking.

2. Briefly warm flatbreads in a preheated oven, frying pan or in the microwave.

3. To serve, spread some hummus on each flatbread, and top with scrambled eggs and diced tomato. Crumble over feta and sprinkle over chilli flakes and sumac, if using. Wrap up and eat!

SERVES: 2

PREP TIME: 5 MINUTES

COOK TIME: 3 MINUTES

olive oil 1½ teaspoons
free-range eggs 2, lightly beaten with a good pinch of **salt**
flat-leaf parsley 3–4 tablespoons chopped
spinach leaves 1½ cups chopped
Lebanese flatbreads or **wraps** 2 medium-sized
hummus 2–3 tablespoons (store-bought, or see page 270)
tomatoes 1–2, diced
feta 30g
chilli flakes ¼ teaspoon (optional)
sumac sprinkle of (optional)

DAIRY FREE   VEG

Dairy-free without feta

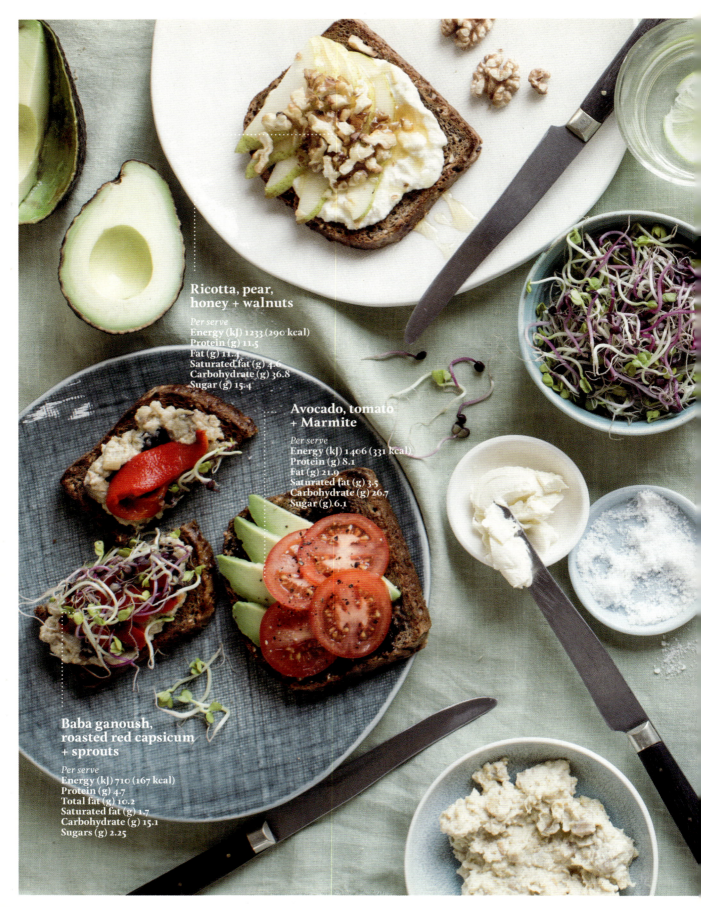

Ricotta, pear, honey + walnuts

Per serve
Energy (kJ) 1233 (290 kcal)
Protein (g) 11.5
Fat (g) 11.4
Saturated fat (g) 4.6
Carbohydrate (g) 36.8
Sugar (g) 15.4

Avocado, tomato + Marmite

Per serve
Energy (kJ) 1406 (331 kcal)
Protein (g) 8.1
Fat (g) 21.9
Saturated fat (g) 3.5
Carbohydrate (g) 26.7
Sugar (g) 6.1

Baba ganoush, roasted red capsicum + sprouts

Per serve
Energy (kJ) 710 (167 kcal)
Protein (g) 4.7
Total fat (g) 10.2
Saturated fat (g) 1.7
Carbohydrate (g) 15.1
Sugars (g) 2.25

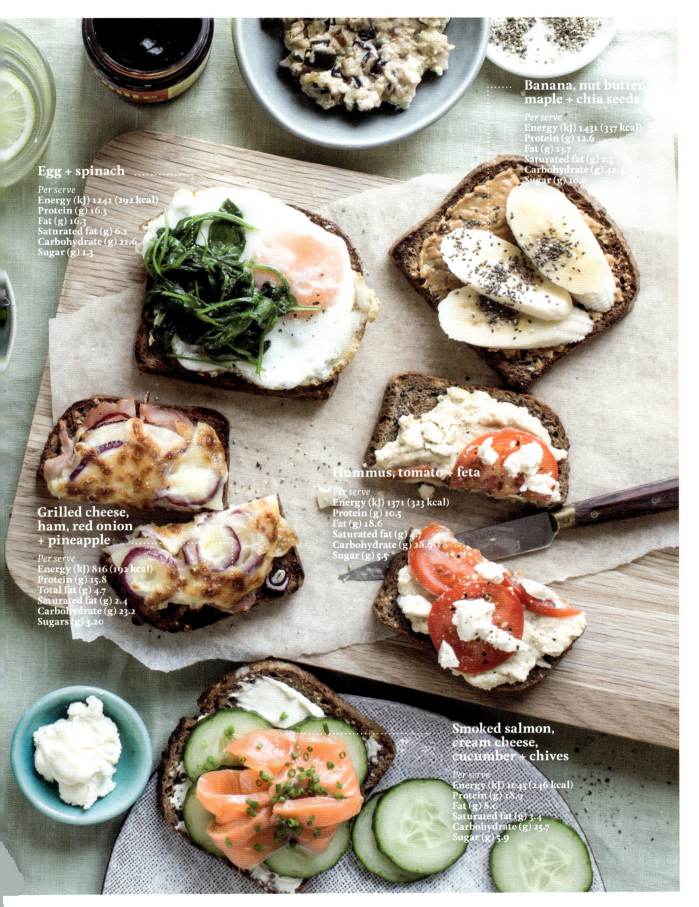

Banana, nut butter, maple + chia seeds
Per serve
Energy (kJ) 1431 (337 kcal)
Protein (g) 12.6
Fat (g) 13.7
Saturated fat (g) 2.3
Carbohydrate (g) 42.4
Sugar (g) 10.6

Egg + spinach
Per serve
Energy (kJ) 1241 (292 kcal)
Protein (g) 16.3
Fat (g) 16.3
Saturated fat (g) 6.1
Carbohydrate (g) 21.6
Sugar (g) 1.3

Hummus, tomato + feta
Per serve
Energy (kJ) 1371 (323 kcal)
Protein (g) 10.5
Fat (g) 18.6
Saturated fat (g) 4.7
Carbohydrate (g) 28.9
Sugar (g) 5.5

Grilled cheese, ham, red onion + pineapple
Per serve
Energy (kJ) 816 (192 kcal)
Protein (g) 15.8
Total fat (g) 4.7
Saturated fat (g) 2.4
Carbohydrate (g) 23.2
Sugars (g) 3.20

Smoked salmon, cream cheese, cucumber + chives
Per serve
Energy (kJ) 1045 (246 kcal)
Protein (g) 18.9
Fat (g) 8.6
Saturated fat (g) 3.4
Carbohydrate (g) 25.7
Sugar (g) 5.9

TOAST TOPPINGS

Wholegrain toast can make a good breakfast or lunch if you load it up with nutritious toppings. Make sure you include some protein and/or healthy fats to help keep you going until the next meal.

AVOCADO, TOMATO + MARMITE

SERVES: 1 **PREP TIME:** 3-5 MINUTES

Spread 2 thin slices **wholegrain toast** with a little **Marmite** and top with ½ **avocado** sliced and 1 sliced **tomato**. Season with a little **salt**, grind over **black pepper** and squeeze over a little **lemon juice**.

(GLUTEN FREE) (DAIRY FREE) (VEG)

Use dairy-free milk + gluten-free bread

SMOKED SALMON, CREAM CHEESE, CUCUMBER + CHIVES

SERVES: 1 **PREP TIME:** 3-5 MINUTES

Spread 2 thin slices **wholegrain toast** with 2 tablespoons **cream cheese** and top with 8 slices **cucumber**, 4 slices **cold smoked salmon** and sprinkle over 1 teaspoon chopped **chives**.

(GLUTEN FREE)

Use gluten-free bread

BANANA, NUT BUTTER, MAPLE + CHIA SEEDS

SERVES: 1 **PREP TIME:** 3-5 MINUTES

Spread 2 thin slices **wholegrain toast** with 2 tablespoons **nut butter** (e.g. almond or peanut butter) and ½ sliced ripe **banana**. Sprinkle over ½ teaspoon **chia seeds** and drizzle over 1 teaspoon **pure maple syrup**.

(GLUTEN FREE) (DAIRY FREE) (VEG)

Use gluten-free bread

BABA GANOUSH, ROASTED RED CAPSICUM + SPROUTS

SERVES: 1 **PREP TIME:** 3-5 MINUTES

Spread 2 thin slices **wholegrain toast** with 4 tablespoons **baba ganoush** and top with a few slices of **roasted red capsicum** (from a jar or the deli) and a small handful of **sprouts**.

(GLUTEN FREE) (DAIRY FREE) (VEG)

Use gluten-free bread

HUMMUS, TOMATO + FETA

SERVES: 1   **PREP TIME:** 3-5 MINUTES

Spread 2 thin slices **wholegrain toast** with 4 tablespoons **hummus**, top with 1 sliced **tomato** and crumble over 15g **feta** (1 tablespoon). Grind over **black pepper** and squeeze over a little **lemon juice**.

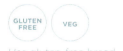

Use gluten-free bread

RICOTTA, PEAR, HONEY + WALNUTS

SERVES: 1   **PREP TIME:** 3-5 MINUTES

Top 2 thin slices **wholegrain toast** with 4 tablespoons **soft ricotta**, ½ sliced ripe **pear**, 1 tablespoon chopped **walnuts** and drizzle over 1 teaspoon **honey**.

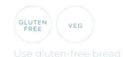

Use gluten-free bread

EGG + SPINACH

SERVES: 1   **PREP TIME:** 3-5 MINUTES

Spread 2 thin slices **wholegrain toast** with 1 teaspoon **butter** and top with a handful of wilted **spinach** and 2 poached, scrambled or fried **free-range eggs**.

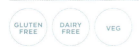

Use gluten-free bread
+ olive oil instead of butter

GRILLED CHEESE, HAM, RED ONION + PINEAPPLE

SERVES: 1   **PREP TIME:** 3-5 MINUTES

Preheat oven grill. Spread 1 teaspoon **butter** or **mayonnaise** on 2 thin slices **wholegrain bread** and top with 2 slices (60-80g) **ham**, 1 drained **pineapple ring** (from a can) and 8-10 slices **red onion**. Sprinkle over 4 tablespoons grated **mozzarella**. Cook under the grill for about 5 minutes or until bread is lightly toasted and cheese is melted and bubbly.

Use gluten-free bread

BREAKFAST

COCONANA BREAD

A delicious loaf with banana and coconut that you can top with peanut butter, yoghurt or a smear of butter for breakfast. Warm up a slice in the microwave or toaster.

1 Preheat oven to 180°C. Lightly grease and line a large loaf tin with baking paper. Combine melted coconut oil or butter in saucepan with honey or maple syrup and heat gently.

2 Add mashed bananas, coconut, eggs, baking soda mixture, lemon zest and juice and salt and mix until well combined.

3 Sift flour into wet mixture and use a large metal spoon to fold the mixtures together until well combined (but be careful not to over-mix).

4 Pour into prepared loaf tin and sprinkle over thread coconut, if using. Bake for about 1 hour, or until a skewer inserted into the middle comes out clean. Leave to cool in the tin for 5 minutes before turning out onto a wire rack to cool.

5 Spread a slice of warm loaf with butter or nut butter. Once cooled, store in an airtight container.

TIP This loaf will keep in the fridge for up to a week. It also freezes well — pre-slice and freeze in a sealed bag. To make baking soda mixture, warm 1 tablespoon milk in a small bowl in the microwave for 10–15 seconds, then stir in baking soda and it will froth up.

MAKES: 1 LARGE LOAF (10 SERVES)

PREP TIME: 5–10 MINUTES

COOK TIME: 1 HOUR

coconut oil or **butter** ½ cup melted (120g)

liquid honey or **pure maple syrup** ½ cup

bananas 3 large ripe, mashed

desiccated coconut 1½ cups

free-range eggs 4

baking soda 1½ teaspoons mixed with 1 tablespoon **warm milk**

lemons finely grated zest of 2

lemon juice 2 tablespoons

salt pinch of

wholemeal or gluten-free flour or **ground almonds** 1¼ cups

thread coconut 2 tablespoons (optional)

TO SERVE

butter ½ teaspoon per slice, or **nut butter** 1 teaspoon per slice

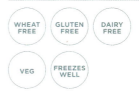

Use dairy-free milk + coconut oil. For wheat-free use gluten-free flour or ground almonds

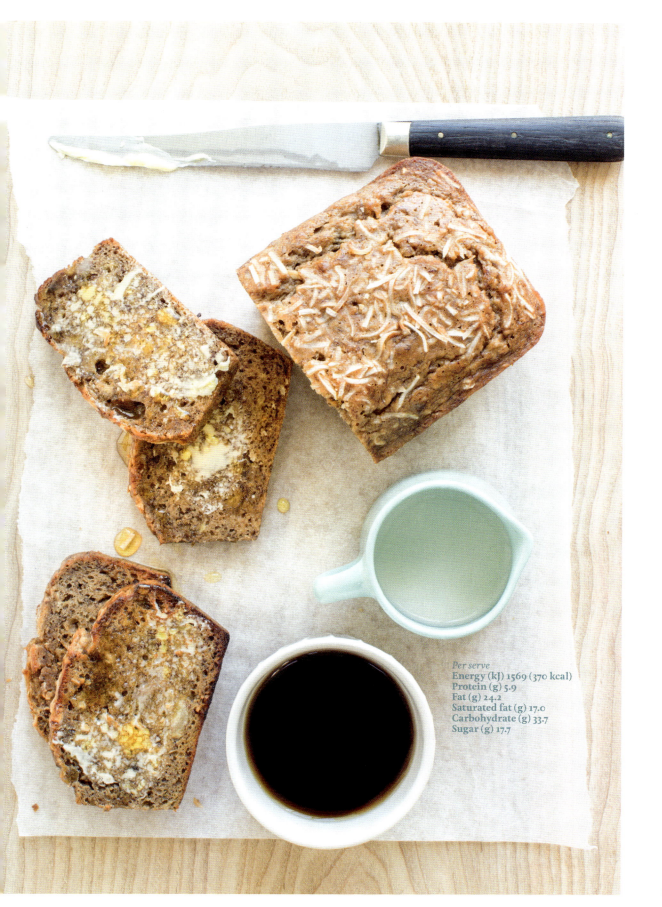

BREAKFAST

Per serve
Energy (kJ) 1569 (370 kcal)
Protein (g) 5.9
Fat (g) 24.2
Saturated fat (g) 17.0
Carbohydrate (g) 33.7
Sugar (g) 17.7

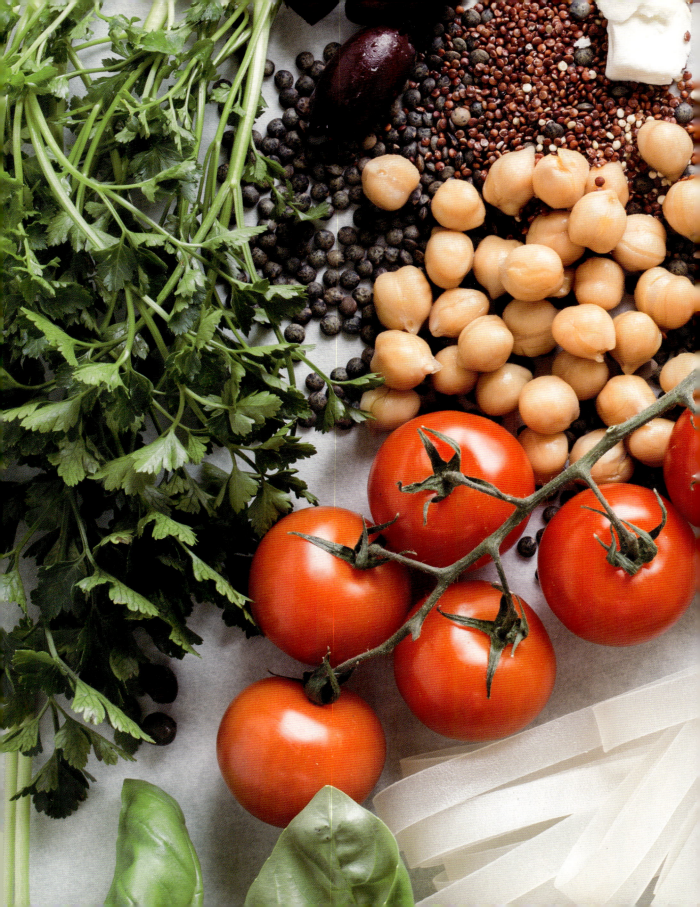

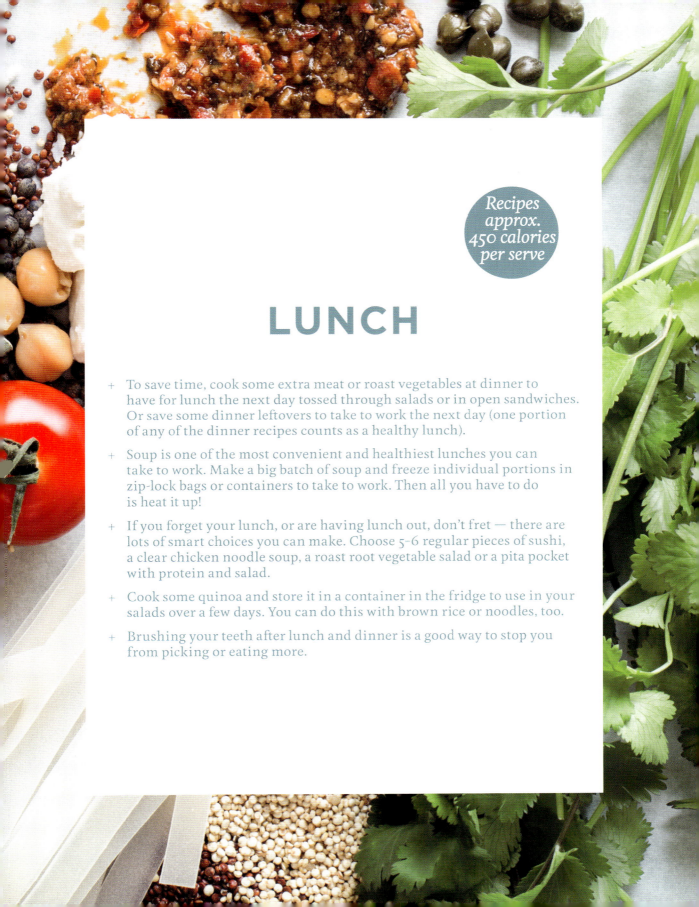

Recipes approx. 450 calories per serve

LUNCH

+ To save time, cook some extra meat or roast vegetables at dinner to have for lunch the next day tossed through salads or in open sandwiches. Or save some dinner leftovers to take to work the next day (one portion of any of the dinner recipes counts as a healthy lunch).

+ Soup is one of the most convenient and healthiest lunches you can take to work. Make a big batch of soup and freeze individual portions in zip-lock bags or containers to take to work. Then all you have to do is heat it up!

+ If you forget your lunch, or are having lunch out, don't fret — there are lots of smart choices you can make. Choose 5-6 regular pieces of sushi, a clear chicken noodle soup, a roast root vegetable salad or a pita pocket with protein and salad.

+ Cook some quinoa and store it in a container in the fridge to use in your salads over a few days. You can do this with brown rice or noodles, too.

+ Brushing your teeth after lunch and dinner is a good way to stop you from picking or eating more.

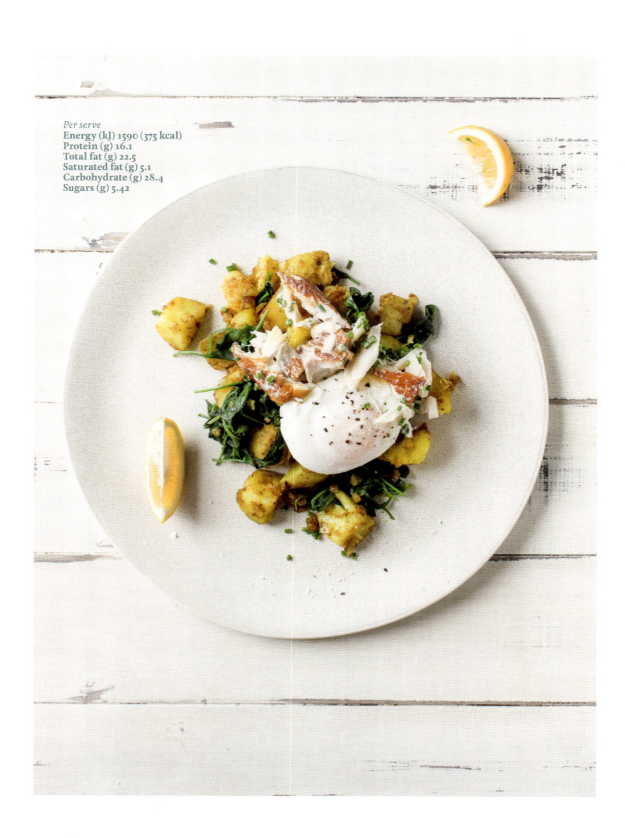

Per serve
Energy (kJ) 1590 (375 kcal)
Protein (g) 16.1
Total fat (g) 22.5
Saturated fat (g) 5.1
Carbohydrate (g) 28.4
Sugars (g) 5.42

CURRIED POTATO + SPINACH HASH WITH SMOKED FISH

This is one of those versatile dishes that can triple as a brunch, lunch or a simple dinner. These curry-spiced potatoes are incredibly savoury and moreish. I turn to them time and time again for a delicious, simple, satisfying dinner, sometimes with a few slices of pan-fried haloumi instead of smoked fish.

1. Bring a medium-sized saucepan of salted water to the boil. Cook potato cubes until tender, 8–10 minutes. Drain well, return to the pan and place back onto low heat to steam for a few minutes — this will help the potatoes dry out a bit.

2. Heat olive oil in a large non-stick frying pan on medium heat and sauté onion until soft, 3–4 minutes. Add potatoes, curry powder and salt. Fry potatoes, moving them around the pan frequently, until they start to break up and go a little bit crispy on the bottom. This will take 5–10 minutes. Toss through spinach until just wilted.

3. Bring a small saucepan of water to a gentle simmer to poach the eggs. In a bowl, mix flaked smoked fish gently with mayonnaise, lemon juice and chives or spring onion. Season to taste with salt and pepper.

4. Carefully crack eggs into simmering water and poach for 1–2 minutes until whites are just set, but yolks are still runny.

5. To serve, divide curried potato and spinach hash between plates, top with some smoked fish mixture and a poached egg. Garnish with more chives or spring onion, and a wedge of lemon to squeeze over just before eating.

TIP The most important tip for perfect poached eggs is to use really fresh eggs. The fresher they are, the 'tighter' the white will be around the yolk. You can use kumara or sweet potato instead of potato, and kale or silverbeet instead of spinach.

SERVES: 2

PREP TIME: 10 MINUTES

COOK TIME: 20 MINUTES

CURRIED POTATO + SPINACH HASH

Agria potatoes 300g, skin on, scrubbed, cut into 2.5cm cubes
olive oil 1 tablespoon
onion 1 diced
curry powder ½–¾ teaspoon
salt good pinch of
baby spinach or **chopped spinach leaves** 2 handfuls

POACHED EGGS + SMOKED FISH

smoked fish (e.g. kahawai, sardines, salmon, mackerel) 70–80g, flaked
good-quality mayonnaise 1½ tablespoons
lemon juice 1 tablespoon
chives or **spring onion** 2 tablespoons chopped + extra to garnish
salt
freshly ground black pepper
free-range eggs 2
lemon ½, cut into wedges to serve

WHEAT FREE   GLUTEN FREE   DAIRY FREE

LUNCH

CREAMY SPICED PARSNIP SOUP WITH CRISPY BACON

Parsnips make a deliciously thick, creamy soup, with a sweet, earthy flavour. Add some warming ginger and spices, a squeeze of lemon, and crispy, salty bacon, and you've got a tasty autumn or winter meal.

1. Heat olive oil in a medium-sized saucepan over medium heat. Cook onion, garlic and ginger until soft, 2–3 minutes. Add cumin, coriander and turmeric and continue to cook for 1 minute further.

2. Add parsnips, potatoes, thyme, chicken or vegetable stock and milk and bring to a gentle boil. Reduce heat and simmer until parsnips and potatoes are very soft, about 25 minutes. Use a hand blender to blend the soup until smooth. Season to taste with salt and pepper, and lemon juice.

3. Heat olive oil in a small frying pan over high heat. Add bacon and cook for a few minutes until crispy.

4. To serve, divide parsnip soup between bowls, and garnish with crispy bacon and parsley.

TIP Freeze individual portions of soup in plastic containers or ziplock bags, ready to 'heat and eat' — great for a quick, convenient work lunch.

SERVES: 4

PREP TIME: 12 MINUTES

COOK TIME: 30 MINUTES

olive oil 1 tablespoon
onion 1, finely diced
garlic 2 cloves, minced
ginger 2cm piece, peeled, finely chopped (about 2 teaspoons)
ground cumin 1 teaspoon
ground coriander ½ teaspoon
ground turmeric ¼ teaspoon
parsnips 650g, peeled, chopped
potatoes 250g, peeled, chopped
thyme leaves 1 tablespoon chopped
good-quality chicken or vegetable stock 3 cups
milk 1½ cups
salt
freshly ground black pepper
lemon juice 1–2 tablespoons

TO SERVE

olive oil 1 teaspoon
lean shoulder or middle bacon 100g, diced
flat-leaf parsley 3 tablespoons finely chopped

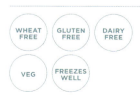

Use dairy-free milk + omit bacon + use vegetable stock

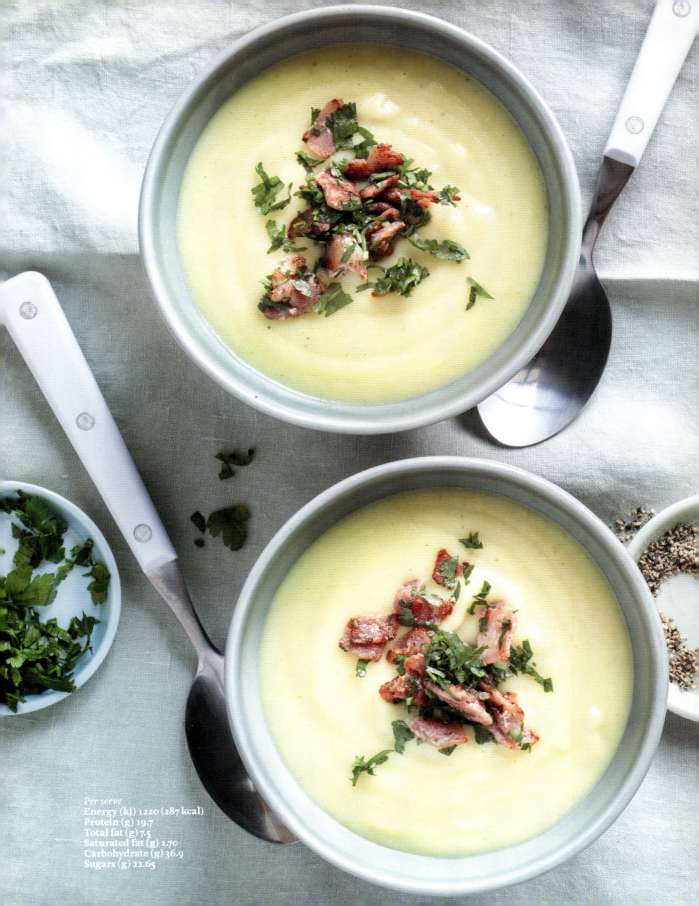

Per serve
Energy (kJ) 1220 (287 kcal)
Protein (g) 19.7
Total fat (g) 7.5
Saturated fat (g) 1.70
Carbohydrate (g) 36.9
Sugars (g) 22.65

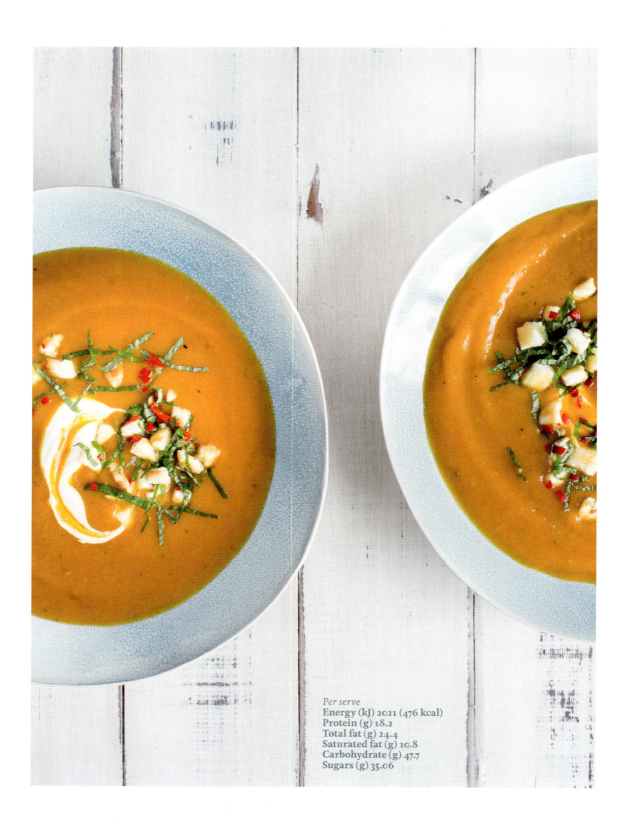

Per serve
Energy (kJ) 2021 (476 kcal)
Protein (g) 18.2
Total fat (g) 24.4
Saturated fat (g) 10.8
Carbohydrate (g) 47.7
Sugars (g) 35.06

MAPLE-ROASTED PUMPKIN + ONION SOUP WITH HALOUMI, MINT AND CHILLI

Roasting the butternut or pumpkin and onions for this soup intensifies their flavour and brings out their natural sweetness. The result is a tastier soup than if you were to boil the vegetables. I love the salty little cubes of haloumi and the freshness of the mint and chilli on top, but you can garnish with whatever you like — a swirl of coconut cream is yummy too.

1. Preheat oven to 220°C. Line an oven tray with baking paper. Toss butternut or pumpkin and onion with maple syrup, olive oil, cumin and thyme. Season well with salt and pepper and roast for 40-45 minutes or until vegetables are soft and caramelised.

2. Transfer roast butternut or pumpkin and onion to a saucepan. Add chicken or vegetable stock. Blend with a stick blender until smooth. Add more stock if needed to get the consistency you want. Heat on the stovetop and season to taste with lemon juice, salt and pepper.

3. Heat olive oil in a non-stick frying pan over medium heat and cook haloumi for a few minutes, tossing frequently, until golden brown.

4. To serve, ladle soup into bowls and serve with a dollop of natural yoghurt and haloumi, chilli and mint on top.

TIP Freeze individual portions of soup in plastic containers or ziplock bags, ready to 'heat and eat' — great for a quick, convenient work lunch. Try chopped up crispy bacon and parsley, or a swirl of coconut cream and coriander instead of haloumi.

SERVES: 2

PREP TIME: 10-15 MINUTES

COOK TIME: 45 MINUTES

butternut or **pumpkin** 1-1.2kg, peeled, cut into 3cm chunks
red onion 1, cut into 2cm-thick wedges
pure maple syrup 1 tablespoon
olive oil 1 tablespoon
ground cumin 1 teaspoon
thyme leaves 1½ teaspoons chopped
salt
freshly ground black pepper
chicken or vegetable stock 1½-2 cups
lemon juice 2-3 tablespoons

TO SERVE
olive oil 1 teaspoon
haloumi 100g, diced into small cubes
red chilli ½, finely chopped
mint leaves 2 tablespoons finely chopped
natural unsweetened thick Greek yoghurt 2-3 tablespoons

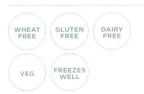

Dairy-free without haloumi + yoghurt + use vegetable stock

LUNCH

MOROCCAN CHICKPEA SOUP (HARIRA)

This hearty soup is full of flavour, and also makes a great light dinner. Chickpeas and lentils are great foods — they're high in protein and have a low glycaemic index, so they help keep you fuller for longer.

1. Heat olive oil in a large saucepan over medium heat. Cook onion, carrots, celery, garlic and ginger until soft, about 6 minutes.

2. Add harissa, tomato paste, cumin, coriander and smoked paprika and cook until fragrant, about 2 minutes.

3. Add thyme, tomatoes, honey, lentils and stock and bring to a boil. Simmer for about 25 minutes, then add chickpeas and continue simmering for a further 10-15 minutes or until lentils are cooked through. They should be tender, but still keep their shape.

4. Season soup to taste with salt and pepper. To serve, garnish with yoghurt, coriander and parsley.

TIP Freeze individual portions of soup in plastic containers or ziplock bags, ready to 'heat and eat' — great for a quick, convenient work lunch.

SERVES: 4
PREP TIME: 10 MINUTES
COOK TIME: 50 MINUTES

olive oil 1 tablespoon
onion 1, finely diced
carrots 2, peeled, finely diced
celery 2 stalks, finely diced
garlic 2 cloves, minced
ginger 1 tablespoon finely chopped
harissa paste (store-bought or see page 276) 2 tablespoons
tomato paste 1 tablespoon
ground cumin 1 tablespoon
ground coriander 2 teaspoons
smoked paprika 2 teaspoons
thyme leaves 1 tablespoon chopped
crushed tomatoes 1 x 400g can
honey ½ teaspoon
puy or French green lentils ½ cup, rinsed
chicken or vegetable stock 1 litre
chickpeas 1 x 400g can, rinsed, drained
salt
freshly ground black pepper

TO SERVE
natural unsweetened yoghurt 2-3 tablespoons
coriander ¼ cup chopped
flat-leaf parsley ¼ cup chopped

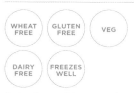

Dairy-free without yoghurt + use vegetable stock

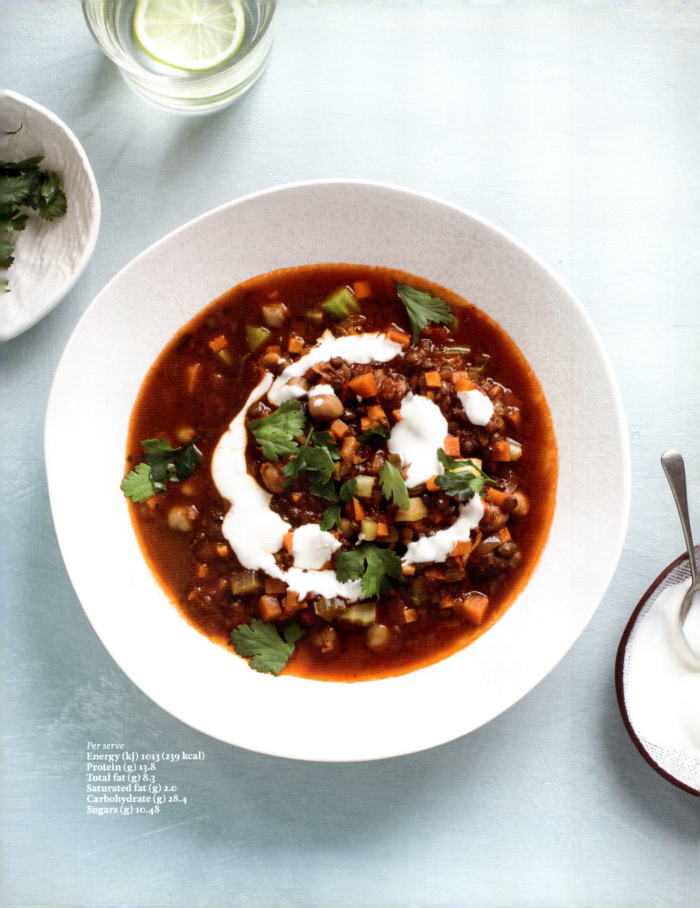

Per serve
Energy (kJ) 1013 (239 kcal)
Protein (g) 13.8
Total fat (g) 8.3
Saturated fat (g) 2.0
Carbohydrate (g) 28.4
Sugars (g) 10.48

MOZZARELLA QUESADILLAS

Mexican quesadillas (pronounced kay-sa-dee-a) are the ultimate casual finger food, perfect for sharing. The tomato jalapeño jam is out of this world tasty, and you can use it as an accompaniment to lots of other Mexican-style dishes.

1. Heat 1 teaspoon olive oil in a frying pan over medium heat. Cook onion until soft, 3-4 minutes. Add garlic, paprika and cumin and cook for 1 minute further. Add tomato paste and cook for 1 minute further. Take off heat and mix in spring onion, beans, chipotle sauce and spinach. Use a fork to roughly crush everything together. Season to taste with salt and pepper.

2. Lay a tortilla wrap on a clean dry surface. Sprinkle over 3 tablespoons mozzarella, then spoon about ⅔ cup of the bean mixture on top, and sprinkle over another 3 tablespoons mozzarella. Top with another tortilla and press down gently but firmly. Repeat for remaining tortillas and filling.

3. Heat 1 teaspoon olive oil in a non-stick frying pan on medium heat. Place one quesadilla in the pan and cook for 2-3 minutes until golden brown and slightly crispy on the outside, and cheese has melted inside. Press down on the quesadilla with a fish slice to help flatten it and make sure the filling sticks to the tortillas. Carefully flip quesadilla over and cook for 2 minutes on the other side until golden brown and cheese has melted. Repeat with remaining quesadillas.

4. Place all tomato jalapeño jam ingredients in a frying pan and simmer rapidly for 8-10 minutes until of a thick consistency. Season with salt and pepper.

5. Mix Greek yoghurt and chives together.

6. To serve, cut each quesadilla into four and pile onto a large plate or wooden board. Garnish with coriander and serve with tomato jalapeño jam and chive yoghurt on the side.

TIP If you can't find chipotle sauce (a Mexican smoked chilli sauce), substitute 1½ tablespoons tomato sauce, 1½ tablespoons chilli sauce and ½ teaspoon smoked paprika.

SERVES: 4-6

PREP TIME: 15 MINUTES

COOK TIME: 15 MINUTES

QUESADILLAS

olive oil 5 teaspoons
onion 1, finely diced
garlic 1 clove, chopped
smoked paprika 1 teaspoon
ground cumin 1 teaspoon
tomato paste 1 tablespoon
spring onions 2, finely sliced
beans (e.g. black beans, pinto beans, haricot beans, etc.) 1 x 400g can, rinsed, drained
chipotle sauce 2-3 tablespoons
spinach leaves 2 handfuls, chopped
salt
freshly ground black pepper
corn or wheat tortillas 8 small
grated mozzarella 1½ cups
coriander ½ cup chopped, to garnish

TOMATO JALAPEÑO JAM

crushed tomatoes 1 x 400g can
pickled jalapeños 2-4 tablespoons chopped or **large red chilli** 1, chopped
brown sugar 1 teaspoon
extra virgin olive oil drizzle of

CHIVE YOGHURT

natural unsweetened thick Greek yoghurt ½ cup
chives 2-3 tablespoons finely chopped

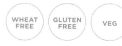

Use corn tortillas

Per serve
Energy (kJ) 1968 (464 kcal)
Protein (g) 21.1
Total fat (g) 16.4
Saturated fat (g) 4.8
Carbohydrate (g) 60.2
Sugars (g) 9.17

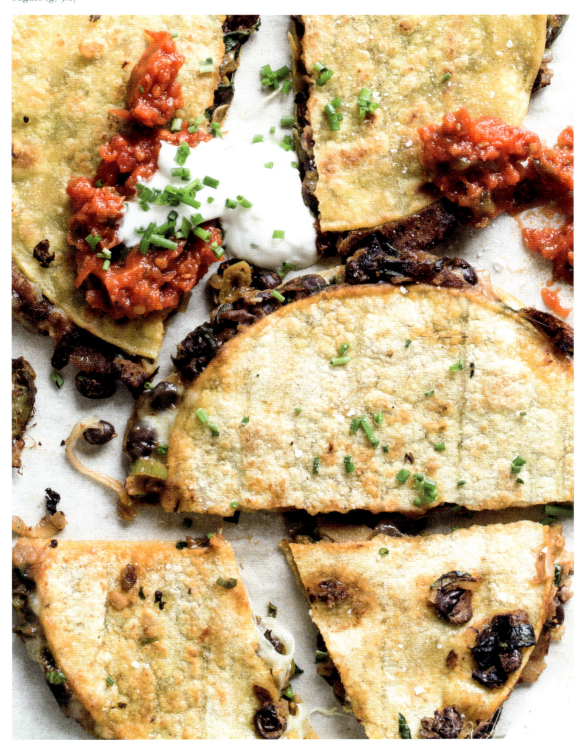

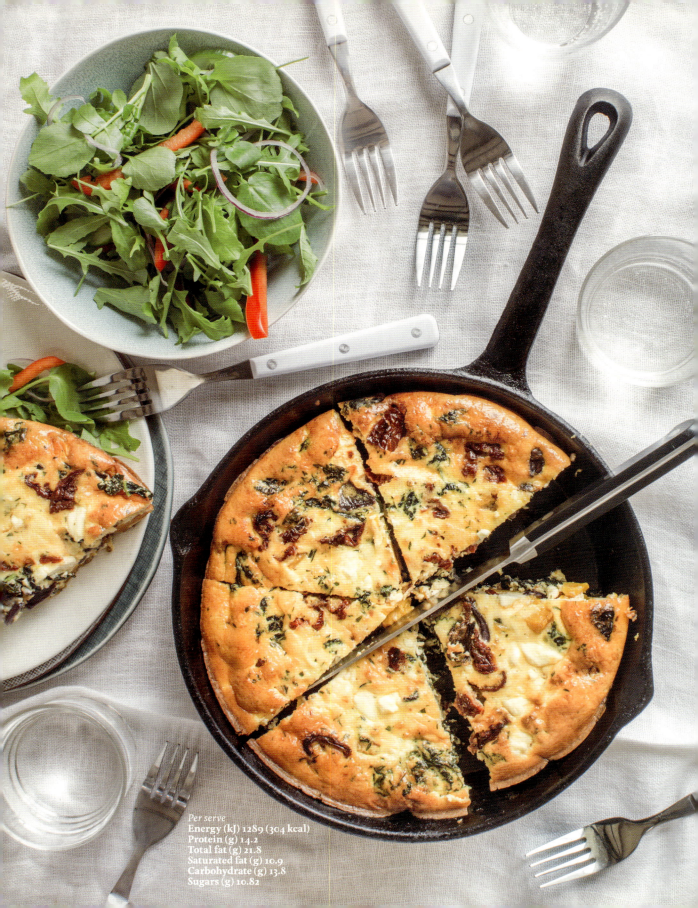

Per serve
Energy (kJ) 1289 (304 kcal)
Protein (g) 14.2
Total fat (g) 21.8
Saturated fat (g) 10.9
Carbohydrate (g) 13.8
Sugars (g) 10.82

PUMPKIN, KALE + FETA FRITTATA

There's no denying eggs are a nutritious food — they contain everything needed to build new life! With the addition of dark, leafy greens and pumpkin, a slice of this frittata makes a very nutritious, delicious lunch.

1. Preheat oven to 200°C. Line an oven tray with baking paper. Toss pumpkin or butternut and red onion with olive oil. Season with salt and pepper and roast for 20–30 minutes or until soft and slightly caramelised.

2. When pumpkin is almost ready, heat a drizzle of olive oil in a large ovenproof heavy-based frying pan with high sides (this is what you use to cook the frittata in). Sizzle garlic for 30 seconds, then add kale, cavolo nero, spinach or silverbeet and cook for a further 2–3 minutes or until wilted. Add a couple of tablespoons of water and place a lid on top of the pan to help create steam to cook the kale through. Continue to cook with the lid off until all the moisture has evaporated (this is important to avoid a soggy frittata).

3. In a bowl lightly whisk together eggs, milk, cream, a good pinch of salt, feta, thyme and chilli flakes, if using.

4. Toss roast butternut or pumpkin and onion with kale in the frying pan, then pour over the egg mixture. Scatter over sundried tomatoes. Bake for 20–30 minutes or until frittata is puffed and golden. Stand in the pan for about 10 minutes before cutting.

5. To serve, cut frittata into wedges and serve with a big leafy green salad and a dollop of chutney on the side.

TIP The frittata will keep in the fridge for a couple of days — just reheat in the microwave or oven. It's great to take to work for lunch.

SERVES: 6

PREP TIME: 12 MINUTES

COOK TIME: 50–60 MINUTES

pumpkin or **butternut** 500g, peeled, cut into 1–2cm cubes
red onion 1 large, cut into 2cm chunks
olive oil 1 tablespoon
salt
freshly ground black pepper
garlic 2 cloves, chopped
curly kale, cavolo nero, spinach or **silverbeet** 120g, tough stalks removed, leaves chopped
free-range eggs 6
milk ½ cup
cream ½ cup
feta 150g, crumbled
thyme leaves 2 teaspoons chopped
chilli flakes ½–¾ teaspoon (optional)
sundried tomatoes ½ cup sliced

TO SERVE

leafy green salad (see page 277) 6 servings
tomato chutney

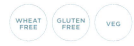

LUNCH

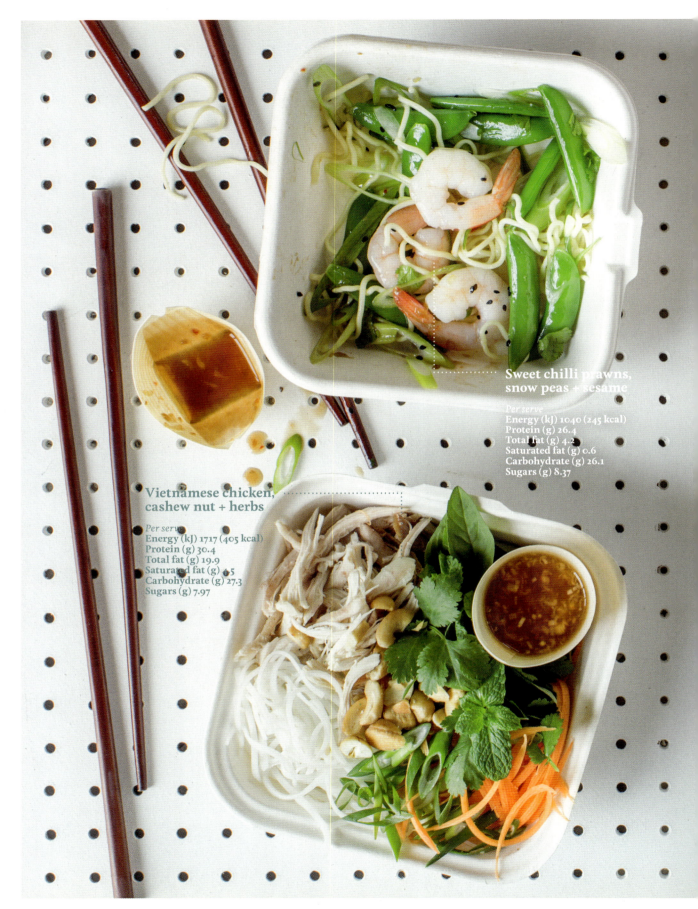

Sweet chilli prawns, snow peas + sesame

Per serve
Energy (kJ) 1040 (245 kcal)
Protein (g) 26.4
Total fat (g) 4.2
Saturated fat (g) 0.6
Carbohydrate (g) 26.1
Sugars (g) 8.37

Vietnamese chicken, cashew nut + herbs

Per serve
Energy (kJ) 1717 (405 kcal)
Protein (g) 30.4
Total fat (g) 19.9
Saturated fat (g) 4.5
Carbohydrate (g) 27.3
Sugars (g) 7.97

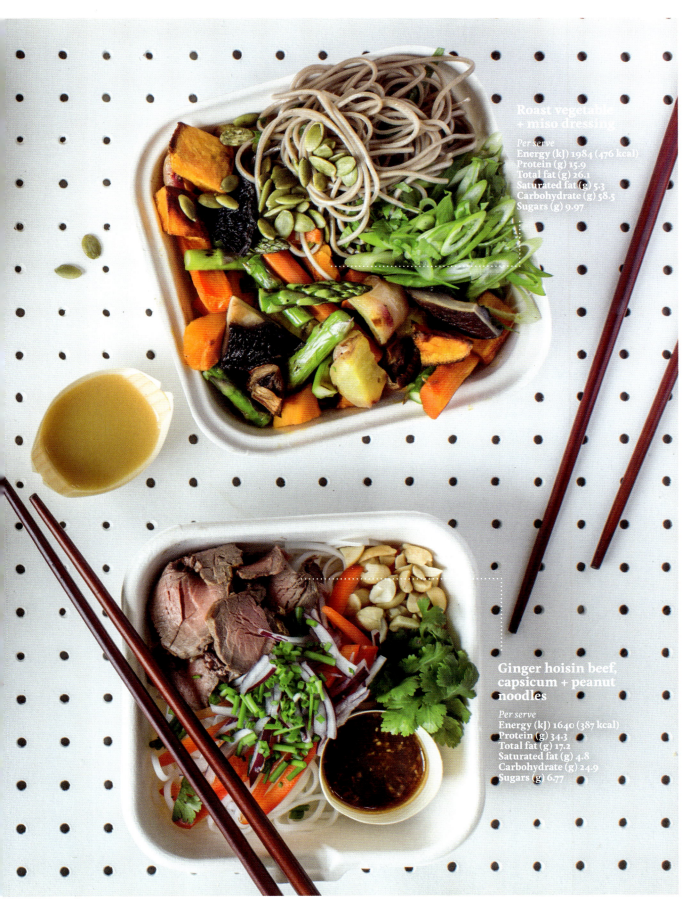

Roast vegetable + miso dressing

Per serve
Energy (kJ) 1984 (476 kcal)
Protein (g) 15.9
Total fat (g) 26.1
Saturated fat (g) 5.3
Carbohydrate (g) 58.5
Sugars (g) 9.97

Ginger hoisin beef, capsicum + peanut noodles

Per serve
Energy (kJ) 1640 (387 kcal)
Protein (g) 34.3
Total fat (g) 17.2
Saturated fat (g) 4.8
Carbohydrate (g) 24.9
Sugars (g) 6.77

NOODLE BOXES

These noodle salads are fast, fresh and tasty, using leftover cooked chicken, meat, vegetables or quick-to-cook prawns. Swap out the suggested protein for whatever you have on hand and double up the quantities to serve two people. These are great to take to work for lunch.

VIETNAMESE CHICKEN, CASHEW NUT + HERBS

1. Cook rice noodles in boiling salted water until soft, about 5 minutes. Drain and rinse under cold water to stop the cooking process and prevent noodles sticking together. Use scissors to snip in a few places to shorten noodles and make them easier to eat.

2. Mix all dressing ingredients together and toss with noodles and remaining ingredients just before eating.

TIP If taking to work as a lunch box, pack the dressing separately and toss with noodle salad ingredients just before eating. To mix it up, you can use any other protein, e.g. prawns, tofu, pork, lamb or beef, in place of chicken.

SERVES: 1

PREP TIME: 10 MINUTES

COOK TIME: 5 MINUTES

thin dried rice stick noodles 50g
cooked chicken 100g (about ¾ cup), shredded
mesclun leaves 1 handful
roasted cashew nuts 2 tablespoons chopped
carrot 1 small, peeled, shredded
spring onion 1, finely sliced
mint, coriander and **Vietnamese mint** or **Thai or aniseed basil** ¼ cup total, chopped
red chilli ½, finely chopped (optional)

DRESSING

sweet chilli sauce 2 teaspoons
fish sauce 1½ teaspoons
lime or lemon juice 1 tablespoon
sesame oil ½ teaspoon
lemongrass 1 teaspoon finely chopped

GINGER HOISIN BEEF, CAPSICUM + PEANUT NOODLES

1. Cook rice noodles in boiling salted water until soft, about 5 minutes. Drain and rinse under cold water to stop the cooking process and prevent noodles sticking together. Use scissors to snip in a few places to shorten noodles and make them easier to eat.

2. Mix all dressing ingredients together and toss with noodles and remaining ingredients just before eating.

TIP If taking to work as a lunch box, pack the dressing separately and toss with noodle salad ingredients just before eating. To mix it up, you can use any other protein, e.g. chicken, pork, prawns or tofu, in place of the beef or lamb.

SERVES: 1

PREP TIME: 10 MINUTES

COOK TIME: 5 MINUTES

thin dried rice stick noodles 50g
cooked beef or lamb 100g (about ¾ cup), sliced
roasted peanuts 1½ tablespoons chopped
red capsicum ½, thinly sliced
coriander 3–4 tablespoons chopped
mint 3–4 tablespoons chopped
red onion 2 tablespoons diced
chives 1 tablespoon chopped
mint, coriander and **Vietnamese mint** or **Thai or aniseed basil** ¼ cup total chopped

DRESSING
hoisin sauce 2 teaspoons
ginger ½ teaspoon finely minced or grated
soy sauce 1 teaspoon
lime or lemon juice 1 tablespoon
sesame oil ½ teaspoon

DAIRY FREE

LUNCH

ROAST VEGETABLE + MISO DRESSING

1. Cook soba noodles in boiling water until just cooked through, about 4 minutes (be careful not to overcook). Drain and rinse under cold water to stop cooking process and prevent noodles sticking together.

2. Mix all dressing ingredients together. Toss dressing with noodles and remaining ingredients just before eating.

TIP If taking to work as a lunch box, pack the dressing separately and toss with noodle salad ingredients just before eating.

SERVES: 1

PREP TIME: 10 MINUTES

COOK TIME: 5 MINUTES

dried soba noodles 50g
roasted vegetables (e.g. pumpkin, carrot, parsnip, mushrooms, yams, leek, onion) 1½ cups chopped
spring onions 1–2, finely sliced
coriander 3–4 tablespoons chopped
pumpkin seeds 2 teaspoons

DRESSING

white miso paste 1 tablespoon
rice vinegar 1 teaspoon
brown sugar 1 teaspoon
sesame oil 1 teaspoon
lime or lemon juice 1 tablespoon

DAIRY FREE   VEG

SWEET CHILLI PRAWNS, SNOW PEAS + SESAME

1. Cook egg noodles in boiling water until just cooked through, 4-5 minutes (be careful not to overcook). Drop prawns and snow peas into the noodles halfway through cooking time.

2. Drain noodles, prawns and snow peas, and rinse noodles under cold water to cool and prevent noodles sticking together.

3. Mix all dressing ingredients together. Toss dressing with noodles, prawns and remaining ingredients just before eating.

TIP If taking to work as a lunch box, pack the dressing separately and toss with noodle salad ingredients just before eating. If you prefer not to use prawns, try chicken, pork, beef or tofu.

SERVES: 1
PREP TIME: 10 MINUTES
COOK TIME: 5 MINUTES

dried egg noodles 50g
frozen raw prawn cutlets 100g (about 10 prawns cutlets), defrosted
snow peas 100g
spring onion 1, finely sliced
coriander ¼ cup chopped
white or black sesame seeds ½ teaspoon

DRESSING
sweet chilli sauce 1 tablespoon
sesame oil ½ teaspoon
lemon or lime juice 1 tablespoon
soy sauce 1 teaspoon

DAIRY FREE

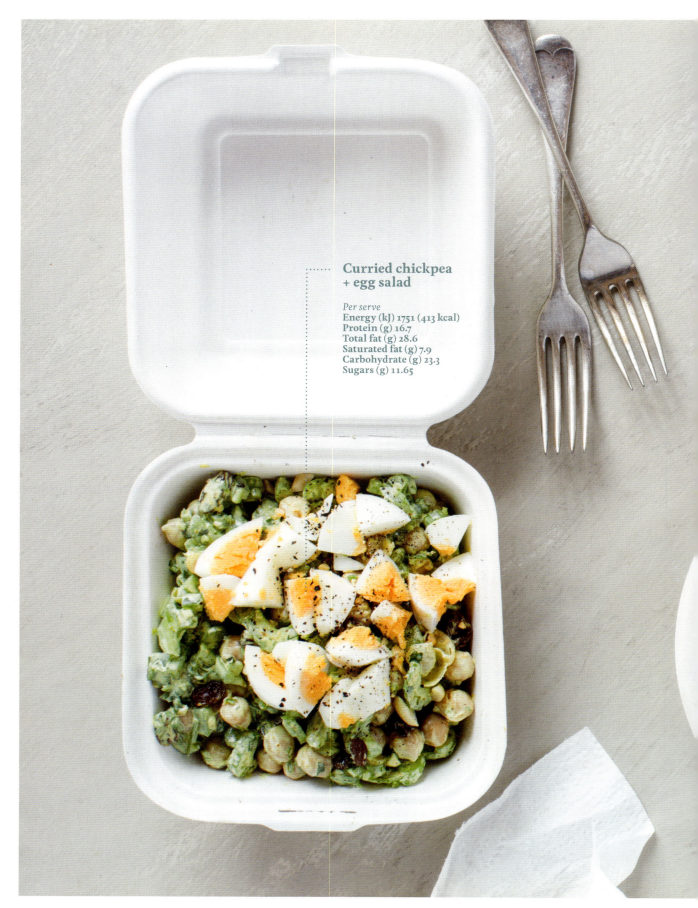

Curried chickpea + egg salad

Per serve
Energy (kJ) 1751 (413 kcal)
Protein (g) 16.7
Total fat (g) 28.6
Saturated fat (g) 7.9
Carbohydrate (g) 23.3
Sugars (g) 11.65

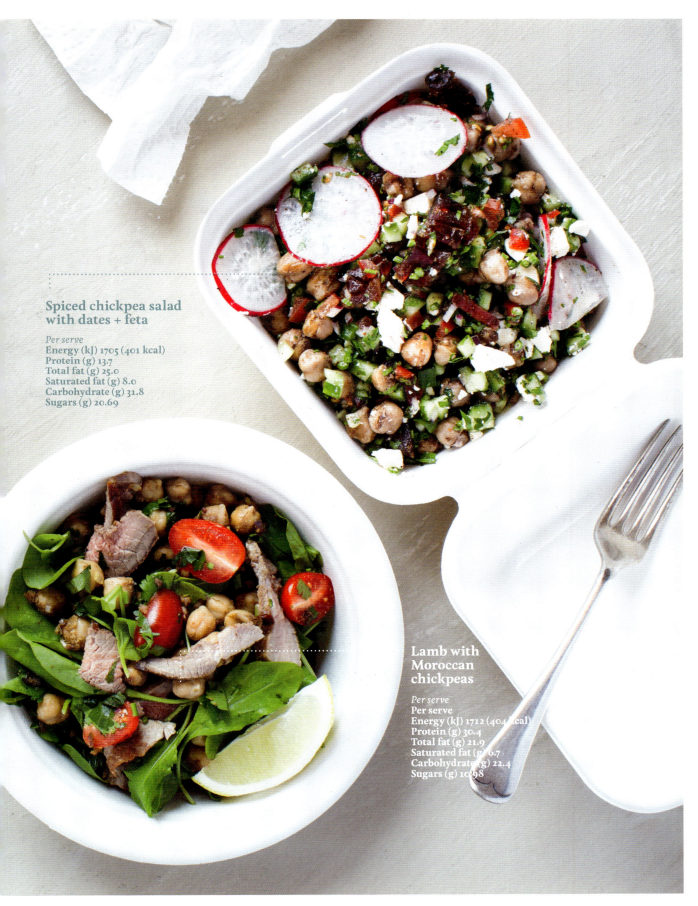

Spiced chickpea salad with dates + feta

Per serve
Energy (kJ) 1705 (401 kcal)
Protein (g) 13.7
Total fat (g) 25.0
Saturated fat (g) 8.0
Carbohydrate (g) 31.8
Sugars (g) 20.69

Lamb with Moroccan chickpeas

Per serve
Per serve
Energy (kJ) 1712 (404 kcal)
Protein (g) 30.4
Total fat (g) 21.9
Saturated fat (g) 6.7
Carbohydrate (g) 22.4
Sugars (g) 10.98

CHICKPEA LUNCH BOXES

By themselves, chickpeas can be bland and boring, but add a few Indian, Moroccan or Middle Eastern spices and boom!, you've got the base for a healthy, flavour-packed meal. The ingredient quantities in these recipes can easily be doubled to serve two people. These are great to take to work.

LAMB WITH MOROCCAN CHICKPEAS

1. Heat olive oil in a small frying pan over medium heat. Cook red onion for 3-4 minutes until soft. Add garlic, chickpeas, cumin and coriander and cook for another 1-2 minutes until chickpeas are warmed through and coated in spices.

2. Remove from heat and toss with preserved lemon or lemon zest, lamb, cherry tomatoes, herbs and baby rocket or spinach.

3. Just before serving, dress with a squeeze of lemon juice and extra virgin olive oil, and season with a little salt and pepper if needed.

SERVES: 1

PREP TIME: 10 MINUTES

COOK TIME: 3-4 MINUTES

olive oil 1 teaspoon
red onion ½ small, finely diced
garlic 1 small clove, minced
chickpeas ½ × 400g can, drained, rinsed
ground cumin 1 teaspoon
ground coriander ½ teaspoon
preserved lemon ½ teaspoon finely chopped, or **lemon** zest of ½
cooked lamb 80g, thinly sliced (about ¾ cup)
cherry tomatoes 4-5, halved
coriander, flat-leaf parsley and **mint** ¼ cup total
baby rocket or **spinach** 1 handful
lemon juice squeeze of
extra virgin olive oil 1 teaspoon
salt
freshly ground black pepper

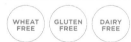

WHEAT FREE · GLUTEN FREE · DAIRY FREE

SPICED CHICKPEA SALAD WITH DATES + FETA

SERVES: 1   **PREP TIME:** 10 MINUTES
COOK TIME: 2-3 MINUTES

olive oil 2 teaspoons
chickpeas ½ x 400g can, drained, rinsed
ground allspice ½ teaspoon
ground cumin ¼ teaspoon
chilli flakes ¼ teaspoon
vine-ripened tomato 1 small, diced
Lebanese cucumber ½, diced
baby radish 1, thinly sliced
red onion 2 tablespoons finely diced
feta 25g, crumbled
medjool dates 2, pitted, chopped
flat-leaf parsley ¼ cup chopped
lemon juice of ½
extra virgin olive oil 1 teaspoon
salt
freshly ground black pepper

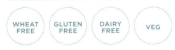

Dairy-free without feta

Heat olive oil in a frying pan over medium heat. Cook chickpeas, allspice, cumin and chilli for 2-3 minutes, gently shaking the pan so they cook evenly and don't stick to the base. To serve, toss spiced chickpeas with remaining ingredients. Season with salt and pepper.

CURRIED CHICKPEA + EGG SALAD

SERVES: 1   **PREP TIME:** 10 MINUTES

good-quality mayonnaise 1 tablespoon
natural unsweetened thick Greek yoghurt 1½ tablespoons
curry powder ½ teaspoon
chickpeas ½ x 400g can, drained, rinsed
hardboiled free-range egg 1, roughly chopped
celery 1 stalk, finely sliced
sultanas 1 tablespoon
peanuts 1 tablespoon roughly chopped
green capsicum ¼, diced
coriander ¼ cup chopped
salt
freshly ground black pepper

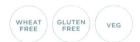

Mix mayonnaise, yoghurt and curry powder together. To serve, toss with remaining ingredients and season to taste with salt and pepper.

LUNCH

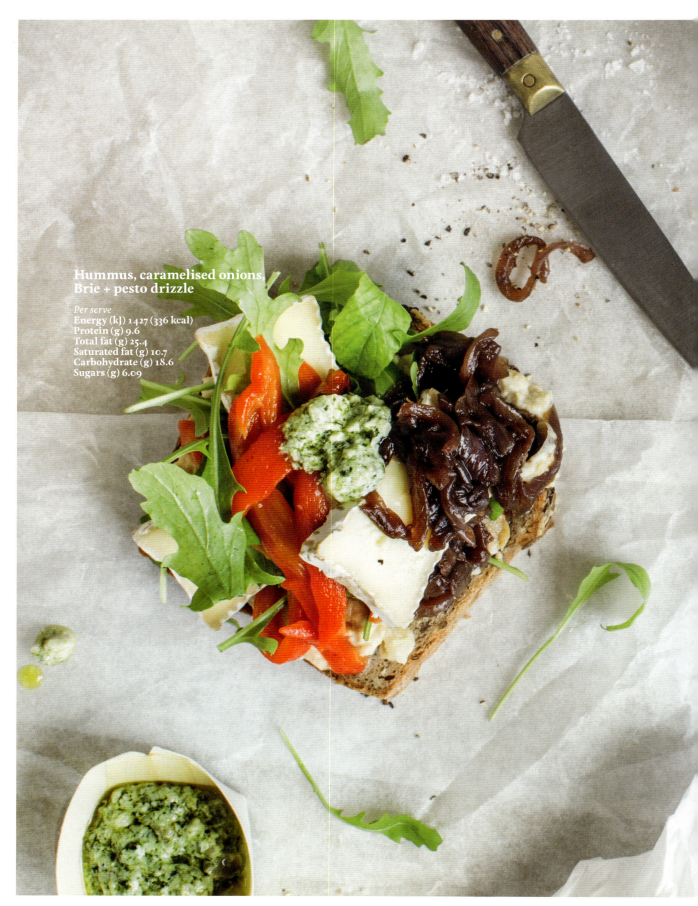

Hummus, caramelised onions, Brie + pesto drizzle

Per serve
Energy (kJ) 1427 (336 kcal)
Protein (g) 9.6
Total fat (g) 25.4
Saturated fat (g) 10.7
Carbohydrate (g) 18.6
Sugars (g) 6.09

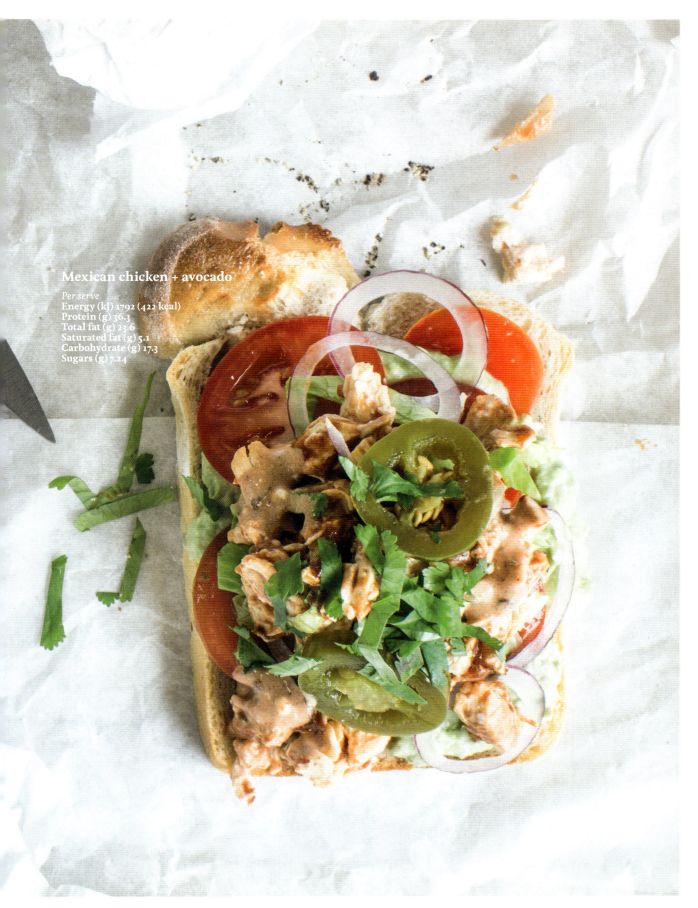

Mexican chicken + avocado

Per serve
Energy (kJ) 1792 (422 kcal)
Protein (g) 36.3
Total fat (g) 23.6
Saturated fat (g) 5.1
Carbohydrate (g) 17.3
Sugars (g) 7.24

French tuna, egg + caper pan bagnat

Per serve
Energy (kJ) 1669 (394 kcal)
Protein (g) 31.8
Total fat (g) 22.0
Saturated fat (g) 5.3
Carbohydrate (g) 19.8
Sugars (g) 9.50

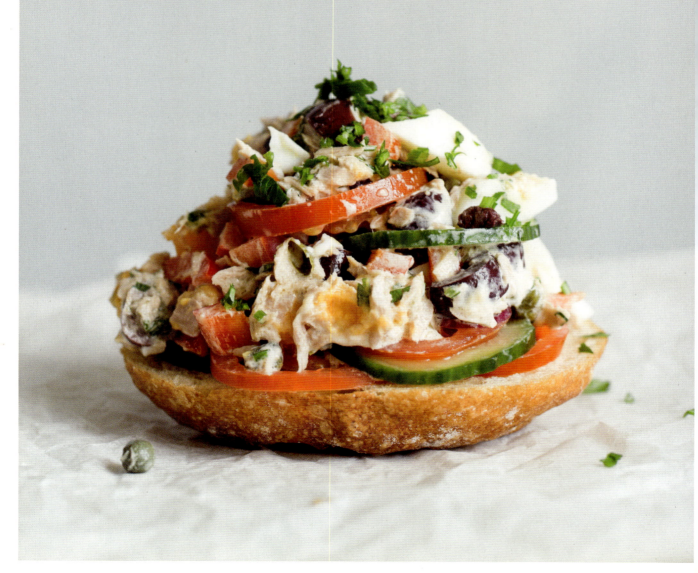

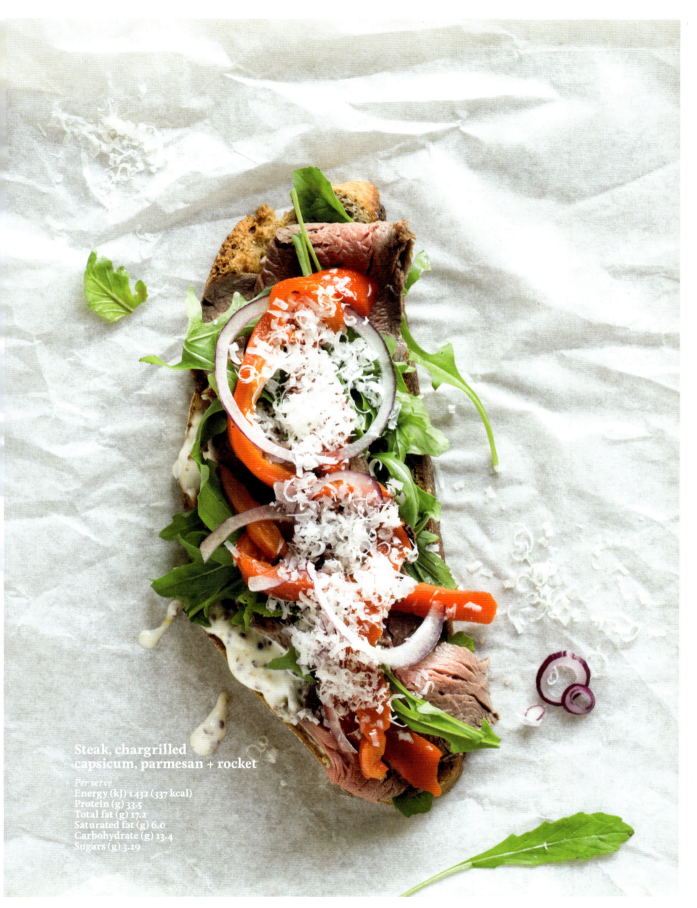

Steak, chargrilled capsicum, parmesan + rocket

Per serve
Energy (kJ) 1,432 (337 kcal)
Protein (g) 33.5
Total fat (g) 17.2
Saturated fat (g) 6.0
Carbohydrate (g) 13.4
Sugars (g) 3.29

OPEN SANDWICHES

Open sandwiches consist of just one piece of bread loaded up with lots of tasty, nutritious ingredients, so you fill up on the good stuff instead of carbs. If you prefer all the fillings to be contained, you can always substitute the bread for a small pita pocket. Feel free to toast your bread if you prefer.

HUMMUS, CARAMELISED ONIONS, BRIE + PESTO DRIZZLE

SERVES: 1   PREP TIME: 5 MINUTES

hummus 2 tablespoons (store-bought or see page 270)
wholegrain bread 1 slice
baby rocket leaves 1 small handful
caramelised onions (home-made, see page 276, or store-bought) 1½–2 tablespoons
roasted red capsicum (from a jar) 1 small or ½ large, sliced
Brie 30g (about 3 slices), sliced
natural unsweetened yoghurt 2 teaspoons
basil pesto 2 teaspoons

Spread hummus over bread. Top with rocket leaves, caramelised onions, capsicum and slices of Brie. Mix yoghurt and pesto together and drizzle over the top.

Use gluten-free bread

MEXICAN CHICKEN + AVOCADO

SERVES: 1   PREP TIME: 5 MINUTES

chipotle sauce 1–2 teaspoons
good-quality mayonnaise 2 teaspoons
leftover cooked chicken 100g (about ¾ cup), shredded
avocado ¼ ripe
lime juice of ½
salt
freshly ground black pepper
wholegrain or rye bread 1 slice (about 50g)
vine-ripened tomato 1, sliced
red onion a few thin slices
shredded lettuce 1 small handful
coriander 2 tablespoons chopped
pickled jalapeños 2–3 slices (optional, but highly recommended!)

Mix chipotle sauce with mayonnaise and toss with cooked chicken. Use a fork to roughly mash avocado and lime juice together and season with salt and pepper. Spread avocado over bread and top with tomato, red onion, lettuce, chipotle chicken, coriander and jalapeños, if using.

GLUTEN FREE   DAIRY FREE

Use gluten-free bread

Here are some of my favourite combos, but you can get creative and mix it up however you like; just stick to having one slice of bread or a small pita pocket, 80-100g protein and a handful of salad or vegetables, plus one or two tasty accompaniments.

FRENCH TUNA, EGG + CAPER PAN BAGNAT

SERVES: 1 **PREP TIME:** 5 MINUTES

canned tuna in spring water or oil 80g, drained, flaked
good-quality mayonnaise 1 tablespoon
capers 1 teaspoon chopped
Kalamata olives 3-4, pitted, chopped
red capsicum ½, finely diced
flat-leaf parsley 1 tablespoon finely chopped
hardboiled egg 1, peeled, chopped
salt
freshly ground black pepper
wholegrain bread or **bread roll** 1 slice (about 50g)
cucumber 6-8 thin slices
tomato 1, sliced
red onion a few very thin slices

Combine tuna, mayonnaise, capers, olives, capsicum, parsley and egg, and season to taste with salt and pepper. Top bread with slices of cucumber, tomato and red onion, and pile on tuna mixture. Season with more pepper.

Use gluten-free bread

STEAK, CHARGRILLED CAPSICUM, PARMESAN + ROCKET

SERVES: 1 **PREP TIME:** 5 MINUTES

good-quality mayonnaise 2 teaspoons
wholegrain mustard 1 teaspoon
wholegrain or rye bread 1 slice (about 50g), toasted
rocket leaves 1 handful
leftover cooked lamb or beef steak 100g, sliced
roasted red capsicum (from a jar) 1 small or ½ large, sliced
red onion a few thin slices
parmesan 1 tablespoon grated

Mix mayonnaise with mustard and spread over toasted bread. Top with rocket leaves, slices of cooked meat, capsicum, red onion and parmesan.

Use gluten-free bread + omit parmesan

LUNCH

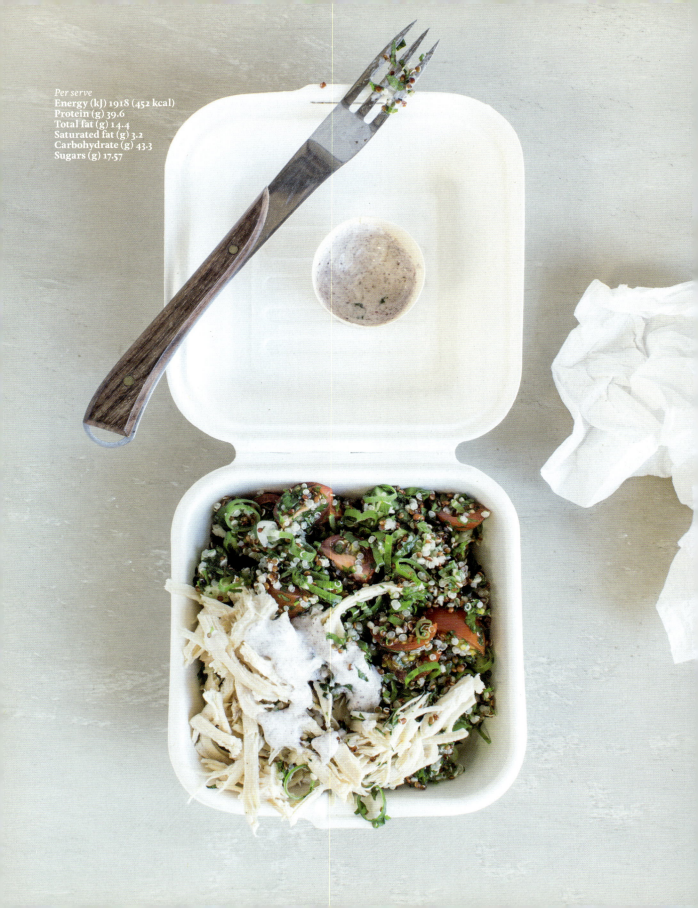

Per serve
Energy (kJ) 1918 (452 kcal)
Protein (g) 39.6
Total fat (g) 14.4
Saturated fat (g) 3.2
Carbohydrate (g) 43.3
Sugars (g) 17.57

QUINOA LUNCH BOXES

Quinoa is a very high-protein grain, so it has a very low glycaemic index, with slow releasing energy, helping to keep you fuller for longer. You cook quinoa as you would rice. My preferred method is: bring 1 cup quinoa and 1½ cups water with a good pinch of salt to the boil in a small pot. As soon as it boils, cover with a tight-fitting lid, reduce to lowest heat and cook for 15 minutes. Then turn off the heat and leave to steam for a further 8–10 minutes (without taking off the lid). Cooked quinoa will keep in the fridge for a few days, so you can use it across several meals. It has a great texture and a nutty, slightly earthy flavour, and works well in salads.

CHICKEN QUINOA TABOULEH WITH YOGHURT DRESSING

1. Toss cooked quinoa, cherry tomatoes, cucumber, spring onion, parsley, mint, lemon zest and juice, and extra virgin olive oil together. Season with salt and pepper to taste.
2. To serve, gently toss shredded chicken with quinoa tabouleh. If using sumac, mix with yoghurt and drizzle over quinoa tabouleh just before eating.

SERVES: 1

PREP TIME: 5–10 MINUTES

cooked quinoa ½ cup
cherry tomatoes ½ punnet, halved
Lebanese cucumber ½, diced
spring onion 1, finely sliced
flat-leaf parsley 3 tablespoons chopped
mint leaves 3 tablespoons chopped
lemon zest and juice of ½
extra virgin olive oil 1 teaspoon
salt
freshly ground black pepper
cooked chicken 90g (¾ cup), shredded
sumac ½ teaspoon (optional)
natural unsweetened yoghurt 2 tablespoons

WHEAT FREE · GLUTEN FREE · DAIRY FREE

Dairy-free without yoghurt

PRAWN, EDAMAME + QUINOA STIR-FRY

1. Heat oil in a wok or large frying pan over high heat. Pat prawns dry with paper towels, season with salt and add to hot pan. Stir-fry for 2–3 minutes until just cooked through. Remove prawns from pan and set aside. Keep pan on the heat.

2. Add carrot, celery, spring onion, bok choy, edamame beans or peas, ginger and garlic and stir-fry for about 2 minutes until just cooked through. Add quinoa and continue to cook for 1 minute to heat the quinoa through. Add cooked prawns back into the pan, along with soy sauce, sesame oil and coriander. Toss briefly to combine, then serve.

TIP See page 99 for quinoa cooking instructions.

SERVES: 1
PREP TIME: 10 MINUTES
COOK TIME: 10 MINUTES

oil 2 teaspoons
frozen raw prawns 80g (about 8), shelled with tails left on, defrosted
salt
carrot ½ small, peeled, finely diced
celery ½ stalk, finely sliced
spring onion 1, finely sliced
baby bok choy 1, finely sliced
frozen podded edamame beans or **peas** ¼ cup, defrosted
ginger 1 teaspoon minced
garlic 1 clove, minced
cooked quinoa ½ cup
soy sauce 2 teaspoons
sesame oil 1 teaspoon
coriander ¼ cup chopped

(WHEAT FREE) (GLUTEN FREE) (DAIRY FREE)

Use gluten-free tamari soy sauce

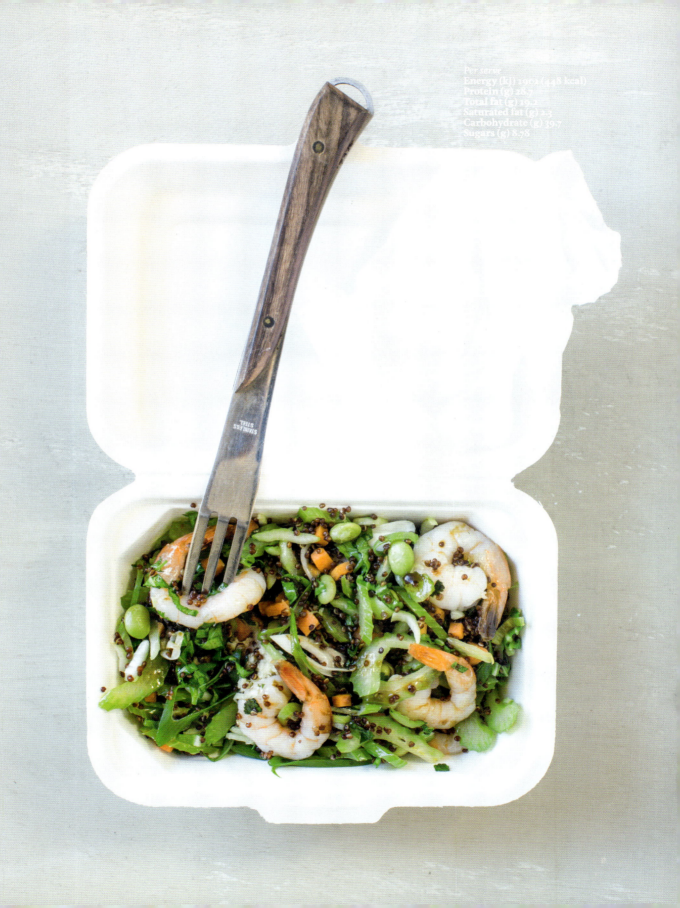

Per serve
Energy (kJ) 1902 (448 kcal)
Protein (g) 28.7
Total fat (g) 19.2
Saturated fat (g) 2.3
Carbohydrate (g) 39.7
Sugars (g) 8.78

AVOCADO, HALOUMI + GRAPE QUINOA SALAD

1. Toss quinoa, avocado, cherry tomatoes, grapes, olives and herbs. Season to taste with salt and pepper.

2. Heat olive oil in a non-stick frying pan over medium-high heat and cook haloumi slices for 1-2 minutes on each side until golden brown and melted on the inside.

3. To serve, mix all dressing ingredients together and toss with quinoa salad. Top with cooked haloumi.

TIP See page 99 for quinoa cooking instructions.

SERVES: 1
PREP TIME: 5-10 MINUTES
COOK TIME: 5 MINUTES

cooked quinoa ½ cup
avocado ¼ ripe, sliced
cherry tomatoes 4-5, halved
seedless grapes ¼ cup, halved
Kalamata olives 4-5, pitted, sliced
flat-leaf parsley and **mint** ¼ cup total chopped
salt
freshly ground black pepper
olive oil ¼ teaspoon
haloumi 50g (about 2 slices), cut into 1cm slices

DRESSING
red wine vinegar 2 teaspoons
wholegrain mustard 1 teaspoon
lemon juice squeeze of
liquid honey ½ teaspoon
extra virgin olive oil 2 teaspoons

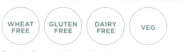

Dairy-free without haloumi

Per serve
Energy (kJ) 2420 (570 kcal)
Protein (g) 19.1
Total fat (g) 38.1
Saturated fat (g) 11.7
Carbohydrate (g) 45.9
Sugars (g) 19.8

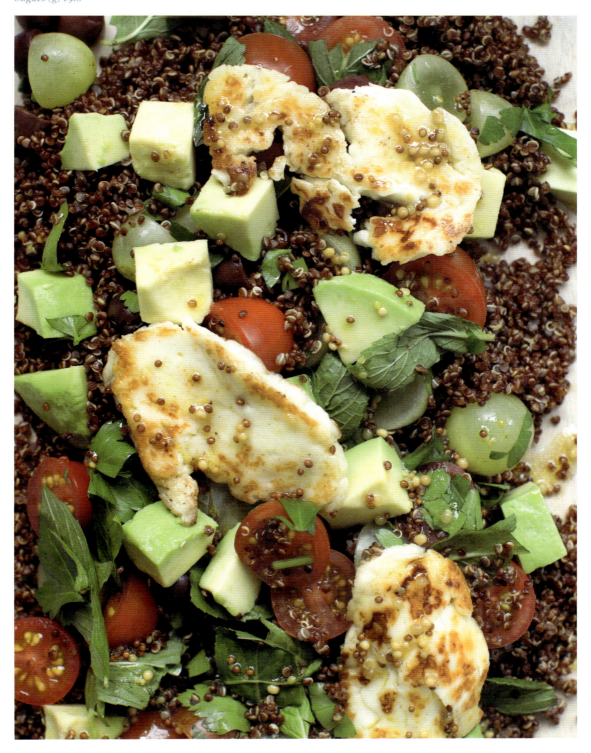

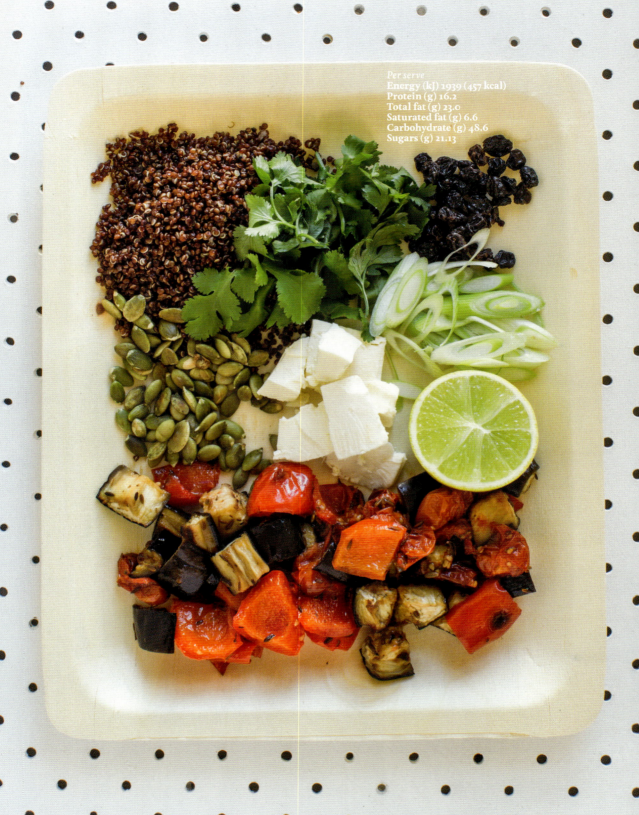

Per serve
Energy (kJ) 1939 (457 kcal)
Protein (g) 16.2
Total fat (g) 23.0
Saturated fat (g) 6.6
Carbohydrate (g) 48.6
Sugars (g) 21.13

ROAST EGGPLANT, TOMATO, FETA + LIME QUINOA SALAD

1. Preheat oven to 200°C. Line an oven tray with baking paper. Drizzle eggplant, capsicum and whole cherry tomatoes with olive oil and toss in prepared tray. Sprinkle over cumin seeds and chilli flakes and season with salt and pepper. Roast for 20-30 minutes until soft and cooked through.

2. To serve, toss roast vegetables with all remaining ingredients except lime juice, and season to taste with salt and pepper. Squeeze lime juice over just before eating.

TIP See page 99 for quinoa cooking instructions.

SERVES: 1

PREP TIME: 5-10 MINUTES

COOK TIME: 30 MINUTES

eggplant ½ small, cut into 2cm chunks
red capsicum ½, cut into 2cm chunks
cherry tomatoes 4-5
olive oil 2 teaspoons
cumin seeds ½ teaspoon, crushed
chilli flakes pinch of (optional)
salt
freshly ground black pepper
cooked quinoa ½ cup
currants 1 tablespoon
spring onion ½, finely sliced
feta 30g, crumbled
coriander and **flat-leaf parsley** ¼ cup total roughly chopped
pumpkin seeds 1 tablespoon
lime juice of ½

LUNCH

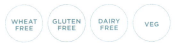

Dairy-free without feta

BAKED CAJUN TORTILLA CHIPS WITH BEANS + GUACAMOLE

Chips with guacamole are my vice. To make my guilty pleasure healthier, I bake my own corn chips. I've used corn tortillas, which go really crispy in the oven, but you could also use wheat tortillas or small pita breads to make baked 'chips'. Serve with some beans and you've got healthy nachos for lunch. Warning: they are quite addictive!

1. Preheat oven to 190°C. Brush tortilla pieces with olive oil on both sides and arrange on a large baking tray in a single layer. Sprinkle with Cajun seasoning and season with salt. Bake for 10-12 minutes or until golden and crispy — watch they don't burn. Set aside to cool. Once cooled, the chips will keep in an air-tight container for a week.

2. Roughly mash all guacamole ingredients together with a fork and season to taste with salt and pepper.

3. Heat bean, corn and kale chilli (or canned chilli beans) in a pot over medium heat or in the microwave.

4. To serve, divide bean chilli between bowls and serve with tortilla chips and guacamole. Garnish with parsley or coriander (if using).

SERVES: 2

PREP TIME: 5-10 MINUTES

COOK TIME: 10 MINUTES

BAKED CAJUN TORTILLA CHIPS

corn tortillas 4 small, cut into sixths
olive oil 1 tablespoon
Cajun seasoning 1 teaspoon
salt

GUACAMOLE

avocado ½ ripe
thick natural unsweetened Greek yoghurt 2 tablespoons
red onion 2 tablespoons finely diced
lime or lemon 1 tablespoon
freshly ground black pepper

TO SERVE

bean, corn and kale chilli (see page 122) or **canned chilli beans** 2 cups
flat-leaf parsley or coriander ¼ cup chopped (optional)

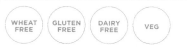

Dairy-free without yoghurt + wheat-free with corn tortillas

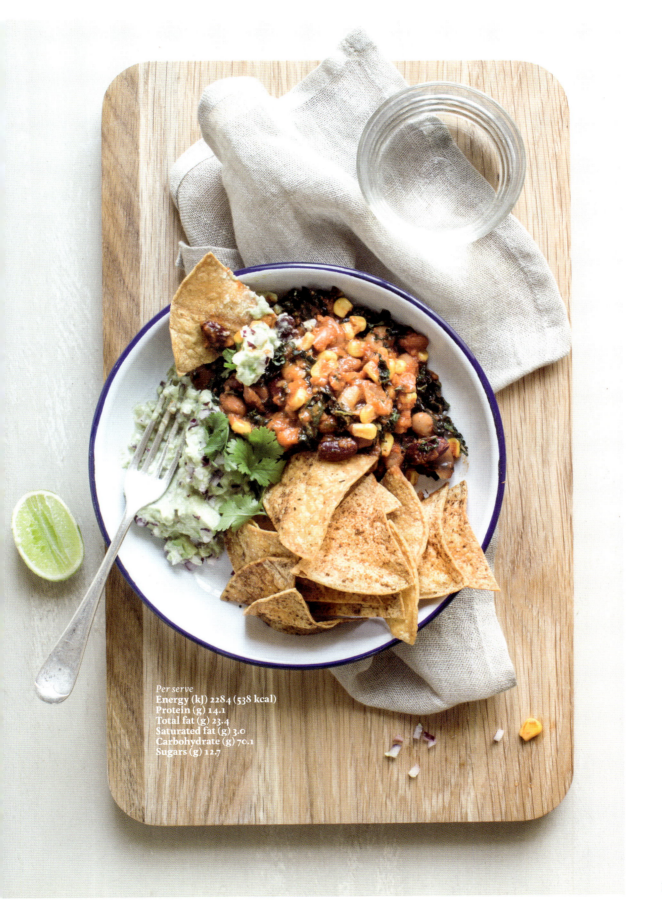

Per serve
Energy (kJ) 2284 (538 kcal)
Protein (g) 14.1
Total fat (g) 23.4
Saturated fat (g) 3.0
Carbohydrate (g) 70.1
Sugars (g) 12.7

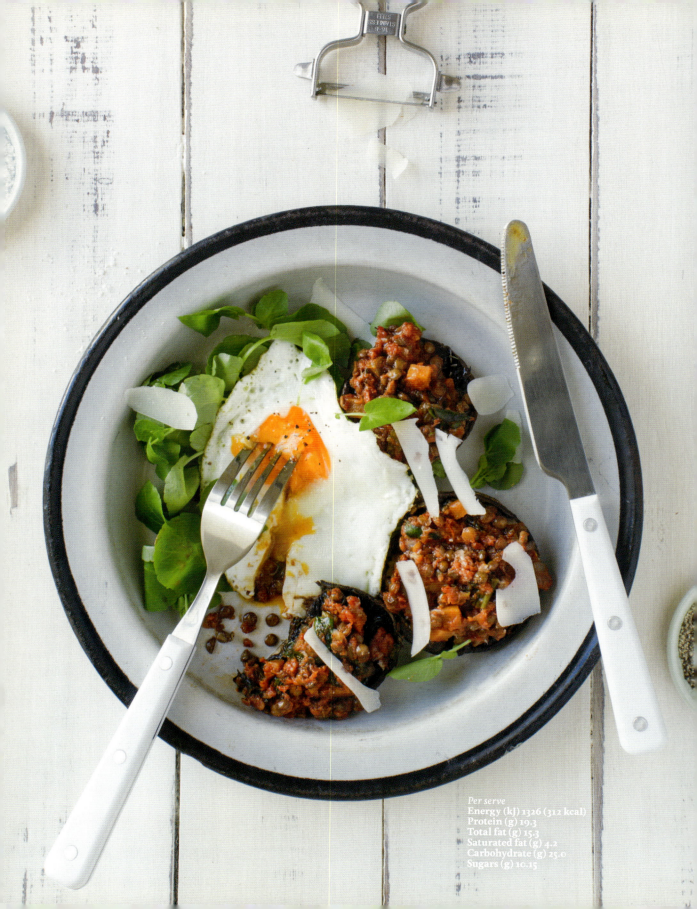

Per serve
Energy (kJ) 1326 (312 kcal)
Protein (g) 19.3
Total fat (g) 15.3
Saturated fat (g) 4.2
Carbohydrate (g) 25.0
Sugars (g) 10.15

LENTIL + PARMESAN MUSHROOM MELTS WITH A FRIED EGG

This hearty, healthy dish is a great way to use up leftover lentil ragu (see page 121). Grilling mushrooms with this thyme and balsamic marinade makes them very tasty indeed.

1. Preheat oven to 200°C. Line an oven tray with baking paper. Mix together extra virgin olive oil, balsamic vinegar, honey and thyme. Arrange mushrooms on prepared oven tray, gill side up. Spoon balsamic mixture over mushrooms and season with salt. Roast for 10–15 minutes until soft.

2. Spoon lentil mixture over cooked mushrooms and sprinkle with parmesan. Return to the oven for a further 5 minutes until parmesan has melted and lentils are hot.

3. Heat olive oil in a large non-stick frying pan over medium-high heat. Carefully crack in eggs and cook for about 2 minutes. Add a splash of water and top with a lid for 1–2 minutes — this will help the eggs steam and cook more evenly.

4. To serve, divide mushrooms between plates and top with a fried egg. Season with salt and pepper, and garnish with parsley and a little more parmesan if desired.

SERVES: 4

PREP TIME: 5 MINUTES

COOK TIME: 20 MINUTES

extra virgin olive oil 1 tablespoon
balsamic vinegar 2 tablespoons
liquid honey 2 teaspoons
thyme leaves 1 tablespoon chopped
portobello mushrooms 12, large, stalks removed
salt
lentil ragu (see page 121) 2 cups
parmesan 1/3 cup grated
olive oil 2 teaspoons
free-range eggs 4
freshly ground black pepper
flat-leaf parsley 1/4 cup chopped

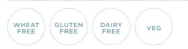

Dairy-free without parmesan

LUNCH

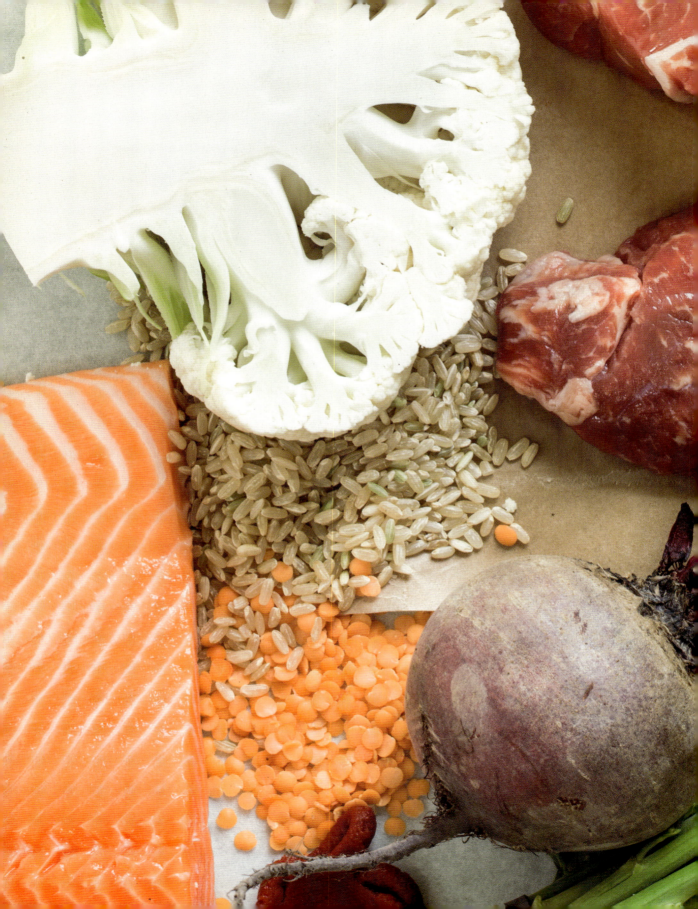

Recipes approx. 550 calories per serve

DINNER

+ Snack on fresh vegetable sticks while you prepare dinner — it will stop you from constantly picking (at the grated cheese!), boost your vegetable intake and avoid you being too ravenous at dinnertime.

+ Eat at the table sitting down, over at least 15-20 minutes — this is the time it takes for the hunger hormone leptin to signal from your stomach to your brain that you are full. If you're a fast eater, chew each bite at least 20 times (eventually that pace of eating will become habit) and put your knife and fork down in between each mouthful.

+ A little bit of organisation and effort up front to prepare and freeze some meals will make healthy eating throughout the week a breeze (look out for the 'freezes well' symbol).

+ Cauliflower can be used as the base for lots of meals as 'rice', 'couscous', 'tabouleh' and even pizza bases! It's high in vitamins and minerals and will help fill you up, and boost your vegetable intake.

+ Eat more root vegetables (kumara, sweet potato, pumpkin, carrots, parsnips, potatoes, etc.) as your carbohydrate base, instead of processed grains (which are fine a couple of times a week, but should not be eaten every night).

CAULIFLOWER-CRUST PIZZA WITH MARGARITA TOPPING

Believe it or not, you can make an amazing-tasting pizza base out of cauliflower! This is gluten free and provides more nutrients than your standard wheat pizza base (and a vege boost!).

1. Preheat oven to 200°C. Line an oven tray with baking paper. Break cauliflower into florets and place in a food processor. Blitz until the cauliflower has a fine, crumbly texture, like rice.

2. Place crumbly cauliflower in a large bowl and microwave uncovered for about 6 minutes or place on prepared oven tray and bake for about 15 minutes or until just tender. Remove and transfer to a clean tea towel. When cool enough to handle, wring tea towel tightly to squeeze out as much water from the cauliflower as you possibly can.

3. Mix cauliflower well with egg, parmesan, garlic, dried herbs and salt and pepper. Transfer mixture back to the same prepared oven tray. Shape and flatten into a circular or rectangular pizza crust, about 0.5cm thick. Bake for 30-40 minutes in the middle of the oven, until the crust is firm and golden brown.

4. Increase oven temperature to 220°C. Remove base and spread with tomato pizza sauce and arrange cherry tomatoes on top. Sprinkle over mozzarella and parmesan, and scatter over half of the basil leaves. Return pizza to the oven for a further 5 minutes until cheese is melted.

5. To serve, scatter over remaining basil leaves and cut into six even pieces. Serve with a big salad on the side.

TIP If you don't have a food processor, you can grate the cauliflower, or even very finely chop it. If you don't have time to make the cauliflower base and just want a quick pizza meal, use large Lebanese flatbreads as the pizza base like the recipe on page 127 (which only take 8-10 minutes to cook).

MAKES: 1 LARGE PIZZA

SERVES: 2

PREP TIME: 15 MINUTES

COOK TIME: 1 HOUR

CAULIFLOWER CRUST BASE

cauliflower 400g (about 2½ cups crumbled)
free-range egg 1 small
parmesan ½ cup grated
garlic 1 clove, minced
dried oregano or **mixed herbs** 1 teaspoon
salt ¼ teaspoon
freshly ground black pepper pinch of

TOPPING

pizza sauce home-made (see page 278) or store-bought ¼ cup
cherry tomatoes 8-10 (about ½ punnet), halved
mozzarella ⅓ cup grated
parmesan 1 tablespoon grated
basil leaves ½ cup

TO SERVE

leafy green salad (see page 277) 2 servings

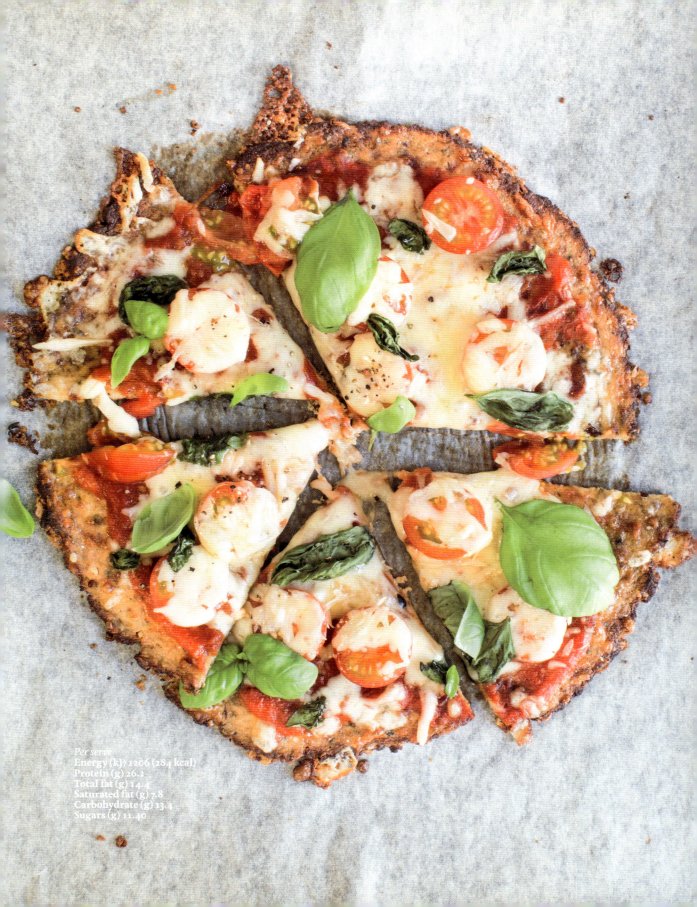

Per serve
Energy (kJ) 1206 (284 kcal)
Protein (g) 26.2
Total fat (g) 14.4
Saturated fat (g) 7.8
Carbohydrate (g) 13.4
Sugars (g) 11.40

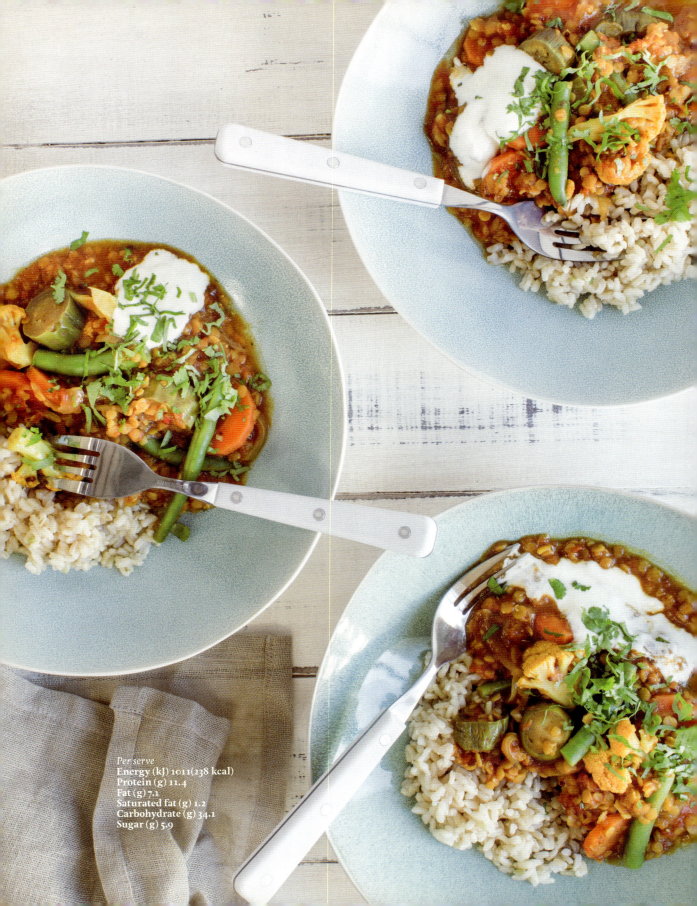

Per serve
Energy (kJ) 1011(238 kcal)
Protein (g) 11.4
Fat (g) 7.1
Saturated fat (g) 1.2
Carbohydrate (g) 34.1
Sugar (g) 5.9

LENTIL + VEGETABLE CURRY

A rich, hearty lentil curry makes a fast, cheap and healthy vegetarian meal that's freezable. Leftovers are great to take to work the next day.

1. Combine lentils and stock in a large saucepan and bring to a boil. Reduce heat, cover and simmer until lentils are tender, about 20 minutes.

2. Heat 2 tablespoons oil in a medium-sized or large frying pan over medium heat. Add onion and cook until golden brown, 6-8 minutes. Add 1 teaspoon oil, garlic, mustard seeds, if using, ginger, cumin, coriander, tumeric and chilli. Cook for a further 2-3 minutes until the mustard seeds start popping.

3. Add onion mixture, tomato paste, tomatoes, salt, carrot, cauliflower and eggplant to the lentils. Cover and simmer for about 20 minutes until vegetables are tender. Add beans with about 10 minutes to go, so they don't overcook. Stir a few times during cooking to avoid the curry catching on the bottom of the pan. Mix in lemon juice at the end, taste and add more salt and pepper to taste.

4. To serve, spoon some rice and curry into each bowl and serve with coconut cream. Garnish with coriander.

TIP Don't skip the step of browning the onions, as it gives the curry lots of flavour.

SERVES: 6

PREP TIME: 15 MINUTES

COOK TIME: 1 HOUR

dried red lentils 1 cup
unsalted chicken or vegetable stock 3½ cups
oil 2 tablespoons + extra 1 teaspoon
onion 1 large, sliced
garlic 3 cloves, minced
black mustard seeds 1 teaspoon (optional)
ginger 2.5cm piece, peeled, grated
ground cumin 1 teaspoon
ground coriander 1 teaspoon
ground turmeric 1 teaspoon
ground chilli ½ teaspoon
tomato paste 1½ tablespoons
crushed tomatoes 1 x 400g can
salt ½ teaspoon
carrot 1 large, sliced into 1cm rounds
cauliflower 1 cup, chopped into florets
eggplant ½ large (or 2 small Japanese), cut into small chunks
green beans 100g, trimmed
lemon juice 1 tablespoon
freshly ground black pepper

TO SERVE

steamed brown rice ½ cup per serving
coconut cream ¼–⅓ cup
coriander ¼ cup chopped

DINNER / VEGETARIAN

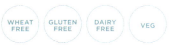

Dairy-free without yoghurt

115

HALOUMI + TOMATO KEBABS WITH ROAST PUMPKIN QUINOA + TAHINI DRESSING

This is one of my favourite vegetarian meals, and one that has won over several carnivores too!

1. Preheat oven to 200°C. Line an oven tray with baking paper. Toss pumpkin or butternut and red onion with fennel and coriander seeds, chilli flakes, if using, olive oil and honey. Season well with salt and pepper and roast for about 20 minutes, turning a few times during cooking, until the pumpkin is soft and caramelised. With a few minutes cooking time to go, toss in chopped garlic. Cook the quinoa.

2. Roll haloumi cubes in sumac, if using, to lightly coat. Skewer haloumi and cherry tomatoes onto bamboo skewers. Make sure the skewers go through the centre of the haloumi and tomatoes so they sit flush and both make contact with the pan when cooking.

3. When ready to cook the kebabs, heat 1 teaspoon olive oil in a large frying pan or on a barbecue hot plate. Cook kebabs in batches for 1-2 minutes on each side until the haloumi is golden and melted inside. Use a fish slice to push down on the kebabs gently for more even cooking. Add 1-2 teaspoons more oil as required.

4. Fluff up quinoa and toss with roast pumpkin and onion, any roasting juices from the tray, baby spinach or kale, olives, lemon and parsley. Season to taste.

5. To serve, divide roast pumpkin quinoa and kebabs between plates and drizzle over tahini dressing.

TIP See page 99 for quinoa cooking instructions. Instead of quinoa you can use couscous if you prefer.

SERVES: 4
PREP TIME: 15 MINUTES
COOK TIME: 25 MINUTES

ROAST PUMPKIN QUINOA
pumpkin or **butternut** 400g skin on, cut into 2cm cubes
red onion 1, cut into 2cm-thick wedges
fennel seeds 1 teaspoon, crushed
coriander seeds 1 teaspoon, crushed
chilli flakes ½ teaspoon (optional)
olive oil 1 tablespoon
liquid honey 1 teaspoon
salt
freshly ground black pepper
garlic 2 cloves, finely chopped
cooked quinoa 1 cup

KEBABS
haloumi 360g, cut into 2cm cubes
sumac 1 tablespoon (optional)
cherry tomatoes 24
bamboo skewers 8
olive oil 1 tablespoon

TO SERVE
baby spinach or **kale** 2 large handfuls
Kalamata olives ¼ cup, pitted, chopped
preserved lemon 1 tablespoon finely chopped or **lemon** grated zest of 1
flat-leaf parsley ¼ cup finely chopped
tahini dressing (see page 279)

WHEAT FREE | GLUTEN FREE | VEG

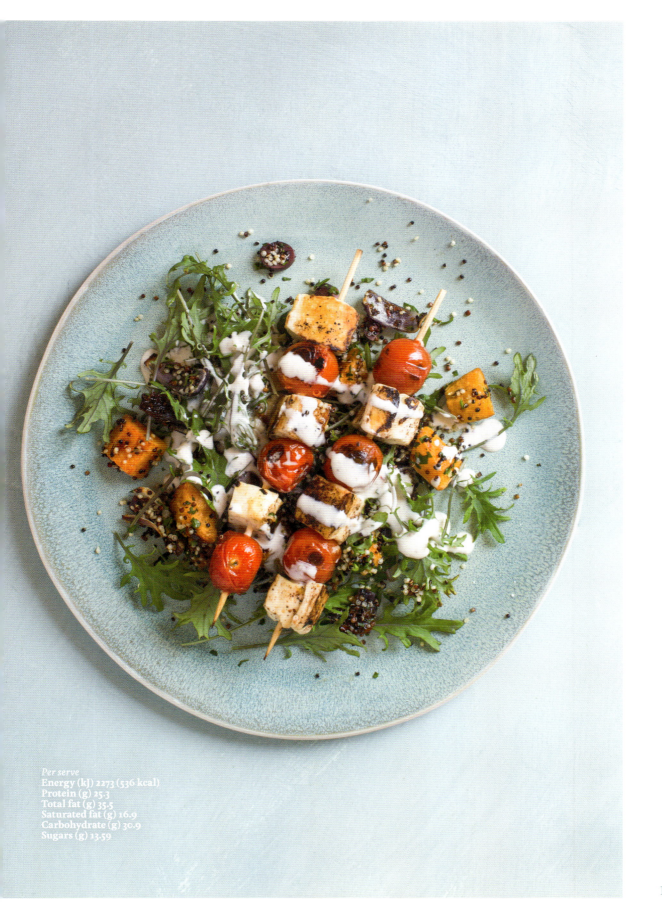

Per serve
Energy (kJ) 2273 (536 kcal)
Protein (g) 25.3
Total fat (g) 35.5
Saturated fat (g) 16.9
Carbohydrate (g) 30.9
Sugars (g) 13.59

DINNER / VEGETARIAN

SUNDRIED TOMATO + CREAM CHEESE-STUFFED MUSHROOMS

I fell in love with stuffed mushrooms the first time I ate them, and this combination of cream cheese, sundried tomatoes, garlic and pine nuts has been a favourite ever since. The mushrooms are 'meaty' and filling enough that you only need a salad with them, but if you like you can add a couple of roast spuds.

1. Preheat oven to 220°C. Mix cream cheese, red onion, thyme, sundried tomatoes, garlic, milk, lemon juice and parsley together. Season with salt and pepper.

2. Trim stalks of the mushrooms. Divide cream cheese mixture evenly and spread on the inside of each mushroom. Arrange mushrooms on an oven tray lined with baking paper and sprinkle over pine nuts and parmesan. Roast for 15-20 minutes or until mushrooms are soft and cream cheese mixture is starting to turn golden on top.

3. Mix all basil dressing ingredients together and season with salt and pepper.

4. To serve, divide courgette salad and rocket or mesclun between plates and dress with creamy basil dressing. Top with stuffed mushrooms. Drizzle over any remaining creamy basil dressing.

SERVES: 2

PREP TIME: 15 MINUTES

COOK TIME: 30 MINUTES

cream cheese ½ cup, softened
red onion 2 tablespoons finely chopped
thyme leaves 1 tablespoon finely chopped
sundried tomatoes 3-4 tablespoons finely chopped
garlic 1 small clove, minced
milk 2 tablespoons
lemon juice of ½
flat-leaf parsley ¼ cup finely chopped
portobello mushrooms 6 large, stalks removed
pinenuts 1 tablespoon
parmesan 2 tablespoons grated

CREAMY BASIL DRESSING

basil leaves ¼ cup very finely chopped
lemon juice 1 tablespoon
mayonnaise 1 tablespoon

COURGETTE RIBBON SALAD

courgette 1 medium-sized, shredded or peeled into thin ribbons
rocket leaves or **mesclun** 2 handfuls

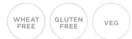

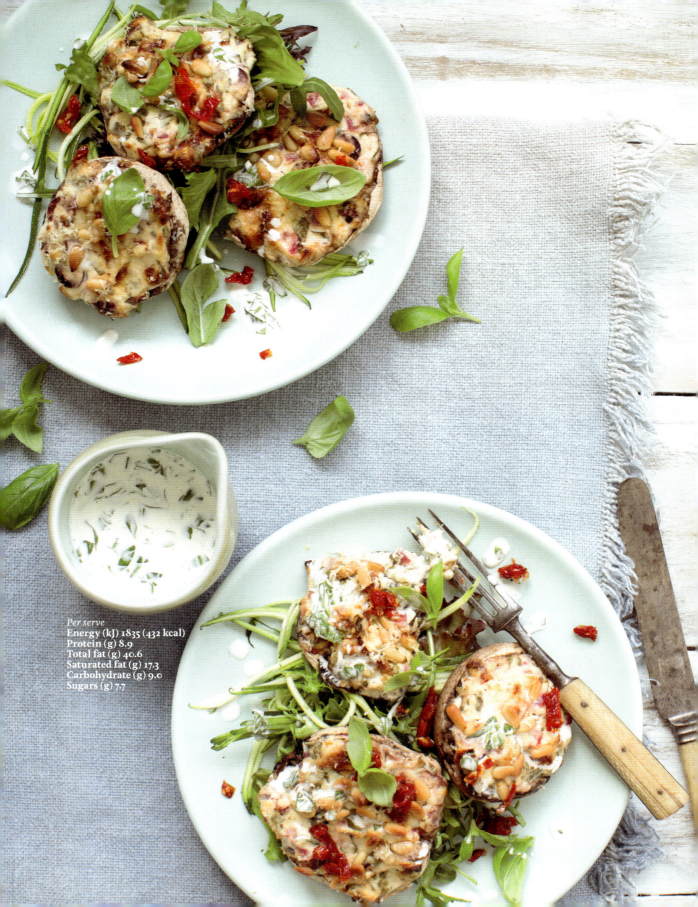

Per serve
Energy (kJ) 1835 (432 kcal)
Protein (g) 8.9
Total fat (g) 40.6
Saturated fat (g) 17.3
Carbohydrate (g) 9.0
Sugars (g) 7.7

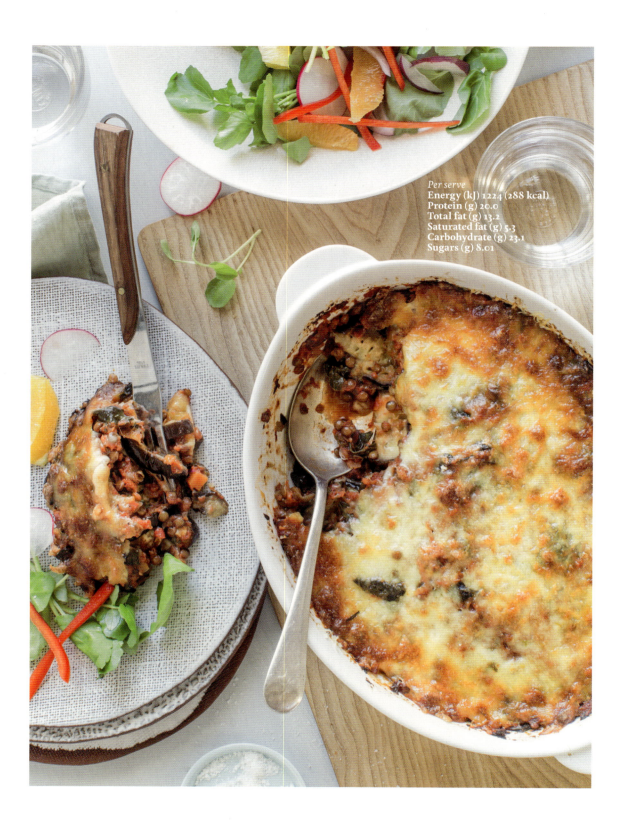

Per serve
Energy (kJ) 1224 (288 kcal)
Protein (g) 20.0
Total fat (g) 13.2
Saturated fat (g) 5.3
Carbohydrate (g) 23.1
Sugars (g) 8.01

LENTIL RAGU + EGGPLANT 'LASAGNE'

If you love lasagne and you love eggplant parmigiana, you'll love this hearty vegetarian meal that's a mix of the two. Slices of baked eggplant are used as the layers in between a rich tomato and lentil sauce, topped with melted mozzarella. This recipe makes a lot of ragu, so you can use leftovers in other recipes such as the lentil and parmesan mushroom melts (see page 109) which are great for breakfast or lunch.

1. Heat olive oil in a large saucepan over medium heat. Cook onion, carrot, celery and garlic for 6-7 minutes until soft. Add all remaining ragu ingredients, except spinach leaves, and bring to a boil. Reduce heat and gently simmer, stirring often, until lentils are tender but still hold their shape and liquid has almost completely evaporated, 35-40 minutes. Add spinach leaves with 5 minutes of cooking time to go and stir through until wilted. Season to taste with salt and pepper. The finished ragu should be very thick.

2. While the ragu is cooking, prepare the eggplant. Preheat oven to 200°C. Line two large oven trays with baking paper. Arrange sliced eggplant on prepared oven trays, brush with olive oil and season with salt and pepper. Bake for 20 minutes or until soft and lightly browned.

3. To assemble lasagne, arrange half of the eggplant slices, slightly overlapping, in a single layer on the bottom of a large baking or casserole dish. Spread over 1½ cups lentil ragu to cover the eggplant. Sprinkle over half of the mozzarella. Cover with another layer of remaining eggplant and remaining ragu. Sprinkle over remaining mozzarella and then parmesan.

4. Bake for about 20 minutes until cheese is melted and golden. Allow to stand for 10 minutes before cutting and serving. Serve with a big leafy green salad on the side.

TIP This recipe can be frozen whole or in individual portions for a quick 'heat and eat' lunch or dinner.

SERVES: 6

PREP TIME: 15 MINUTES

COOK TIME: 80 MINUTES

LENTIL RAGU

olive oil 1 tablespoon
onion 1, diced
carrot 1 medium-sized, peeled, diced
celery 1 stalk, diced
garlic 2 cloves, chopped
thyme leaves 2 teaspoons chopped
bay leaf 1
puy or French green lentils 1 cup
tomato paste 1 tablespoon
crushed tomatoes 3 x 400g cans
vegetable or chicken stock 1½ cups
spinach leaves 3 cups, roughly chopped
salt
freshly ground black pepper

TO ASSEMBLE

eggplants 2 large or 3 medium-sized, sliced into 1cm-thick rounds
olive oil 2 tablespoons
lentil ragu 3 cups (see above)
mozzarella 1½ cups grated
parmesan ¼ cup grated

TO SERVE

leafy green salad (see page 277) 6 servings

WHEAT FREE · GLUTEN FREE · VEG · FREEZES WELL

BEAN, CORN + KALE CHILLI TACOS

An alternative to meat chilli, this quick bean chilli (using canned beans) is just as filling and delicious. I've added kale for extra nutrition. This recipe makes a lot of chilli, so you can freeze it or use up the leftovers in various other dishes like 'The Works' (see page 43) or the bean nachos (see page 106).

1. Heat olive oil in a large heavy-based frying pan over medium heat. Cook onion, celery, carrots and garlic for 5–7 minutes or until soft. Add chilli, cumin, coriander and smoked paprika and cook until fragrant, 1–2 minutes. Add chipotle sauce, tomato paste and sweet chilli sauce, and cook for 1 minute further. Add crushed tomatoes, stock, beans and corn and bring to a simmer. Simmer for about 10 minutes until liquid has reduced and sauce has thickened slightly.

2. Stir through kale, cavolo nero or spinach and cook for a further 5 minutes or so. Season to taste with salt, pepper and lime or lemon juice.

3. Heat taco shells in the oven according to packet instructions until crispy.

4. To serve, place taco shells, bean chilli, salsa and yoghurt in serving dishes in the middle of the table for everyone to help themselves. To build a taco, place a couple of spoonfuls of bean chilli into a taco shell and top with a spoonful of salsa and a dollop of Greek yoghurt.

TIP Instead of crispy corn tacos, you could also use soft corn tortillas or wheat tortillas.

SERVES: 6
PREP TIME: 15 MINUTES
COOK TIME: 25 MINUTES

olive oil 1 tablespoon
onion 1 large, diced
celery 2 stalks, diced (about 1 cup)
carrots 2, peeled, diced (about 1 cup)
garlic 2 cloves, chopped
red chilli 1, chopped
ground cumin 2 tablespoons
ground coriander 1 tablespoon
smoked paprika 2 tablespoons
chipotle sauce ¼ cup
tomato paste ¼ cup
sweet chilli sauce 1 tablespoon
crushed tomatoes 1 x 400g can
vegetable or chicken stock 2 cups
beans (e.g. kidney, pinto, haricot, black beans) 3 x 400g cans
corn kernels 1 x 400g can, drained
curly kale, cavolo nero or **spinach** 2 cups, tough stems removed, shredded
salt
freshly ground black pepper
lime or lemon juice 1–2 tablespoons

TO SERVE
corn taco shells 12
tomato + avocado salsa (see page 279)
natural unsweetened thick Greek yoghurt ½ cup

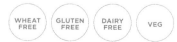

For dairy-free replace yoghurt with avocado

Per serve
Energy (kJ) 1224 (288 kcal)
Protein (g) 20.0
Total fat (g) 13.2
Saturated fat (g) 5.3
Carbohydrate (g) 23.1
Sugars (g) 8.01

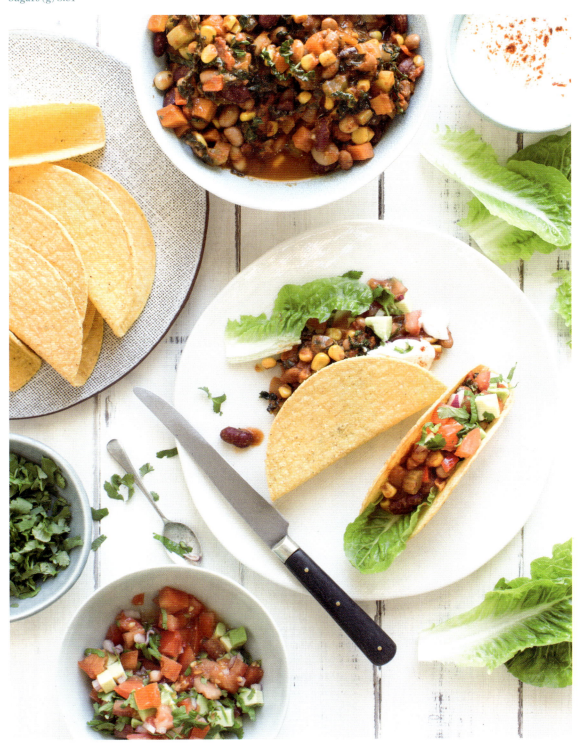

DINNER / VEGETARIAN

VEGETARIAN PAD THAI

This delicious Friday night favourite pad Thai recipe has heaps of flavour and is healthy and really quick to make (so there's no need to buy a takeaway version).

1. Cook noodles in boiling water for 2-3 minutes until just cooked through. Be careful not to overcook them. Drain and rinse under cold water to stop the cooking process and prevent noodles sticking together. Snip with scissors in a few places to shorten noodles. Set aside.

2. Mix all sauce ingredients together and set aside.

3. Heat oil in a wok or large non-stick frying pan over medium-high heat. Fry mushrooms, lemongrass, kaffir lime leaves and white part of spring onions for 1 minute. Add drained noodles, green part of spring onions, bean sprouts, chilli, if using, and sauce. Stir-fry, tossing together, for 4-5 minutes until heated through.

4. Set noodles aside on a serving plate and keep pan on the heat. Add beaten eggs to the pan and cook for about 2 minutes, stirring a few times, or until set as an omelette. Use a fish slice to roughly chop the omelette in the pan.

5. To serve, top noodles with omelette, peanuts and coriander and serve in the middle of the table for everyone to help themselves.

TIP You can also try adding cooked chicken or prawns.

SERVES: 4

PREP TIME: 10 MINUTES

COOK TIME: 5-10 MINUTES

dried rice stick noodles (about 1cm wide) 200g
oil 1 tablespoon
button or portobello mushrooms 150-200g, thinly sliced
lemongrass 1 stalk, tough outer leaves removed, finely chopped
kaffir lime leaves 2 medium-sized, central stem removed, very finely shredded
spring onions 2-3, cut into 2cm lengths
mung bean sprouts 2 large handfuls
red chilli 1 large, finely sliced (optional)
free-range eggs 4, lightly whisked with a good pinch of **salt**

PAD THAI SAUCE

soy sauce 2 tablespoons
sweet chilli sauce 3½ tablespoons
lime or lemon juice 2 teaspoons
sesame oil 2 teaspoons
coconut milk ⅓ cup

TO SERVE

roasted peanuts ¼ cup, chopped
coriander ¼ cup chopped

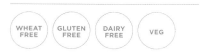

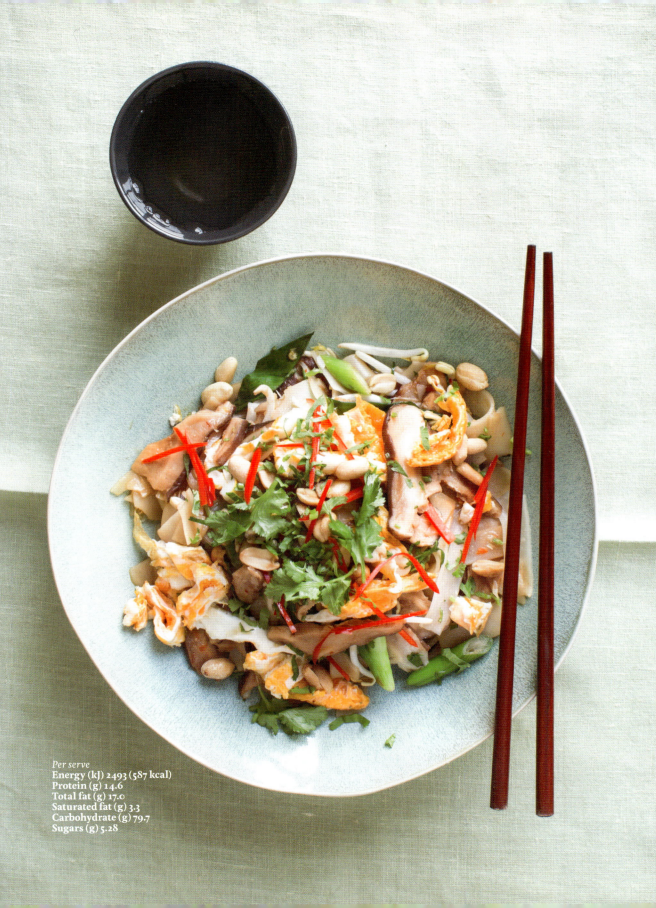

Per serve
Energy (kJ) 2493 (587 kcal)
Protein (g) 14.6
Total fat (g) 17.0
Saturated fat (g) 3.3
Carbohydrate (g) 79.7
Sugars (g) 5.28

Per serve
Energy (kJ) 1263 (298 kcal)
Protein (g) 15.5
Total fat (g) 14.2
Saturated fat (g) 5.4
Carbohydrate (g) 26.0
Sugars (g) 9.44

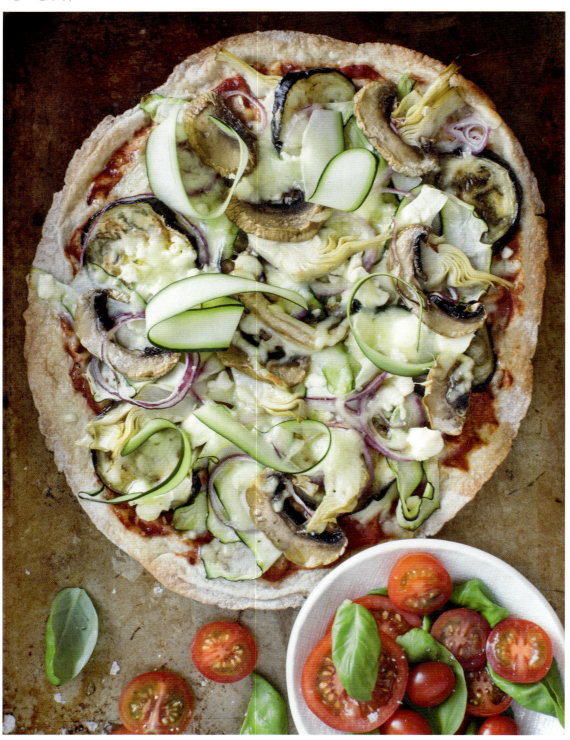

EGGPLANT, MUSHROOM, COURGETTE + ARTICHOKE PIZZA

For a lighter pizza, I use large Lebanese flatbreads (easily found in any supermarket) as the base, which speeds up the cooking time, too. They freeze well, so you can always have a couple on hand.

1. Preheat oven to 200°C. Line an oven tray with baking paper. Arrange eggplant slices on tray and brush with olive oil. Season with salt and bake for 15 minutes until soft and lightly browned.

2. Place Lebanese flatbreads on a large baking tray. Spread with tomato pizza sauce and top with baked eggplant, mushrooms, courgette ribbons (reserving a few for garnish), red onion and artichokes. Crumble over feta and sprinkle over grated mozzarella.

3. Bake for 8-10 minutes until edges are crispy and cheese is melted. Top with reserved courgette ribbons.

4. To serve, cut each pizza into quarters and serve two slices per serving with tomato and basil salad on the side.

TIP For a gluten-free pizza base, use the cauliflower pizza base recipe on page 112.

SERVES: 4

PREP TIME: 10 MINUTES

COOK TIME: 25 MINUTES

eggplant 1 small, sliced into ½ cm-thick rounds
olive oil 1 tablespoon
salt
Lebanese flatbreads 2 large
pizza sauce (home-made, see page 278, or store-bought) 6-8 tablespoons
button mushrooms 150g, sliced
courgettes 2, cut into thin ribbons with a vegetable peeler
red onion 1, thinly sliced
marinated artichokes (from a jar, can or the deli) ⅓ cup sliced
feta 50g
mozzarella ⅔ cup grated

TO SERVE

tomato + basil salad (see page 279) 4 servings

VEG

DINNER / VEGETARIAN

EGGPLANT, TOFU + CARAMELISED CHILLI STIR-FRY WITH CASHEW NUTS

My taste-testers declared this was the best vegetarian stir-fry dish they'd ever had. The caramelised chilli sauce is so darn good, coating each cube of tofu with loads of flavour, topped off with crunchy cashew nuts and fresh herbs.

SERVES: 4–6

PREP TIME: 15 MINUTES

COOK TIME: 15 MINUTES

CARAMELISED CHILLI SAUCE

soy sauce 1 tablespoon
fish sauce 2 teaspoons
sesame oil 1 teaspoon
brown sugar or **coconut sugar** 2 teaspoons
sweet chilli sauce 2 teaspoons
rice vinegar 1½ teaspoons
red chilli 1 large, finely sliced

EGGPLANT + TOFU STIR-FRY

oil 2 tablespoons
firm tofu 300g, cut into 2cm cubes
eggplant 1 small, cut into 2cm cubes, or **Japanese eggplant** 2, cut into 1cm-thick rounds
red onion 1, cut into 1cm-thick wedges
vegetable stock 2–3 tablespoons
spring onions 2, sliced

TO SERVE

roasted cashew nuts ¼ cup chopped
Asian herbs (e.g. coriander, mint, Vietnamese mint, Thai or aniseed basil) ¼ cup to serve
steamed brown rice ½ cup per serving

1. Combine all caramelised chilli sauce ingredients and set aside.

2. Heat 1 tablespoon oil in a wok or large non-stick frying pan over medium-high heat. Pat tofu cubes dry with paper towels. Fry tofu for about 5 minutes until golden, then set aside.

3. Heat remaining tablespoon oil and stir-fry eggplant and red onion for about 4–5 minutes until lightly browned and cooked through, adding 1 tablespoon stock occasionally to prevent the vegetables from sticking and burning. Add spring onion and continue to cook for a further 1–2 minutes.

4. Add tofu back to the pan, along with the caramelised chilli sauce, and cook over high heat for 1–2 minutes, allowing the sauce to bubble and thicken and become sticky. Give everything one final toss and turn off the heat.

5. To serve, garnish with roasted cashew nuts and Asian herbs and serve with steamed brown rice on the side.

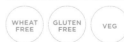

WHEAT FREE | GLUTEN FREE | VEG

Use gluten-free tamari soy sauce

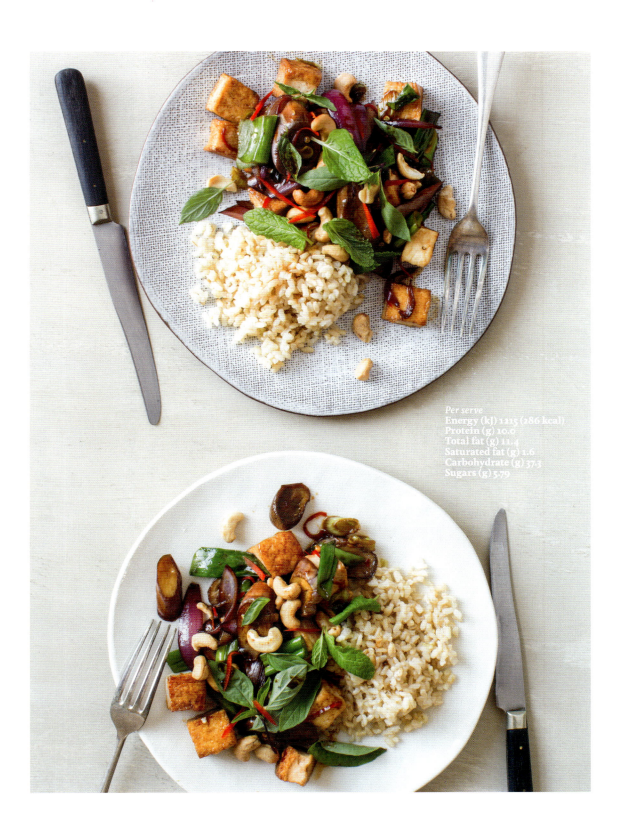

Per serve
Energy (kJ) 1215 (286 kcal)
Protein (g) 10.0
Total fat (g) 11.4
Saturated fat (g) 1.6
Carbohydrate (g) 37.3
Sugars (g) 5.79

DINNER / VEGETARIAN

BAKED SAMOSAS WITH PINEAPPLE SALSA + KASUNDI

Samosas are usually soaked in oil from being deep fried. These ones, however, are baked, not fried, and just as crispy and delicious. They're especially good with the sweet pineapple and coconut salsa and the kasundi, which is an Indian spiced tomato chutney.

1. Preheat oven to 200°C. Line an oven tray with baking paper. Toss kumara, sweet potato or potato and onion with mustard seeds, curry powder and olive oil. Season well with salt and pepper and bake for 15-20 minutes, until tender.

2. Cook spinach until just wilted by either microwaving it, or pouring boiling water over it and leaving it for 1 minute. When cool, squeeze out as much moisture from the spinach as you can by wringing in a clean tea towel. Chop finely.

3. Combine cooked potato mixture with peas, spinach and coriander and roughly crush with a fork to combine. Season with salt and pepper to taste.

4. Place a sheet of filo pastry on a clean, dry bench (keep the remaining sheets covered with a clean, damp tea towel to prevent them drying out). Brush filo sheet lightly with butter. Fold over a third lengthwise and fold over again, so you have a long rectangular strip 3 layers thick.

5. Place long end of pastry strip facing you. Place 2 heaped tablespoonfuls of mixture at the left side of pastry. To enclose filling, fold bottom left corner diagonally to meet top edge of filo strip, making a triangular parcel. Continue folding until pastry is completely used. Continue with remaining 11 filo sheets.

6. Arrange samosas on a baking tray and brush samosas with a little butter on both sides. Sprinkle with sesame seeds and bake in the centre of the oven for about 30 minutes, in the centre of the oven, until pastry is crisp and golden.

7. Serve with pineapple and coconut salsa and kasundi or chutney on the side.

SERVES: 4

MAKES: 12 SAMOSAS

PREP TIME: 15-20 MINUTES

COOK TIME: 45 MINUTES

kumara, sweet potato or **potatoes** (e.g. Agria) 650g, peeled, cut into 1cm cubes
onion 1, chopped
mustard seeds 2 teaspoons (optional)
curry powder 2 tablespoons
olive oil 1 tablespoon
salt
freshly ground black pepper
spinach leaves 3 cups chopped
frozen peas 1½ cups, defrosted
coriander ¼ cup chopped
filo pastry 12 sheets
melted butter 3 tablespoons
sesame seeds 1 teaspoon

TO SERVE

pineapple + coconut salsa (see page 278)
kasundi (see page 277) or **tomato chutney** 2 tablespoons per serving

(VEG)

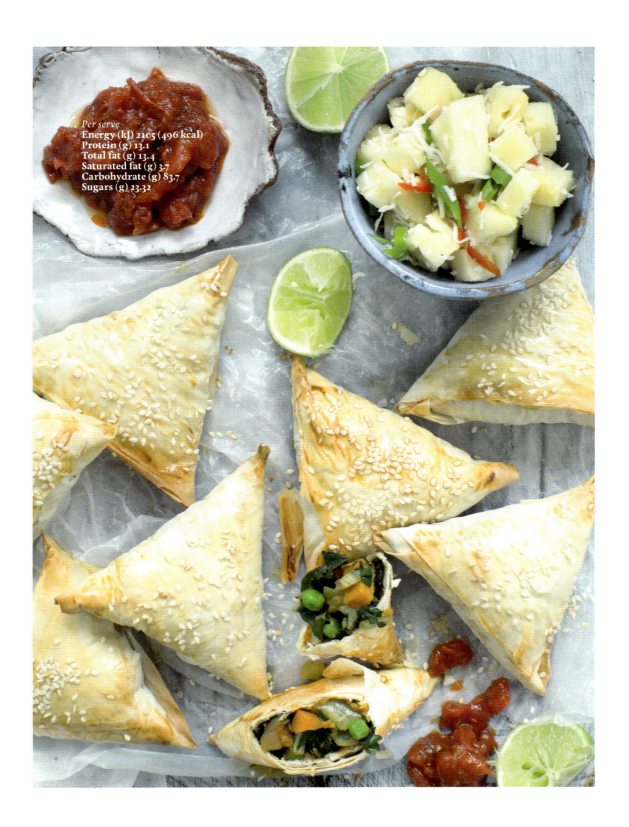

Per serve
Energy (kJ) 2105 (496 kcal)
Protein (g) 13.1
Total fat (g) 13.4
Saturated fat (g) 3.7
Carbohydrate (g) 83.7
Sugars (g) 23.32

DINNER / VEGETARIAN

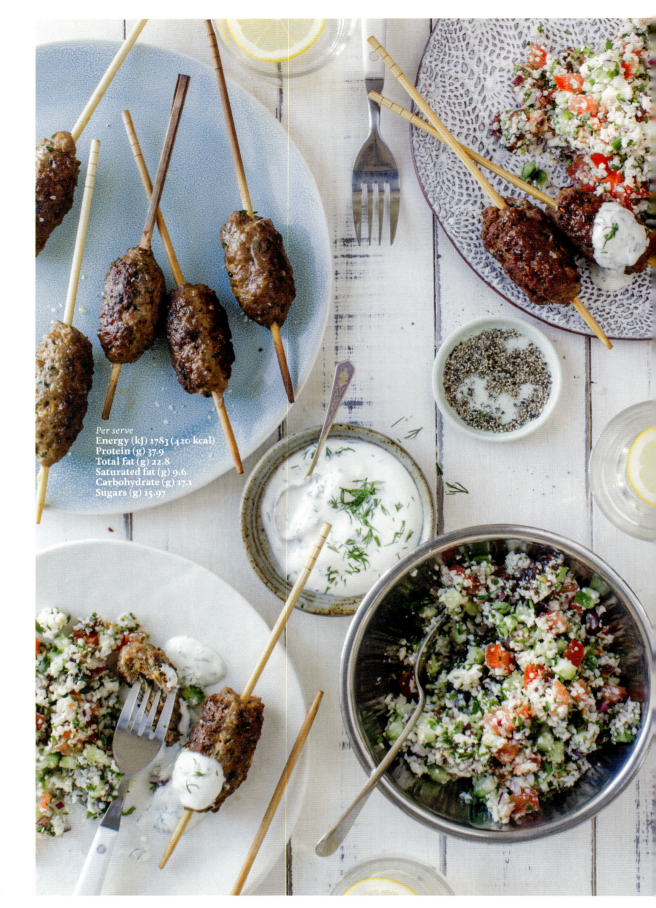

Per serve
**Energy (kJ) 1783 (420 kcal)
Protein (g) 37.9
Total fat (g) 22.8
Saturated fat (g) 9.6
Carbohydrate (g) 17.1
Sugars (g) 15.97**

TURKISH LAMB KOFTE + CAULIFLOWER 'COUSCOUS'

This Turkish spice mix of cinnamon, cumin and paprika is excellent with lamb, especially if barbecued for that subtle smoky flavour. Cauliflower couscous is a revelation — light and fluffy, just like couscous, and quick to make.

1. Preheat oven to 220°C. In a large mixing bowl, with clean hands, mix lamb mince, spices, garlic, parsley, lemon zest, salt and pepper until well combined. Moisten your hands with cold water (to prevent sticking) and roll ¼ cupfuls of mince mixture into meatballs. Poke a bamboo skewer or wooden chopstick through the middle of each meatball and shape around the skewer into a sausage shape.

2. Place cauliflower in a food processor and blitz to a fine, crumbly, couscous-like texture. You may have to do this in batches to avoid overcrowding. Place in a large bowl and microwave for a few minutes, stirring a few times, or spread out on an oven tray and cook for 5 minutes, until cauliflower is very lightly cooked but still slightly crunchy.

3. Brush lamb kofte skewers with olive oil and season with a little salt. Heat a large frying pan, grill pan or barbecue on medium-high heat. Cook kofte for about 3 minutes on each side or until lamb is cooked through. Alternatively, you can cook the kofte in the oven for 12 minutes or until cooked through.

4. Toss cauliflower 'couscous' with cucumber, tomato, red onion, olives, dates, feta, mint, parsley, lemon juice and extra virgin olive oil, and season to taste with salt and pepper.

5. Mix dill and yoghurt together. Serve kofte and tabouleh with a dollop of dill yoghurt on the side.

TIP If you don't have a food processor, you can grate the cauliflower, or even very finely chop it using a large, sharp knife.

SERVES: 4

PREP TIME: 15–20 MINUTES

COOK TIME: 10 MINUTES

TURKISH LAMB KOFTE

lean lamb mince 600g
ground cinnamon 1 teaspoon
ground cumin 1½ teaspoons
smoked paprika 1 teaspoon
chilli flakes ½–1 teaspoon (optional)
garlic 1 clove, crushed
flat-leaf parsley ¼ cup finely chopped
lemon zest of 1
salt 1 teaspoon
freshly ground black pepper ½ teaspoon
bamboo skewers 12
olive oil for brushing

CAULIFLOWER 'COUSCOUS'

cauliflower 1 head (750–800g), cut into florets
telegraph cucumber ½, finely diced
tomatoes 2, diced
red onion ½ small, finely diced
Kalamata olives ¼ cup, chopped
dates ¼ cup finely chopped
feta 50g, crumbled
mint leaves ¼ cup chopped
flat-leaf parsley ¼ cup chopped
lemon juice of 1 (use zested one above)
extra virgin olive oil 1 tablespoon

DILL YOGHURT

dill 1 tablespoon finely chopped
natural unsweetened thick Greek yoghurt ⅓ cup

DINNER / MEAT

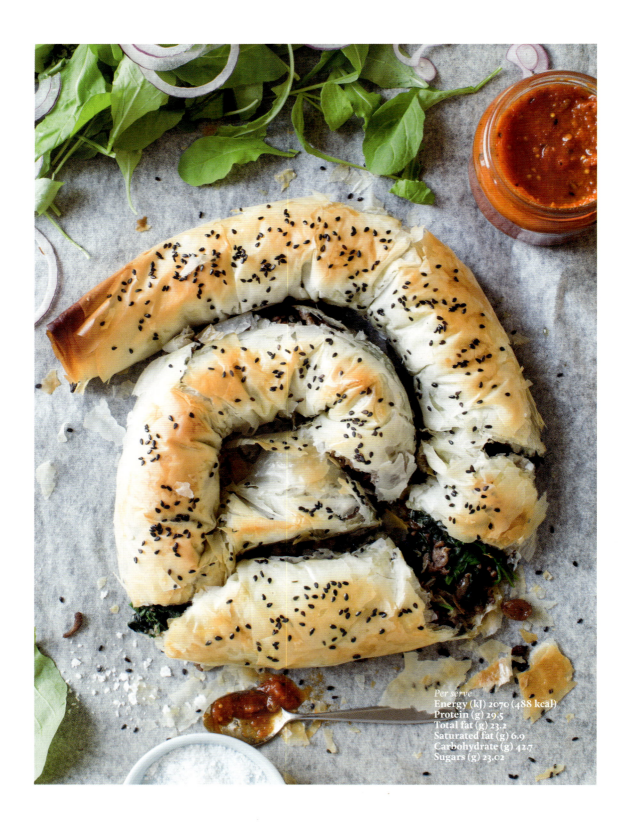

Per serve
Energy (kJ) 2070 (488 kcal)
Protein (g) 29.5
Total fat (g) 23.2
Saturated fat (g) 6.9
Carbohydrate (g) 42.7
Sugars (g) 23.02

GREEK LAMB + SPINACH SPIRAL FILO PIE

It's extremely satisfying to pull this impressive-looking pie out of the oven. Make sure you wring as much water as possible out of the spinach to avoid soggy pastry. Don't worry if the filo pastry cracks or crumbles a little — it's all part of this pie's rustic appeal.

1. Preheat oven to 200°C. Lightly grease an oven tray with oil. Heat 1 tablespoon olive oil in a large frying pan on high heat. Cook lamb mince, onions, garlic, spices, oregano and sultanas for 10-12 minutes until mince is well browned and any moisture has evaporated. Season to taste with salt and pepper.

2. Briefly steam or blanch spinach or silverbeet until wilted. Drain well and squeeze out as much water as you can by wringing it out in a clean tea towel. Finely chop and combine with mince mixture. Season to taste with salt and pepper. Place mixture in the fridge to cool.

3. Place a large sheet of baking paper on a clean, dry work surface. Lay a sheet of filo pastry on top of baking paper and lightly brush with melted butter right up to the edges. Place another sheet of filo next to the first sheet of filo, overlapping it by 2.5cm so that you end up with one large sheet that is twice as long. Brush with butter and repeat layering of remaining sheets of filo until it is 5 sheets thick (and 2 sheets long).

4. Place spoonfuls of lamb mixture down the long side of the filo closest to you, then carefully roll up into a long sausage shape, seam side down. Gently twist into a spiral shape — don't worry if the filo breaks a bit. Carefully lift baking paper and transfer to the oven tray. Slide pie off the baking paper and onto tray, with the help of a fish slice. Brush pastry with butter and sprinkle over sesame seeds. Bake for about 25 minutes or until golden and crispy.

5. To serve, cut into quarters and serve with salad and chutney on the side.

SERVES: 4

PREP TIME: 20 MINUTES

COOK TIME: 30 MINUTES

olive oil 1 tablespoon
lean lamb mince 450g
onions 2, diced
garlic 2 cloves, finely chopped
ground cumin 2 teaspoons
ground allspice 1½ teaspoons
ground cinnamon ¼ teaspoon
chilli flakes ½–1 teaspoon (optional)
dried oregano 1 teaspoon
sultanas ½ cup
salt
freshly ground black pepper
spinach or **silverbeet leaves** 300g, chopped
filo pastry 10 sheets
melted butter 2 tablespoons
white or black sesame seeds 2 teaspoons

TO SERVE

leafy green salad (see page 277) 4 servings
tomato or fruit chutney 1 tablespoon per serving

Use olive oil instead of butter

DINNER / MEAT

LAMB BAHARAT WITH BRAISED VEGETABLES, BARLEY, LEMON + OLIVES

Baharat is a beautiful Arabic spice blend that you can buy pre-made or make yourself (see tip below). The vegetables and barley in this recipe are cooked in chicken stock with lemon and olives until very tender.

1. Preheat oven to 200°C. Heat olive oil in a frying pan over medium heat. Cook onion, garlic, cumin and coriander for 4–5 minutes until onion is just starting to caramelise. If at any time it looks like the onion is catching on the bottom of the pan and burning, just add a tablespoon or two of water or stock to the pan.

2. In a medium-sized baking or casserole dish, combine cooked onion mixture, carrots, parsnips, barley, preserved lemon, olives, chicken stock, thyme and cinnamon stick. Season well with salt and pepper. Cover tightly with tinfoil and bake until the carrots, parsnips and barley are tender, about 40 minutes.

3. Pat lamb steaks dry with paper towels and coat with baharat spice blend. Leave to marinate at room temperature until ready to cook.

4. When vegetables are almost cooked, heat olive oil in a large frying pan over medium-high heat. Cook lamb for 2–3 minutes on each side, depending on thickness of your steaks, for medium-rare, or until cooked to your liking. Cover with tin foil and leave to rest for 5 minutes before slicing against the grain.

5. To serve, arrange slices of lamb on top of braised vegetables and barley and garnish with fresh herbs.

TIP To make baharat spice blend, combine 1½ teaspoons ground cumin, 1 teaspoon freshly ground black pepper, 1 teaspoon ground coriander, ¼ teaspoon ground cloves, 1½ teaspoons paprika, 1 teaspoon ground cinnamon, ½ teaspoon ground nutmeg and 1 teaspoon salt. If you don't have preserved lemon, the zest of ½ fresh lemon will do.

SERVES: 4

PREP TIME: 10 MINUTES

COOK TIME: 45 MINUTES

VEGETABLES
olive oil 2 teaspoons
red onion 1, cut into 1cm-thick wedges
garlic 2 cloves, chopped
ground cumin 2 teaspoons
ground coriander 2 teaspoons
carrots 2 medium-sized, peeled, cut into 3cm-thick batons
parsnips 2 medium-sized, peeled, cut into 3cm-thick batons
pearl barley ⅓ cup
preserved lemon ¼, flesh removed, rind thinly chopped
green olives 1 cup
chicken stock 1½ cups
thyme leaves 1 tablespoon
cinnamon stick 1
salt
freshly ground black pepper

LAMB
lamb steaks (rump, fillet or leg) 600g
baharat spice blend (see tip) 3 tablespoons
olive oil 2 teaspoons

TO SERVE
mixed fresh herbs (e.g. flat-leaf parsley, coriander and mint) 1 cup chopped

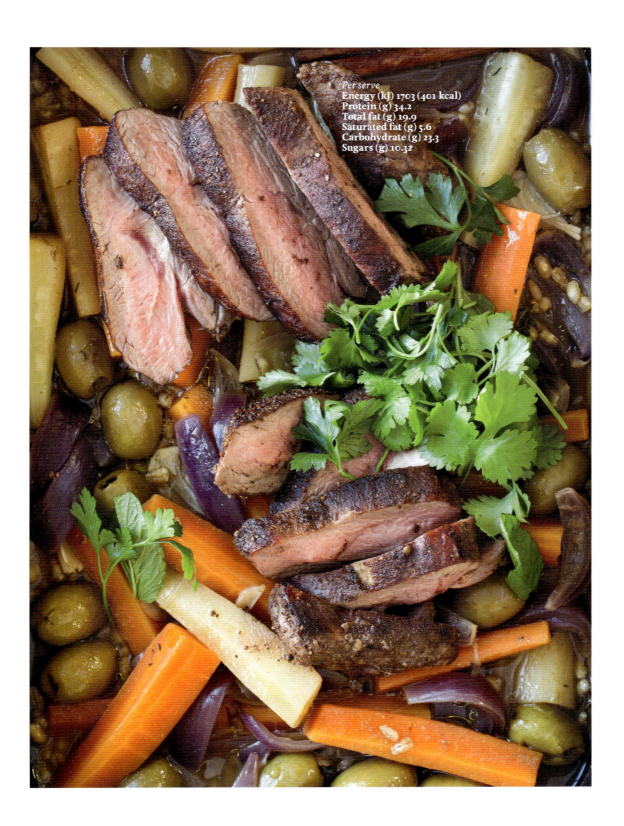

Per serve
Energy (kJ) 1703 (401 kcal)
Protein (g) 34.2
Total fat (g) 19.9
Saturated fat (g) 5.6
Carbohydrate (g) 23.3
Sugars (g) 10.32

DINNER / MEAT

Per serve
Energy (kJ) 1533 (361 kcal)
Protein (g) 43.7
Total fat (g) 16.5
Saturated fat (g) 5.9
Carbohydrate (g) 10.7
Sugars (g) 5.73

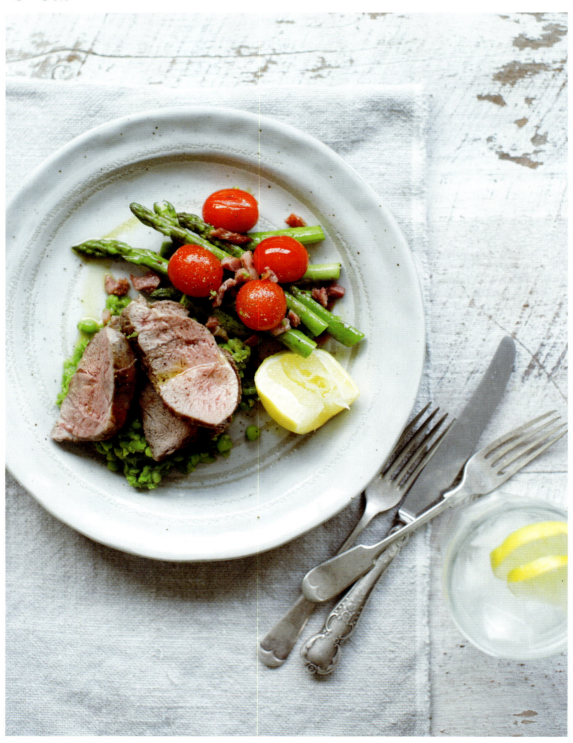

LAMB, CRUSHED MINTED PEAS, SCORCHED TOMATOES, ASPARAGUS + BACON

This is such a tasty dish — all the ingredients are just meant to be together! It's a really quick dish to make, too.

1. Place peas and stock in a saucepan and bring to a simmer. Simmer for 3–5 minutes until peas are tender. Roughly crush or mash peas with a masher or fork and mix in mint. Season to taste with lemon juice, salt and pepper. Keep warm.

2. Heat ½ teaspoon olive oil in a large frying pan over medium-high heat. Cook bacon for 3–4 minutes until crisp. Set aside. Keep pan on the heat.

3. Pat lamb steaks dry with paper towels and season with salt. Heat 2 teaspoons oil in frying pan over high heat. Cook for about 2 minutes on each side for medium-rare, or until cooked to your liking. Set aside to rest for a few minutes. Keep pan on the heat.

4. Add cherry tomatoes and asparagus or beans to the hot pan. Shake around and cook for about 3–4 minutes until the skins of the cherry tomatoes are starting to blister and the asparagus or beans are starting to char a little. Add balsamic vinegar and honey and allow to bubble for 10 seconds before turning off the heat. Shake the pan around to coat tomatoes and asparagus or beans in the glaze.

5. To serve, slice lamb and divide evenly among plates with crushed peas, scorched tomatoes and asparagus or beans. Sprinkle over crispy bacon.

SERVES: 4

PREP TIME: 10 MINUTES

COOK TIME: 15 MINUTES

frozen peas 3 cups
chicken stock 1 cup
mint leaves 2½ tablespoons finely chopped
lemon juice squeeze of
salt
freshly ground black pepper
olive oil 2 teaspoons
streaky bacon 3 rashers, diced
lean lamb leg steaks 600g
cherry tomatoes 1 punnet
asparagus 1 bunch (8–12 spears) or **green beans** 200g, trimmed
balsamic vinegar 1 tablespoon
honey 1 teaspoon

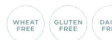

DINNER / MEAT

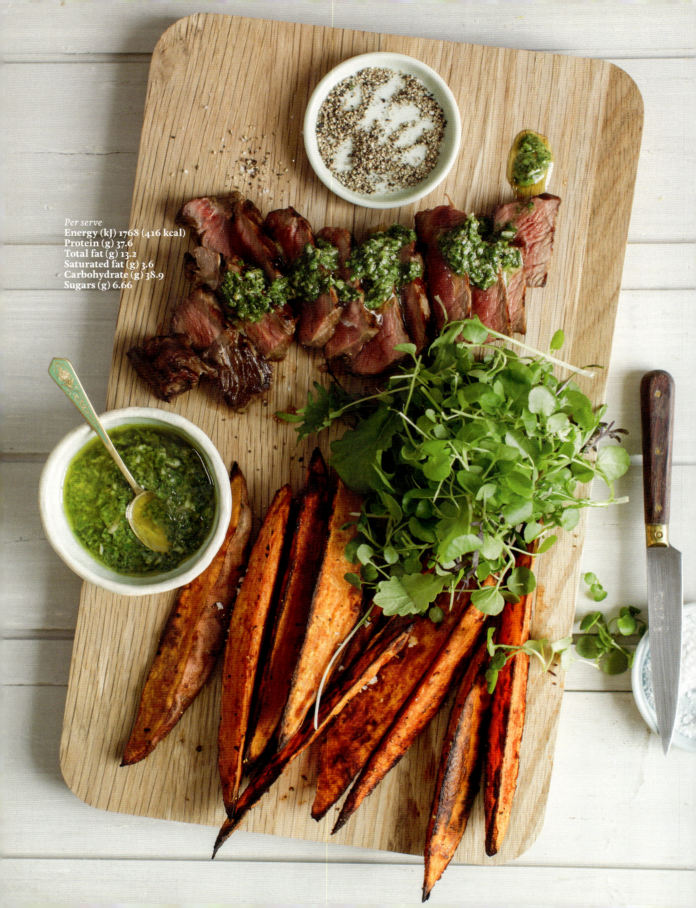

Per serve
Energy (kJ) 1768 (416 kcal)
Protein (g) 37.6
Total fat (g) 13.2
Saturated fat (g) 3.6
Carbohydrate (g) 38.9
Sugars (g) 6.66

STEAK, SMOKY KUMARA FRIES + SALSA VERDE

This is one of my favourite simple meals. It's bursting with flavour — I reckon my salsa verde recipe is one of the best out there!

1. Preheat oven to 200°C. Line an oven tray with baking paper. Combine kumara or sweet potato, olive oil and smoked paprika on prepared oven tray. Season well with salt and pepper and roast for 25-30 minutes until golden and cooked through.

2. Heat olive oil in a large frying pan over high heat. Pat steaks dry with paper towels and season with salt. Cook for about 2 minutes on each side for medium-rare, or until cooked to your liking. Set aside to rest for a few minutes.

3. To serve, slice steak on an angle and divide between plates with smoky kumara fries and a big handful of watercress or baby rocket dressed with a little extra virgin olive oil and lemon juice. Drizzle over salsa verde.

SERVES: 4

PREP TIME: 10 MINUTES

COOK TIME: 25-30 MINUTES

SMOKY KUMARA FRIES

orange kumara (or other kumara or sweet potato) 600g skin on, scrubbed, cut lengthways into 1-2cm-thick wedges

olive oil 1 tablespoon

smoked paprika 1¼ teaspoons

salt

freshly ground black pepper

STEAK

olive oil 2 teaspoons

lean beef or lamb steaks (e.g. sirloin, rump, leg, eye fillet) 600g, trimmed of excess fat (at room temperature)

TO SERVE

watercress or **baby rocket** 4 large handfuls

salsa verde (see page 278)

WHEAT FREE · GLUTEN FREE · DAIRY FREE

MEXICAN SHREDDED BEEF, TOMATO + BARLEY SOUP

This soup is smoky and spicy, with lots of Mexican flavour. If you don't have barley you could use orzo (risoni) pasta or pearl couscous instead (just cook it for about half the time as the barley). If you have some beef left over, make the beef tostadas on page 163.

SERVES: 6

PREP TIME: 10 MINUTES

COOK TIME: 2½–3 HOURS

1. Heat olive oil in a large heavy-based frying pan or saucepan with a lid over medium heat. Cook onion, capsicum, celery, garlic, cumin, coriander and paprika for about 5 minutes until onion is soft.

2. Add chipotle sauce, tomato purée, chicken stock, beef and chilli, if using. Cover with a tight-fitting lid and simmer over low heat for 2–2½ hours until meat is tender. If your lid is not tight-fitting, cover the saucepan with tinfoil before placing the lid on top — this helps to create a seal to keep in the heat and moisture. Alternatively, cook in a preheated 160°C oven for 2–2½ hours in a covered casserole dish.

3. Once the meat is tender, remove the meat from the pan and set aside on a chopping board. Add barley to the pan, cover again and continue to cook for a further 30 minutes until barley is just tender. While the barley is cooking, use two forks to pull apart and shred the meat into strands.

4. Once barley is tender, add shredded beef back to the pan along with corn kernels and warm through. Season to taste with salt and pepper.

5. To serve, ladle some soup into each bowl and top with a dollop of yoghurt or sour cream, some coriander and tortilla or corn chips. Serve with a wedge of lime to squeeze over just before eating.

TIP Chipotle sauce is a Mexican smoked chilli sauce — find it in the international or Mexican food section of the supermarket.

olive oil 1 tablespoon
onion 1, diced
capsicums 2, diced
celery 1 stick, diced
garlic 2 cloves, chopped
ground cumin 2 teaspoons
ground coriander 2 teaspoons
smoked paprika 1 teaspoon
chipotle sauce ¼ cup
tomato purée or **crushed tomatoes** 1 x 400g can
chicken stock 5½ cups
braising beef (e.g. shin meat, brisket, blade, skirt or chuck steak) 500g, trimmed of fat, cut into 5cm pieces
red chilli ½, sliced
pearl barley ½ cup
corn kernels ½ x 400g can, drained
salt
freshly ground black pepper

TO SERVE

natural unsweetened thick Greek yoghurt or **sour cream** 6 tablespoons
coriander ¼–½ cup chopped
tortilla chips (see page 106) or **corn chips** 6 per serving (optional)
lime 1, cut into wedges

Dairy-free without yoghurt

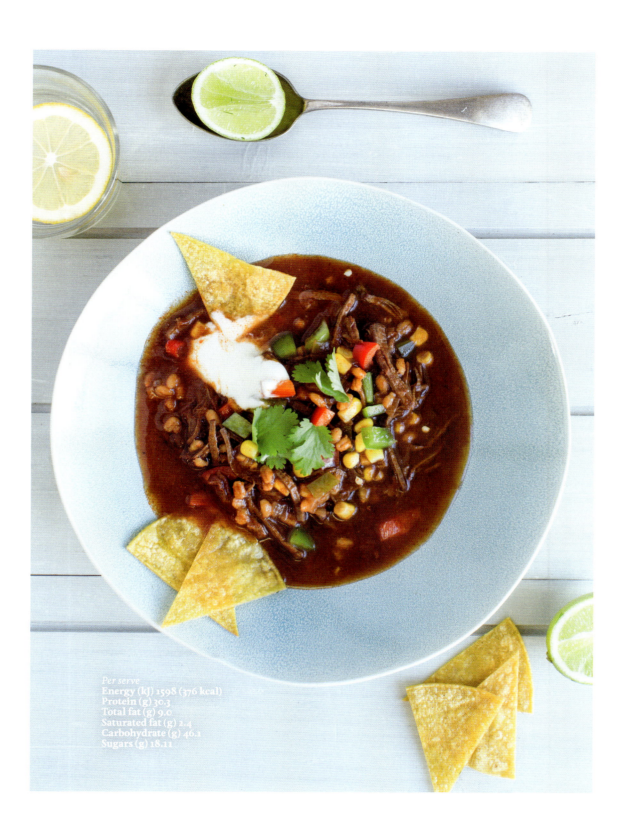

Per serve
Energy (kJ) 1598 (376 kcal)
Protein (g) 30.3
Total fat (g) 9.0
Saturated fat (g) 2.4
Carbohydrate (g) 46.1
Sugars (g) 18.11

DINNER / MEAT

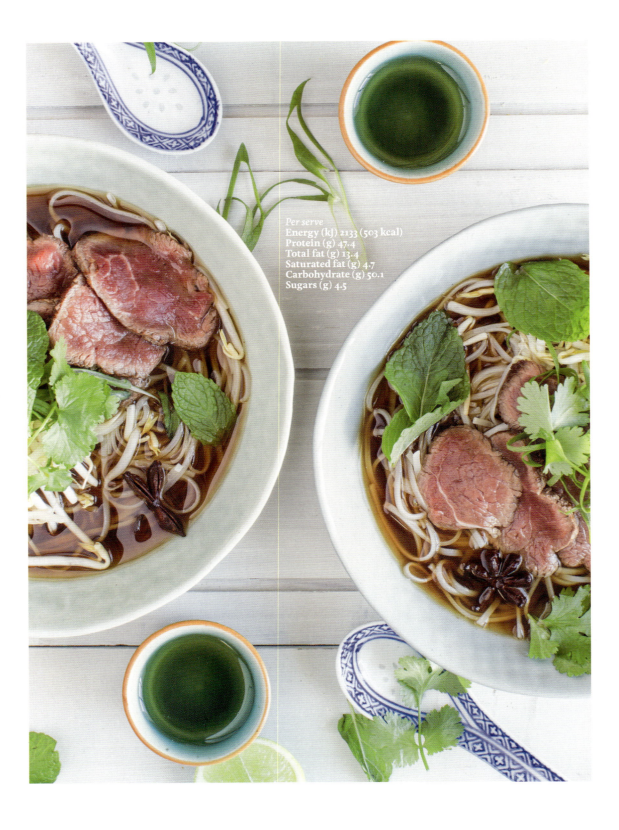

Per serve
Energy (kJ) 2133 (503 kcal)
Protein (g) 47.4
Total fat (g) 13.4
Saturated fat (g) 4.7
Carbohydrate (g) 50.1
Sugars (g) 4.5

RARE BEEF NOODLE SOUP (PHO BO)

*Vietnamese food is naturally light, flavoursome and healthy.
Pho bo is a traditional dish that is great for a quick lunch or dinner.*

1. Combine all broth ingredients in a large saucepan and bring to a gentle simmer. Cover partially with a lid and simmer gently for 5–10 minutes to let all the flavours infuse while you prepare the rest of the meal.

2. Cook rice noodles in salted boiling water for 3–4 minutes or until soft. Drain and divide equally between serving bowls.

3. Pat beef dry with paper towels and season well with salt. Heat oil in a medium-sized frying pan on high heat. Cook beef for about 45 seconds on all sides, so that it is just seared on the outside but still rare in the middle. Set aside to rest for a few minutes before slicing very thinly with a sharp knife.

4. Season broth to taste with more fish sauce or soy sauce if needed. Strain hot broth through a sieve, discarding spices and ginger, etc., bring back to the boil, and ladle over noodles in serving bowls.

5. To serve, place slices of beef and a handful of bean sprouts in the boiling hot soup. The heat of the broth will lightly cook the beef and mung bean sprouts. Top with spring onions and herbs. Serve with chilli or chilli sauce, and a lime wedge to squeeze over just before eating.

TIP Use thin slices of poached chicken breast instead of beef if you prefer.

SERVES: 2

PREP TIME: 5 MINUTES

COOK TIME: 15–20 MINUTES

BROTH

good-quality unsalted beef stock (preferably home-made) 4 cups (1 litre)
Chinese five spice ¼ teaspoon (optional)
whole star anise 2
cinnamon stick 1
whole cloves 3–4
red chilli 1, sliced (optional)
whole black peppercorns 1 teaspoon
ginger 2.5cm piece, peeled, thinly sliced
kaffir lime leaf 1 or **lime** zest of 1
fish sauce or **soy sauce** 2 tablespoons
lime juice of 1

BEEF + NOODLES

thin dried rice stick noodles or **vermicelli** 100–120g
beef eye fillet 300g (at room temperature)
salt
oil 1 teaspoon

TO SERVE

mung bean sprouts 2 small handfuls
spring onions 2–3, finely sliced
Asian herbs (e.g. mint, coriander, Vietnamese mint, Thai or aniseed basil) ½–¾ cup
red chilli 1, finely sliced, or **chilli sauce**
lime 1, cut into wedges

DINNER / MEAT

WHEAT FREE · GLUTEN FREE · DAIRY FREE · FREEZES WELL

BLACK PEPPER STEAK + MUSHROOM PIE

This pie is full of mushrooms and tender chunks of beef, with a rich peppery gravy. It's a lovely way to have your pie and eat it too.

1. Heat olive oil in a large heavy-based frying pan or flameproof casserole dish over medium heat. Cook onion for 3-4 minutes until soft. Add garlic and carrot and continue cooking for 2-3 minutes.

2. Add steak, mushrooms, tomato paste, beef stock, Worcestershire sauce and pepper. Cover with a tight-fitting lid and simmer over low heat for 2-2½ hours or until meat is tender. If you don't have a tight-fitting lid, cover with tinfoil first and then a lid. Check on the meat a few times during cooking, and top up with a little more stock if it looks like it's drying out. Alternatively, cook in the oven at 160°C for 2-2½ hours in a casserole dish, or in a slow cooker.

3. About 30 minutes before the stew is ready, preheat oven to 200°C. Cut pastry sheet into 4 squares. Place on a baking tray and bake for 15-20 minutes until pastry is puffed and golden.

4. Stir cornflour mixture into hot stew and continue to simmer, stirring frequently, until sauce thickens — this may take a few minutes. Season to taste with salt and pepper.

5. To serve, spoon some meat and sauce onto each plate and top with a puff pastry square. Serve with steamed vegetables on the side.

TIP The stewed meat freezes well, so freeze in portions for an easy fast-tracked meal.

SERVES: 4

PREP TIME: 10 MINUTES

COOK TIME: 2-2½ HOURS

olive oil 1 tablespoon
onion 1 large, chopped
garlic 2 cloves, chopped
carrot 1, peeled, diced
lean beef or venison stewing steak (e.g. leg, blade, shoulder) 600g, cut into 2-3cm cubes
mushrooms (e.g. portobello and/or button) 400g, stems removed, sliced
tomato paste 4 tablespoons
beef stock 2-2½ cups
Worcestershire sauce 2 tablespoons
freshly ground black pepper 1 teaspoon
salt
puff pastry 1 sheet (150g), defrosted
cornflour 2 teaspoons mixed with 2 tablespoons **cold water**

TO SERVE
steamed vegetables (e.g. broccoli, asparagus, beans, peas, carrots) 6 cups

Use gluten-free puff pastry

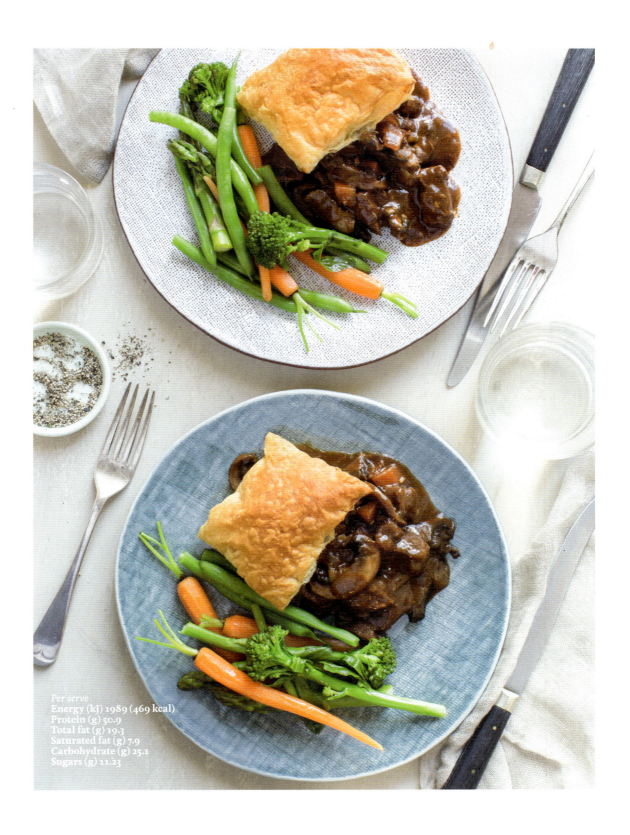

Per serve
Energy (kJ) 1989 (469 kcal)
Protein (g) 50.9
Total fat (g) 19.3
Saturated fat (g) 7.9
Carbohydrate (g) 25.1
Sugars (g) 11.23

DINNER / MEAT

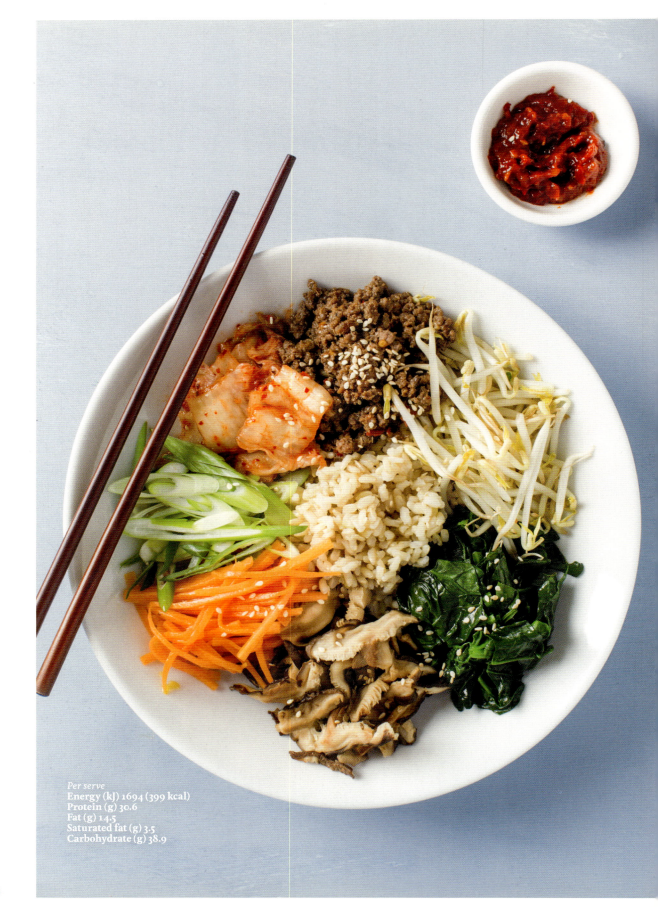

Per serve
Energy (kJ) 1694 (399 kcal)
Protein (g) 30.6
Fat (g) 14.5
Saturated fat (g) 3.5
Carbohydrate (g) 38.9

KOREAN BEEF + VEGETABLE BOWL

This is a fun meal to eat — you can mix everything up together in the bowl, or take turns mixing and matching the different ingredients with the rice.

1. Combine beef mince with soy sauce, chilli sauce, honey, garlic, ginger, sesame oil and black pepper. Set aside to marinate at room temperature for 15 minutes while you prepare the vegetables.

2. Cover dried shiitake mushrooms in boiling water and soak until soft, 5-10 minutes. Drain well, and squeeze mushrooms dry.

3. Heat 1 teaspoon of the oil in a wok or large frying pan over high heat. Add marinated beef mince and stir-fry, breaking up the mince, until well browned and cooked through, 5-10 minutes. Set mince aside. Add mushrooms, with a dash of extra soy sauce and sesame oil, and cook for a few minutes, then set aside with the mince.

4. Clean out the wok and heat the remaining teaspoon oil. Add carrots and stir-fry briefly for 1 minute, then set aside. Add spinach, along with 1-2 tablespoons of water, and briefly stir-fry for 1 minute, then set aside. Add mung bean sprouts and briefly stir-fry for 1 minute, then set aside.

5. To serve, spoon hot rice into the middle of each bowl and top with a small pile of each vegetable and some mince. Arrange some kimchi around the bowl, if using. Garnish with spring onions and sesame seeds.

TIP If you don't have dried shiitake mushrooms, use fresh sliced button mushrooms instead (which you don't have to soak).

SERVES: 4

PREP TIME: 10 MINUTES

COOK TIME: 15 MINUTES

BEEF

lean beef mince 400g
soy sauce 3 tablespoons
chilli sauce 1½ tablespoons
honey 1½ teaspoons
garlic 2-3 cloves, minced
ginger 2 teaspoons minced
sesame oil 1 teaspoon
freshly ground black pepper 1 teaspoon
oil 2 teaspoons

VEGETABLES

dried sliced shiitake mushrooms 2 cups
carrots 2, peeled, cut into thin matchsticks
baby spinach or **chopped spinach leaves** 4 large handfuls
mung bean sprouts 2 large handfuls

TO SERVE

steamed brown rice ½ cup per serving
kimchi (pickled Korean cabbage) ¼ cup (optional)
spring onions 2-3, finely sliced
toasted sesame seeds 1 tablespoon

WHEAT FREE   GLUTEN FREE   DAIRY FREE

Use gluten-free tamari soy sauce

JAPANESE BEEF NOODLE SALAD

This beef noodle dish is super-fast, healthy, fresh and full of flavour.

1. Cook soba noodles in boiling water for 2 minutes, then drop edamame beans in with the noodles for a further 1-2 minutes until noodles are just cooked (be careful not to overcook them). Drain and rinse under cold water to cool and stop the noodles cooking further and sticking together. Set aside.

2. Pat steaks dry with paper towels and season with a little salt. Heat oil in a large frying pan over medium-high heat. Cook steaks for about 2 minutes on each side for medium-rare, or until cooked to your liking. Mix soy sauce, vinegar, honey and sesame oil together and add to the hot pan with the beef — let it bubble for 15-30 seconds until slightly sticky and reduced, then turn off the heat. Spoon sauce over the beef to coat evenly. Leave beef in the pan to rest for 5 minutes while you finish preparing the rest of the meal.

3. Combine all dressing ingredients together.

4. When ready to serve, in a large bowl toss most of the dressing (reserve about 2 tablespoons) with the noodles and salad ingredients except sesame seeds. Slice beef thinly on an angle against the grain.

5. To serve, divide noodle salad between plates and top with slices of beef and any sauce from the pan. Spoon over reserved dressing, sprinkle over sesame seeds and grind over black pepper.

TIP Use thinly sliced pieces of poached chicken breast instead of beef as a variation.

SERVES: 4
PREP TIME: 10 MINUTES
COOK TIME: 10 MINUTES

NOODLES + BEEF
dried soba noodles 200g
frozen podded edamame beans ½ cup, defrosted
lean beef steaks (e.g. sirloin, rump or fillet) 500g, cut into 3cm-thick slices
salt
oil 2 teaspoons
soy sauce 2 tablespoons
rice vinegar 2 teaspoons
honey 1 teaspoon
sesame oil 1 teaspoon

DRESSING
soy sauce 3 tablespoons
liquid honey 2 teaspoons
rice vinegar 1½ tablespoons
lime juice 1½ tablespoons
sesame oil 2 teaspoons
ginger 2 teaspoons minced

SALAD
baby radishes 3-4, finely sliced
spring onions 2, finely sliced
celery 2-3 stalks, finely sliced
leafy greens (e.g. mesclun, baby rocket, watercress, mizuna) 3-4 handfuls
mung bean sprouts 1 cup
toasted sesame seeds 2 teaspoons
freshly ground black pepper

Use thin rice stick noodles instead of soba noodles, and gluten-free tamari soy sauce

Per serve
Energy (kJ) 1922 (453 kcal)
Protein (g) 39.1
Total fat (g) 20.9
Saturated fat (g) 3.2
Carbohydrate (g) 41.7
Sugars (g) 5.90

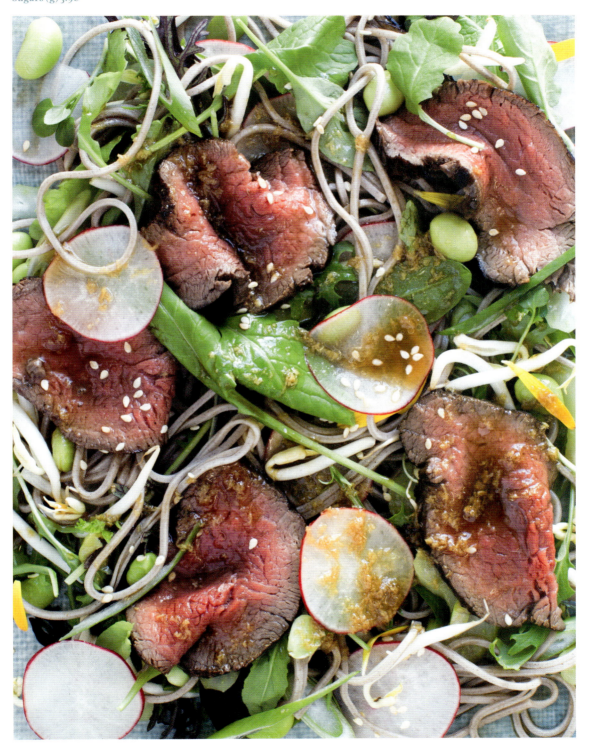

DINNER / MEAT

SPANISH MEATBALLS, BEANS + CAULIFLOWER PARSLEY MASH

Using a mix of chorizo mince and beef mince makes these meatballs juicy and gives them loads of flavour. To bump up the vegetables I use a mix of cauliflower and potato in the mash.

1. Snip the ends of chorizo sausages and squeeze the soft meat into a mixing bowl. Add beef mince, soaked breadcrumbs, egg and salt and mix together, using clean hands, until well combined. Roll tablespoons of mixture into meatballs and set aside in the fridge for 5 minutes to firm up a little.

2. Place cauliflower and potatoes for mash in a large saucepan of salted water and bring to the boil. Cook until soft, 10-12 minutes.

3. Now, make the sauce. Heat olive oil in a large frying pan or saucepan with a lid over medium heat. Cook onion for 3-4 minutes until soft. Add garlic and cook for 1-2 minutes. Stir in tomatoes, stock, paprika, chilli and thyme. Simmer, uncovered, for 8-10 minutes until thickened.

4. Stir beans and spinach through simmering sauce, then add meatballs. Spoon some hot sauce over them, then cover with a lid and simmer for 5-7 minutes or until meatballs are just cooked through. Turn them over once during cooking. (Try not to overcook them — test one by breaking it open.)

5. Drain potatoes and cauliflower well. Tip back into pot and place back over low heat — this will help the potato and cauliflower dry out. Mash with butter, raw garlic and parsley. Season to taste with salt and pepper.

6. To serve, divide mash and meatballs between plates. Spoon over sauce and beans and garnish with more parsley.

SERVES: 4

PREP TIME: 20 MINUTES

COOK TIME: 40 MINUTES

MEATBALLS

good-quality raw soft chorizo sausages or **sausage mince** 250g
lean beef mince 250g
breadcrumbs ½ cup soaked in 2 tablespoons **milk**
egg 1 small
salt ½ teaspoon
olive oil 1 tablespoon
onion 1, finely chopped
garlic 2 cloves, finely chopped
crushed tomatoes 2 x 400g cans
beef or chicken stock 1 cup
smoked paprika 1¼ teaspoons
chilli flakes ¼-½ teaspoon
thyme 1 tablespoon chopped
cannellini or butter beans 1 x 400g can, rinsed, drained
spinach 2 handfuls chopped

CAULIFLOWER PARSLEY MASH

cauliflower 500g, chopped
Agria potatoes 300g, peeled, chopped
butter 1 tablespoon
garlic ½ small clove, very finely minced
flat-leaf parsley ¼-½ cup finely chopped
salt and **freshly ground black pepper**

TO SERVE

flat-leaf parsley 2-3 tablespoons chopped

WHEAT FREE · GLUTEN FREE · DAIRY FREE · FREEZES WELL

Dairy-free without butter + . use gluten-free breadcrumbs

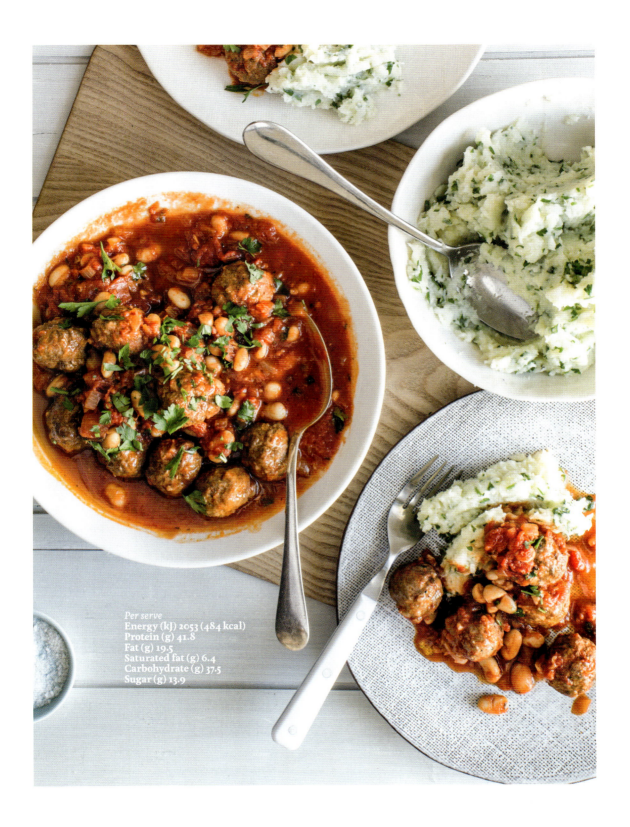

Per serve
Energy (kJ) 2053 (484 kcal)
Protein (g) 41.8
Fat (g) 19.5
Saturated fat (g) 6.4
Carbohydrate (g) 37.5
Sugar (g) 13.9

DINNER / MEAT

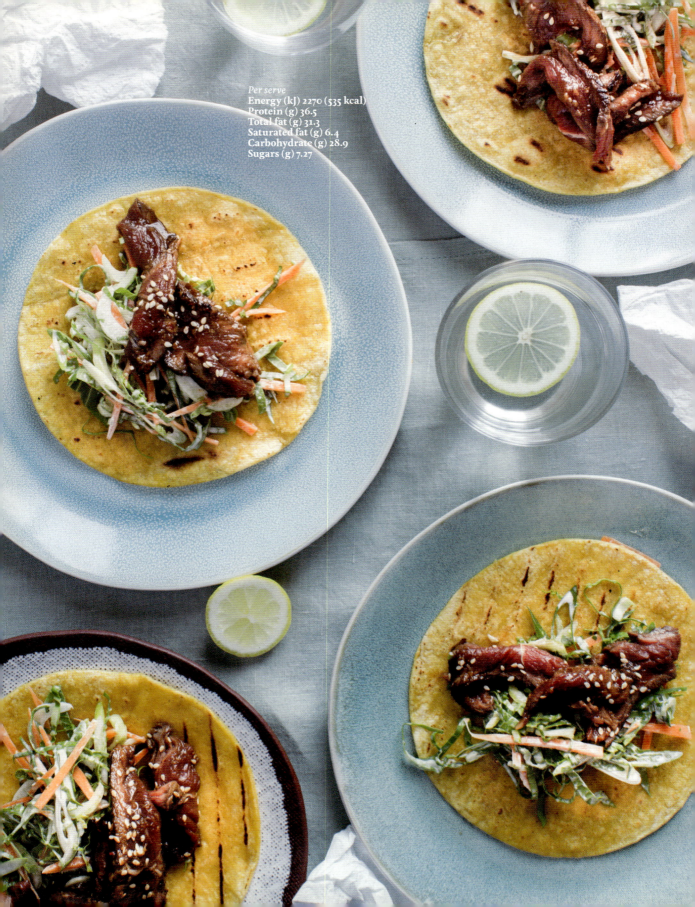

Per serve
Energy (kJ) 2270 (535 kcal)
Protein (g) 36.5
Total fat (g) 31.3
Saturated fat (g) 6.4
Carbohydrate (g) 28.9
Sugars (g) 7.27

ASIAN STEAK TACOS WITH BOK CHOY SLAW

I know it's not conventional, but this Asian spin on a Mexican favourite is so tasty. If you've never tried raw bok choy in a slaw, you're missing out! It makes an excellent alternative to cabbage, with great taste, freshness and crunch.

1. Rub steak all over with Chinese five spice and season with salt. Heat 1 tablespoon oil in a large frying pan over medium-high heat. Cook steaks for about 2 minutes on each side for medium-rare, or until cooked to your liking. Set steaks aside to rest for a few minutes before slicing very thinly against the grain.

2. While the steak is resting make the slaw. Trim 1cm off the stalk ends of the bok choy, then finely slice the stalks and leaves. Mix mayonnaise and lemon juice together and gently toss with bok choy, carrot, spring onion and coriander.

3. Mix together remaining oil, soy sauce, honey, water, chilli, if using, garlic, ginger and sesame oil. Heat the pan the steak was cooked in and add sauce. Let it bubble for 30-60 seconds until reduced and sticky. Turn off the heat and add sliced steak to the pan, quickly tossing it in the sauce to coat evenly. Sprinkle over sesame seeds.

4. Heat tortillas according to packet instructions.

5. To serve, place tortillas, bok choy slaw and steak in dishes in the middle of the table for everyone to help themselves. To build a taco add spoonfuls of beef and sauce to the tortilla and top with slaw. Roll up and eat.

SERVES: 4

PREP TIME: 15-20 MINUTES

COOK TIME: 10 MINUTES

STEAK + SAUCE

lean beef steak (e.g. sirloin or rump) 500g, trimmed of excess fat
Chinese five spice 1 teaspoon
salt
oil 2 tablespoons
soy sauce 3 tablespoons
liquid honey 2 teaspoons
water 2 tablespoons
chilli paste or sauce 1-2 teaspoons (optional)
garlic 2 small cloves, crushed
ginger 2 teaspoons finely minced
sesame oil 2 teaspoons
sesame seeds 2 teaspoons

BOK CHOY SLAW

baby bok choy 3 (2½-3 cups shredded)
good-quality mayonnaise 4 tablespoons
lemon juice of ½
carrot 1, peeled, shredded or coarsely grated
spring onions 2, finely sliced
coriander ½ cup chopped

TO SERVE

soft corn or wheat tortillas 8 small

DINNER / MEAT

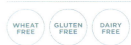

Use gluten-free tamari soy sauce

VEGE-PACKED SPAGHETTI BOLOGNESE

Spaghetti Bolognese is one of those comfort food dishes I love, so I just had to include it. This version is extra good for you, with its hidden vegetables and wholemeal pasta.

1. Heat 1 tablespoon olive oil in a large frying pan or saucepan over medium heat. Add mince and salt and cook until well browned, about 5 minutes. Set cooked mince aside. Wipe out pan.

2. Heat remaining olive oil in the pan over medium heat. Cook onion, garlic and butternut or pumpkin until soft, about 5 minutes. Add courgette, carrot, tomato passata or crushed tomatoes, dried herbs, cream, if using, and cooked mince, and simmer uncovered for about 5 minutes until slightly thickened and vegetables are cooked through. Season to taste with salt and pepper.

3. Cook spaghetti in boiling salted water until al dente (just cooked), 10-12 minutes. Drain and divide between serving bowls.

4. To serve, spoon Bolognese sauce over spaghetti and garnish with a little parmesan, if using. Serve with a leafy green salad on the side.

SERVES: 6

PREP TIME: 20 MINUTES

COOK TIME: 15 MINUTES

olive oil 2 tablespoons
lean beef mince (or a mixture of pork and beef) 500g
salt 1 teaspoon
onion 1 large, grated
garlic 2 cloves, minced
butternut or **pumpkin** 1 cup, grated
courgettes 2 medium-sized, grated
carrot 1 medium-sized, peeled, grated
tomato passata sauce or **canned crushed tomatoes** 3½–4 cups
dried oregano or **mixed herbs** ¼ teaspoon
cream, mascarpone or **crème fraîche** ⅓ cup (optional)
freshly ground black pepper
dried wholemeal or **quinoa spaghetti** 480g

TO SERVE

parmesan ⅓ cup grated (optional)
leafy green salad (see page 277) 6 servings

Use gluten-free quinoa spaghetti

Per serve
Energy (kJ) 2336 (551 kcal)
Protein (g) 34.7
Total fat (g) 19.1
Saturated fat (g) 7.3
Carbohydrate (g) 62.5
Sugars (g) 8.89

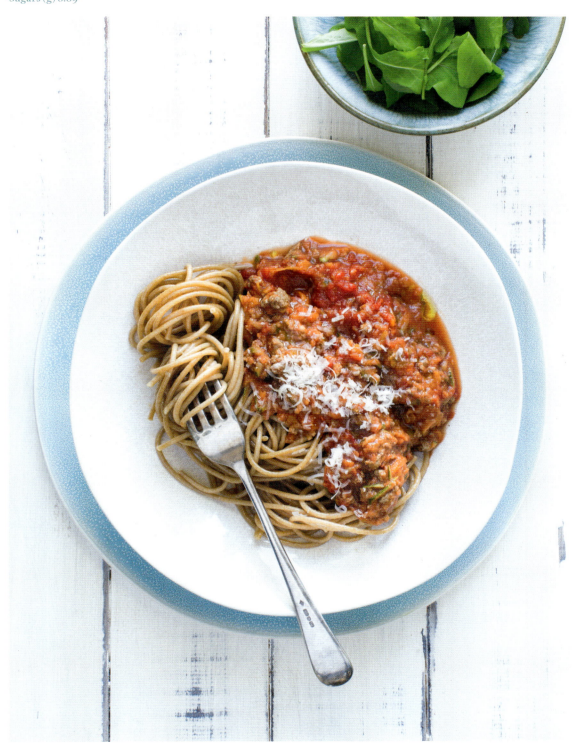

DINNER / MEAT

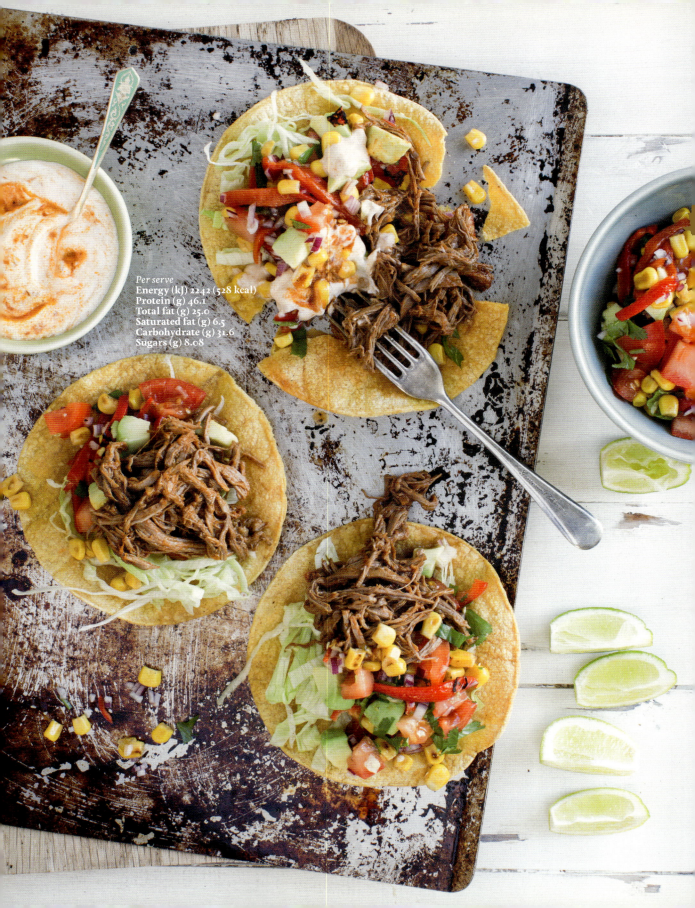

Per serve
Energy (kJ) 2242 (528 kcal)
Protein (g) 46.1
Total fat (g) 25.0
Saturated fat (g) 6.5
Carbohydrate (g) 31.6
Sugars (g) 8.08

BEEF TOSTADAS WITH CHARRED CORN SALSA

This recipe uses leftover slow-cooked Mexican shredded beef from page 142, but if you havn't got any you could use beef mince fried with some chipotle sauce. Tostadas are crunchy, deep-fried tortillas, but I bake mine in the oven until golden and crisp. This is a fun (and messy) meal to eat — use your hands to break off pieces of tostada, pile on some beef and salsa, eat and enjoy!

1. Preheat oven to 200°C. Cut the kernels off the corn cob with a sharp knife. Heat olive oil in a medium-sized frying pan over medium-high heat. Cook the corn kernels, tossing occasionally, until charred and cooked through, about 5 minutes. Remove from the heat and let cool. Combine charred corn with tomatoes, roast capsicum, avocado, red onion, coriander, lemon or lime juice and chilli, if using. Season to taste with salt and pepper.

2. Mix yoghurt and chipotle sauce together.

3. Very lightly brush tortillas with a little olive oil and place on an oven tray in a single layer. Bake for 10-12 minutes until golden and crisp. Watch they don't burn.

4. Warm up Mexican shredded beef on the stovetop or in the microwave.

5. To serve, pile some salsa, shredded lettuce and Mexican shredded beef on each tostada and drizzle over chipotle yoghurt.

SERVES: 4

PREP TIME: 10 MINUTES

COOK TIME: 15 MINUTES

SALSA

corn cob 1, husked or **corn kernels** ½ x 400g can drained, rinsed
olive oil 1 teaspoon
tomatoes 2, diced
roasted red capsicum (from a jar or the deli) 1, thinly sliced
avocado ½ medium-sized ripe, diced
red onion ½ small, finely diced
coriander ¼ cup roughly chopped
lemon juice of ½ or **lime** juice of 1
red chilli ½, finely chopped (optional)
salt
freshly ground black pepper

CHIPOTLE YOGHURT

natural unsweetened thick Greek yoghurt 4 tablespoons
chipotle sauce 2-3 teaspoons

TO SERVE

corn tortillas 8 small
olive oil 1 tablespoon
Mexican shredded beef (see page 142) 4 cups
iceberg lettuce 4 handfuls shredded

DINNER / MEAT

WHEAT FREE | GLUTEN FREE | DAIRY FREE

Dairy-free without yoghurt

VIETNAMESE PORK MEATBALLS WITH RICE NOODLE SALAD

This was the first meal I had when I arrived in Vietnam, where it's called bun cha. It's simple, fresh, full of flavour and healthy, like most Vietnamese dishes. It's served with lots of lovely fresh herbs and you can eat it in a relaxed style by rolling up the meatballs in lettuce leaves and dipping them into the nuoc cham (chilli and fish sauce) dressing.

1. Mix pork mince, fish sauce, salt, sugar, pepper, shallot, garlic and ginger together. Roll teaspoons of mixture into small meatballs and flatten slightly (this will make them easier to cook). Set aside in the fridge for 5 minutes to firm up a bit.

2. Mix all nuoc cham dressing ingredients together and set aside.

3. Pour boiling water over vermicelli noodles and leave to soak for about 5 minutes. Drain and run under cold water to prevent noodles sticking together. Use scissors to snip noodles into shorter lengths (which make them easier to eat).

4. Heat a large non-stick frying pan over medium heat. Brown meatballs all over until cooked through.

5. To serve, place noodles, lettuce leaves, spring onions, bean sprouts, herbs and nuoc cham dressing in the middle of the table. To assemble, pile a small amount of noodles, spring onion, bean sprouts, herbs and 1–2 meatballs in each lettuce leaf. Spoon over some dressing, wrap up and eat.

TIP You can make chicken mince meatballs instead of pork if you prefer.

SERVES: 4

PREP TIME: 15 MINUTES

COOK TIME: 20 MINUTES

MEATBALLS
pork mince 500g
fish sauce 2 teaspoons
salt 1 teaspoon
brown sugar 1 teaspoon
freshly ground black pepper 1 teaspoon
shallot 1, finely minced
garlic 2 cloves, minced
ginger 1 teaspoon minced
oil 1 tablespoon

NUOC CHAM DRESSING
lime or lemon juice ¼ cup
sweet chilli sauce 2 tablespoons
fish sauce 2 tablespoons
water 2–3 tablespoons
garlic 1 small clove, finely minced
red chilli ½, finely chopped

RICE NOODLE SALAD
dried vermicelli rice noodles 100g
lettuce (coral or cos) about 20 leaves
spring onions 2–3, finely sliced
mung bean sprouts 1½ cups
mint leaves ¼–½ cup sliced
coriander ¼–½ cup chopped
Thai or aniseed basil and **Vietnamese mint** ¼ cup total sliced (optional)

WHEAT FREE · GLUTEN FREE · DAIRY FREE

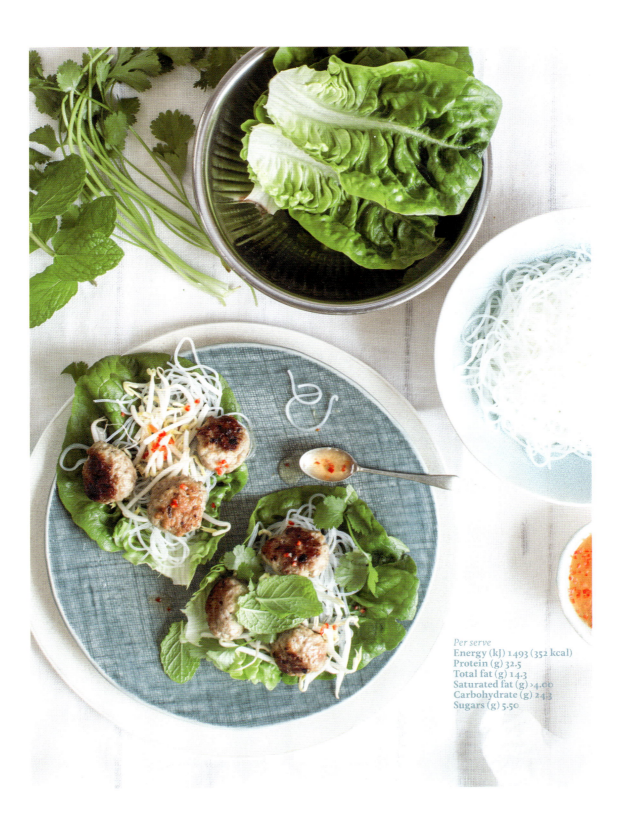

Per serve
Energy (kJ) 1493 (352 kcal)
Protein (g) 32.5
Total fat (g) 14.3
Saturated fat (g) >4.00
Carbohydrate (g) 24.3
Sugars (g) 5.50

HOISIN PORK + VEGE STIR-FRY

A quick, simple stir-fry meal using lean pork, but you could substitute beef or chicken.

1. Mix all sauce ingredients together and set aside.

2. Heat 1 tablespoon oil in a wok or large frying pan over high heat. Pat pork dry with paper towels and season with salt. Stir-fry pork for 2-3 minutes until browned. Set aside.

3. Add remaining oil to the pan and stir-fry ginger, garlic, red onion, celery, courgette and capsicum and stir-fry for 2-3 minutes until vegetables are just cooked. If the garlic, ginger or vegetables are sticking to the bottom of the pan and burning, just add 1-2 tablespoons chicken stock.

4. Add cooked pork back to the pan along with the sauce, and bring the sauce to a boil. Toss a few times to evenly coat meat and vegetables in sauce, then turn off the heat.

5. To serve, divide pork stir-fry and rice between bowls. Garnish with coriander, if using.

SERVES: 2

PREP TIME: 10 MINUTES

COOK TIME: 10 MINUTES

SAUCE

hoisin sauce 1 tablespoon

chilli ½ –1 teaspoon minced or **chilli paste** 1 teaspoon

sesame oil 1 teaspoon

sherry or **Chinese cooking wine** 2 tablespoons

chicken stock ⅓ cup

cornflour 1 teaspoon mixed with **water** 1½ tablespoons

PORK STIR-FRY

oil 1½ tablespoons

free-range lean pork fillet or rump 300g, thinly sliced (at room temperature)

salt

ginger 1cm piece, peeled, cut into thin matchsticks

garlic 2 cloves, chopped

red onion ½, sliced

celery 1 stalk

courgette 1 small, sliced

red, green or yellow capsicum 1, sliced

TO SERVE

steamed brown rice ½ cup per serving

coriander ¼ cup chopped (optional)

For wheat-free, substitute hoisin sauce for 1 tablespoon tamari sauce + ¼ teaspoon Chinese five spice + 1 teaspoon brown sugar

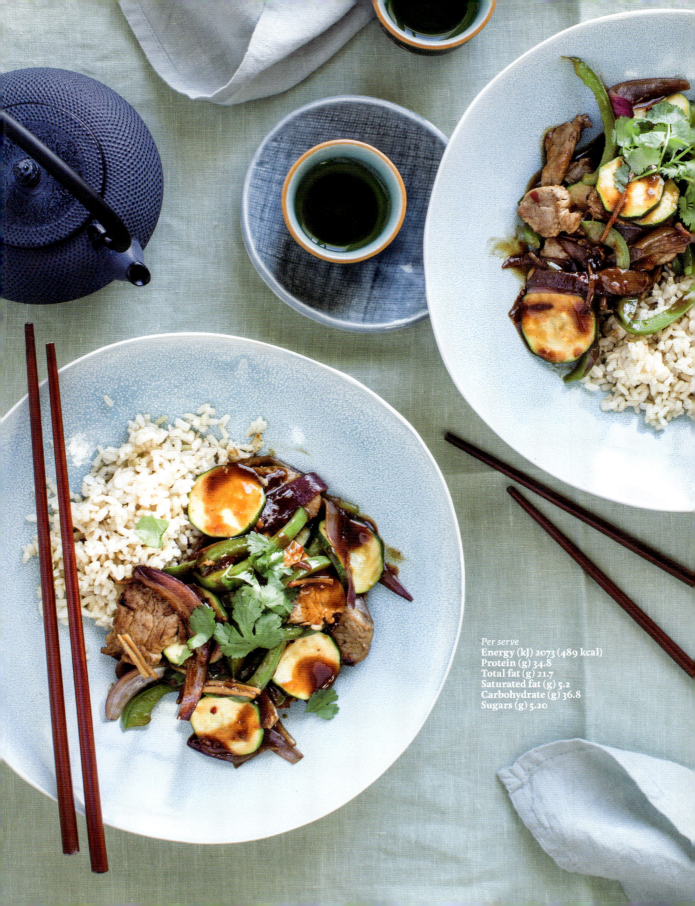

Per serve
Energy (kJ) 2073 (489 kcal)
Protein (g) 34.8
Total fat (g) 21.7
Saturated fat (g) 5.2
Carbohydrate (g) 36.8
Sugars (g) 5.20

NAKED BURGERS WITH QUICK BEETROOT RELISH + KUMARA CHIPS

You don't need a bun to have a burger. 'Naked' burgers (everything but the bread bun) are the way to go to get all the flavour, all the nutrition, but half the calories.

1. Preheat oven to 200°C. Line an oven tray with baking paper. Toss kumara or sweet potato and olive oil together on prepared tray. Season well with salt and pepper and bake for 25-30 minutes until golden and crispy.

2. Mix together all burger ingredients, except olive oil. Divide mixture into eight portions and shape into eight burger patties 1-2cm thick. Heat a large frying pan or barbecue grill to medium. Rub olive oil all over the burgers. Brown burgers for 1-2 minutes on each side until half-cooked then transfer to the oven to finish cooking for 3-4 minutes. Set burgers aside to rest for a few minutes.

3. While you are cooking and resting the burgers, make the relish.

4. Mix yoghurt with wholegrain mustard and horseradish, if using.

5. To serve, place two burgers on each plate and divide kumara chips, rocket leaves, tomato and red onion between plates. Serve with a good spoonful or two of beetroot relish and yoghurt on the side.

TIP The burger patties can be frozen (uncooked). When you want to cook one, just take it out of the freezer and allow to defrost first.

SERVES: 4
PREP TIME: 15 MINUTES
COOK TIME: 25-30 MINUTES

KUMARA CHIPS
red or gold kumara (or other sweet potato) 600g skin on, scrubbed, cut into 2cm-thick wedges
olive oil 1 tablespoon
salt
freshly ground black pepper

VENISON BURGERS
breadcrumbs ¼ cup soaked in 2 tablespoons milk
venison or beef mince 600g
free-range egg 1
onion 1, grated
garlic 2 cloves, finely minced
ground cumin 1 teaspoon
ground coriander 1 teaspoon
ground allspice 1 teaspoon
salt 1 teaspoon
olive oil 1 tablespoon

TO SERVE
quick beetroot relish (see page 278) 1 cup
natural unsweetened thick Greek yoghurt ⅓ cup
wholegrain mustard 2 teaspoons
horseradish sauce 1-2 teaspoons (optional)
baby rocket 4 handfuls
tomatoes 2-3, sliced
red onion ½ small, thinly sliced into rings

WHEAT FREE | GLUTEN FREE | DAIRY FREE | FREEZES WELL

Use gluten-free breadcrumbs + omit yoghurt

Per serve
Energy (kJ) 2403 (566 kcal)
Protein (g) 42.0
Total fat (g) 22.5
Saturated fat (g) 6.4
Carbohydrate (g) 51.4
Sugars (g) 14.98

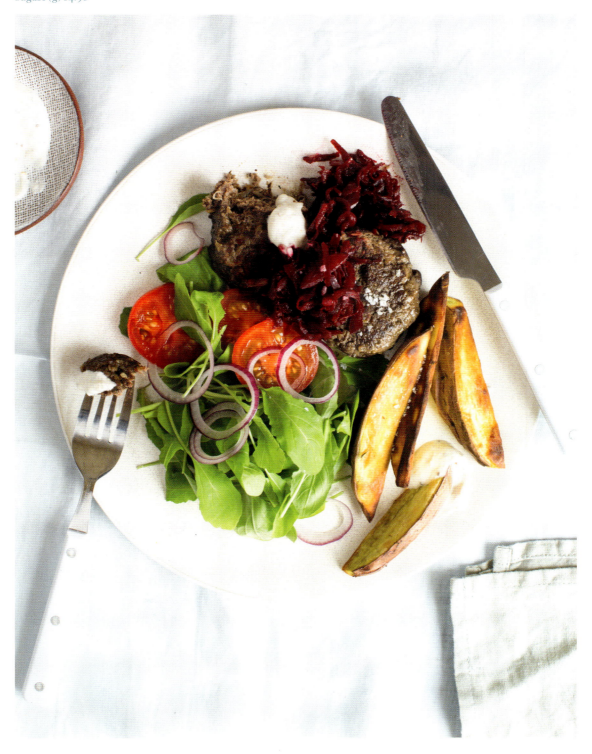

DINNER / MEAT

165

CHICKEN + MINT SALAD ROLLS WITH PEANUT DIPPING SAUCE

Just like the ones you get in Vietnamese restaurants. You can either cook fresh chicken mince or use leftover cooked shredded chicken. These rolls make a light dinner and they're great to take for lunch, too.

1. Heat oil in a wok or large frying pan over high heat. Stir-fry chicken mince until browned, about 10 minutes. Season with salt and pepper and set aside to cool to room temperature.

2. Mix cooked chicken mince, carrot, cabbage, mint and coriander together in a large bowl.

3. To assemble the rice paper rolls, fill a large shallow dish with warm water and place a flat, damp tea towel on the bench. Place a few rice paper wrappers at a time in the warm water and soak for 10–20 seconds until soft and pliable. Carefully transfer one wrapper to tea towel. Smear ½ teaspoon hoisin sauce on each wrapper, then place a small handful of chicken mixture in the centre (be careful not to overfill). Fold the bottom edge of the rice paper over the filling, then fold each side in and roll up. Repeat with remaining wrappers.

4. Mix peanut butter with boiling water to loosen, then mix with remaining dipping sauce ingredients.

5. Serve five rolls per person with 2 tablespoons dipping sauce. Alternatively, serve the rice paper wrappers, hoisin sauce and chicken filling on the table for everyone to make their own rolls.

TIP Use pork mince or prawns instead of chicken as a variation.

SERVES: 4
PREP TIME: 20–30 MINUTES
COOK TIME: 10 MINUTES

CHICKEN ROLLS
oil 1 tablespoon
chicken mince 400g
salt
freshly ground black pepper
carrot 2 cups grated
cabbage 2 cups finely shredded
mint leaves 1 cup
coriander ¾ cup chopped
large dried rice paper wrappers 1 packet (about 25 large wrappers)
hoisin sauce ⅓ cup

PEANUT DIPPING SAUCE
crunchy peanut butter 3 tablespoons
boiling water 1 tablespoon
sweet chilli sauce 3 tablespoons
lime juice 3 tablespoons
soy sauce or **fish sauce** 1 teaspoon

DAIRY FREE

Per serve
Energy (kJ) 1642 (387 kcal)
Protein (g) 4.7
Total fat (g) 5.5
Saturated fat (g) 0.9
Carbohydrate (g) 10.8
Sugars (g) 9.78

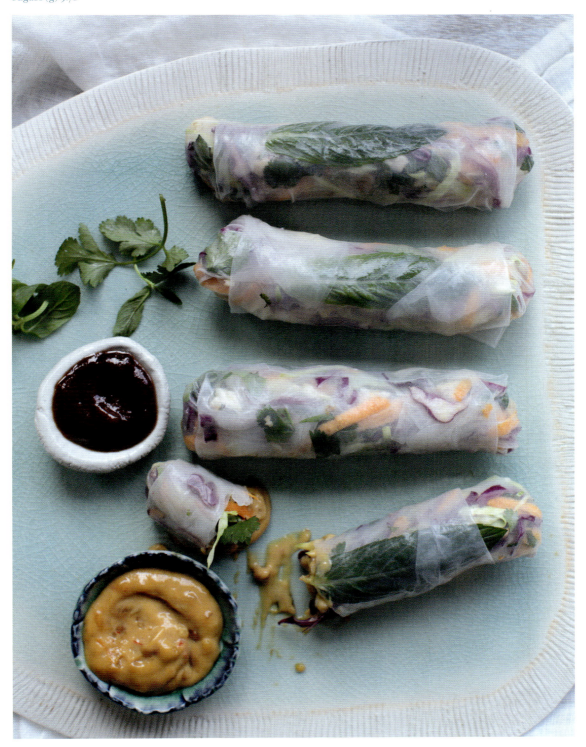

CHICKEN + SPINACH TIKKA MASALA WITH BUTTERED LEMON CAULIFLOWER 'RICE'

This curry has all the flavour but not the fat or sugar that most takeaways do. Cauliflower 'rice' is genius — it has the same light, fluffy texture as rice, but a fraction of the calories and it bumps up your vege intake, too.

SERVES: 4

PREP TIME: 20 MINUTES

COOK TIME: 20–25 MINUTES

CHICKEN AND SPINACH TIKKA MASALA

oil 1 tablespoon
onion 1 large, chopped
garam masala 2 teaspoons
ground cumin 1 tablespoon
smoked paprika 1 tablespoon
ground turmeric 1½ teaspoons
ground chilli 1 teaspoon
garlic 2 cloves, minced
fresh ginger 2 teaspoons finely chopped or grated
lemon zest of ½
salt 1 teaspoon
boneless skinless chicken thighs 600g, cut into 2-3cm pieces
crushed/chopped tomatoes 1 x 400g can
sweet chilli sauce 1 tablespoon
lemon juice of ½
cream ½ cup
baby spinach 3 large handfuls, chopped
natural unsweetened yoghurt 3-4 tablespoons, to serve
coriander ¼–½ cup chopped, to serve

BUTTERED CAULIFLOWER RICE

cauliflower 1 head (about 750-800g including the stem), cut into florets
butter 1 tablespoon
lemon zest of ½
coriander or **flat-leaf parsley** ¼–½ cup chopped

1. Heat oil in a large, heavy-based frying pan over medium heat. Cook onion for 6-8 minutes until soft and starting to turn golden brown. Add spices, garlic, ginger, lemon zest and salt and continue cooking for a further 1-2 minutes. If at any time the onion or spices are catching on the bottom of the pan and burning, just add a tablespoon or two of water, stir, and it should lift from the bottom of the pan.

2. Add chicken, tomatoes, sweet chilli sauce, lemon juice and cream, cover and simmer for 5-10 minutes until chicken is cooked through and sauce has slightly thickened. Stir through spinach until wilted, and season to taste with salt and pepper. Gently swirl through yoghurt.

3. To make the cauliflower rice, briefly blitz cauliflower in a food processor until it resembles the texture of rice or couscous. You may have to do this in batches to avoid overcrowding the food processor. Transfer to a glass or microwavable bowl and microwave on high, uncovered, for a few minutes (this steams the cauliflower and evaporates extra moisture to make it fluffy). Toss hot cauliflower rice with butter and coriander or parsley, and season to taste with salt and pepper.

4. To serve, spoon some cauliflower rice and chicken tikka masala onto each plate. Garnish with a little yoghurt and coriander.

TIP If you don't have a food processor, you can coarsley grate the cauliflower to resemble rice, or even very finely chop it using a large, sharp knife.

WHEAT FREE • GLUTEN FREE • FREEZES WELL

Per serve
Energy (kJ) 1503.6 (354 kcal)
Protein (g) 35.3
Total fat (g) 17.9
Saturated fat (g) 8.6
Carbohydrate (g) 14.0
Sugars (g) 12.4

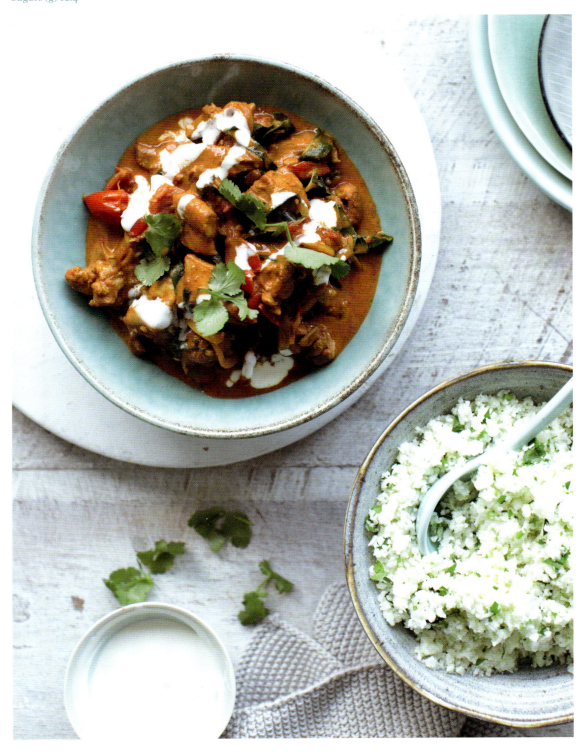

DINNER / CHICKEN

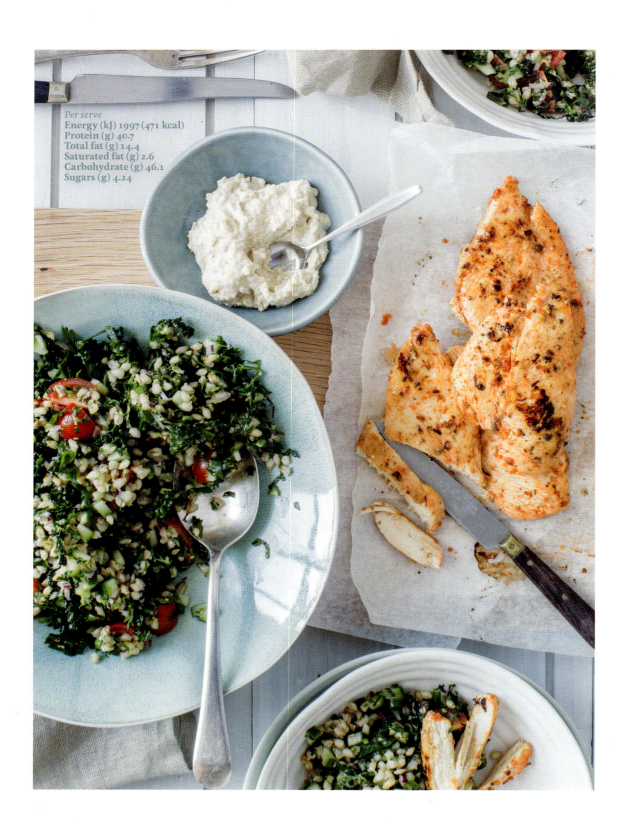

Per serve
Energy (kJ) 1997 (471 kcal)
Protein (g) 40.7
Total fat (g) 14.4
Saturated fat (g) 2.6
Carbohydrate (g) 46.1
Sugars (g) 4.24

HARISSA CHICKEN STEAKS WITH KALE + BARLEY TABOULEH

Harissa, a spice mix from North Africa, packs a real flavour punch and is great for marinating any meat. I love using barley in salads — it adds texture and a lovely nutty flavour. 'Massaging' the kale with olive oil and lemon juice helps soften it and take away some of its bitterness.

1. Preheat oven to 200°C. Bring a small saucepan of salted water to the boil. Cook barley in boiling water until tender but still a little firm to the bite, 15–20 minutes. Drain barley and rinse under the tap to cool slightly. Drain well.

2. Cut chicken breasts in half horizontally so you have two thinner chicken steaks. To do this, place a chicken breast flat on a chopping board. Place one hand on top of the chicken breast and, using a sharp knife, slice through the chicken breast horizontally, trying to keep an equal thickness either side.

3. Coat chicken steaks well with harissa paste, rubbing it all over. Place chicken in a small roasting or oven dish, season with salt and roast for 8–10 minutes until cooked through but still moist and succulent on the inside. Rest chicken for a few minutes after cooking.

4. Drizzle kale with lemon juice and olive oil and sprinkle with a pinch of salt. Use your fingertips to gently massage the kale — it helps soften it. Toss kale with barley, red onion, cucumber, cherry tomatoes, parsley, mint and dukkah or roasted almonds. Season to taste with salt and pepper.

5. To serve, place a chicken steak on each plate and top with tabouleh. Spoon over any cooking juices from the chicken. Serve with a dollop of hummus on the side.

TIP Harissa paste adds so much flavour to any meat dish — make it up in bulk and store it in the fridge with a very thin layer of oil on top (it will keep for a few weeks) or freeze it. You can use bulgur wheat as an alternative to barley if you prefer.

SERVES: 4

PREP TIME: 15 MINUTES

COOK TIME: 20 MINUTES

pearl barley 1 cup
chicken breast 600g boneless, skinless
harissa paste (store-bought or see page 276) 2 tablespoons
salt
curly kale, cavolo nero, spinach or **rocket** about 100g, tough stalks removed, leaves chopped
lemon juice of 1
extra virgin olive oil 1 tablespoon
red onion ½, finely diced
telegraph cucumber ½, halved, deseeded and finely diced
cherry tomatoes 1 punnet, halved
flat-leaf parsley ½ cup chopped
mint leaves ½ cup sliced
dukkah or **chopped roasted almonds** 2 tablespoons
freshly ground black pepper

TO SERVE

hummus ½ cup (store-bought or see page 270)

WHEAT FREE   DAIRY FREE

DINNER / CHICKEN

CHICKEN, SILVERBEET, LEMON + PARSLEY MACARONI SOUP

This chicken soup will make you feel good from the inside out — especially if you've got the winter chills! A whole chicken cooked in the pot to make a flavourful stock, with fresh, zesty and clean flavours of lemon and parsley.

SERVES: 6

PREP TIME: 15 MINUTES

COOK TIME: 1 HOUR 15 MINUTES

free-range chicken 1 whole size 16
thyme 4–5 sprigs
carrot 1, peeled, chopped
celery 2 stalks, chopped
onion 1, chopped
garlic 2 cloves, chopped
whole black peppercorns 1 teaspoon
salt 1 teaspoon
chicken stock 1.5 litres
water 2 litres
orzo, risoni or **macaroni elbows pasta** 1¾ cups
freshly ground black pepper
lemon juice of 1
silverbeet or **spinach** 1 bunch (about 450g), tough stems removed, chopped
flat-leaf parsley ½ cup chopped

1. Wash chicken inside and out, making sure the gut cavity is clean. Pat dry. Place whole chicken, thyme, carrot, celery, onion, garlic, black peppercorns and salt in a large stockpot and pour over stock and water to just cover. Cover with a lid and bring to a gentle boil. Reduce heat and simmer, partially covered, for 1 hour or until chicken is cooked through (check by cutting between the drum and thigh with the tip of a sharp knife).

2. Remove chicken from pot and set aside. Strain stock, discarding all vegetables. Return stock to the pot and bring to the boil. Add pasta, stir, and boil until just cooked, but still a little firm to the bite, about 8 minutes. Season to taste with salt and pepper.

3. While pasta is cooking, shred chicken meat, discarding the skin. Add shredded chicken, lemon juice, silverbeet and parsley to the soup and simmer for a further 2 minutes until heated through.

4. To serve, ladle soup into bowls and serve piping hot.

TIP Freeze in individual portions for a quick 'heat and eat' lunch or dinner.

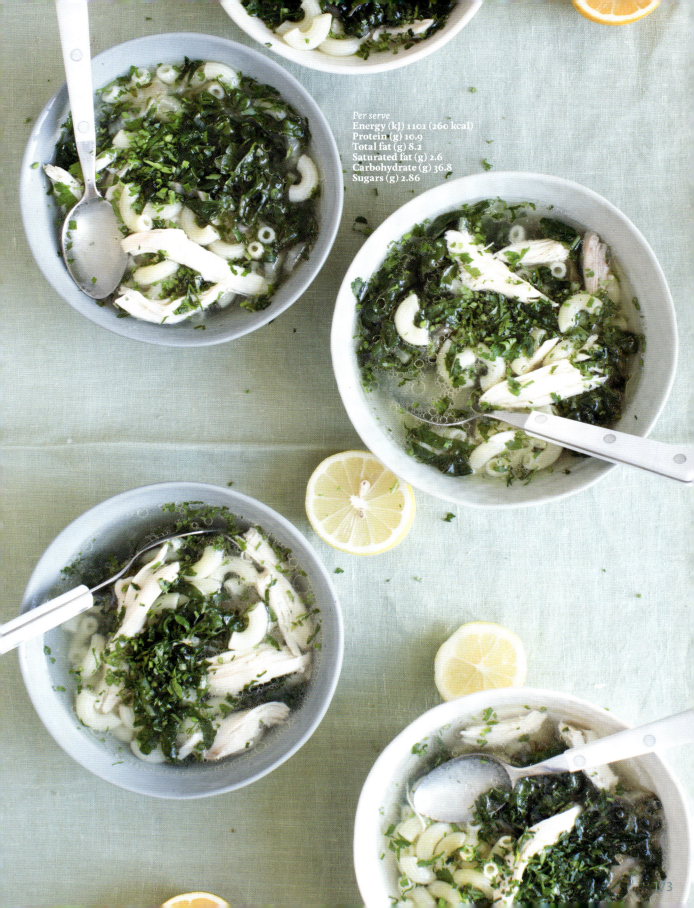

Per serve
Energy (kJ) 1101 (260 kcal)
Protein (g) 10.9
Total fat (g) 8.2
Saturated fat (g) 2.6
Carbohydrate (g) 36.8
Sugars (g) 2.86

SPICY JAMAICAN JERK CHICKEN, MANGO SALSA + ALLSPICE FRIES

Your taste buds will be dancing to the tropical flavours of the Caribbean when you eat this.

1. Combine chicken, Jamaican jerk paste and honey in a bowl. If you have time, set aside in the fridge to marinate for a few hours or overnight.

2. Preheat oven to 220°C. Line two oven trays with baking paper. Season chicken with salt. Heat a drizzle of oil in a large frying pan over medium-high heat and brown chicken for 2-3 minutes, then transfer to one of the prepared trays.

3. Toss kumara, olive oil, allspice and chilli flakes, if using, in the other tray. Bake both trays for about 20 minutes until fries are golden and chicken is cooked through. (Place fries above the chicken in the oven.)

4. While fries and chicken are cooking, mix all salsa ingredients together and season to taste with salt and pepper.

5. To serve, divide fries, salsa and chicken equally between plates.

TIP Make this tasty, spicy Jamaican jerk paste up in bulk and store it in the fridge with a very thin layer of oil on top (it will keep for a few weeks) or freeze it. You can use chicken thighs instead of breast if you prefer — just cook for 10-15 minutes only.

SERVES: 4
PREP TIME: 15 MINUTES
COOK TIME: 20-30 MINUTES

JERK CHICKEN
chicken breast 600g boneless, skinless
Jamaican jerk paste (store-bought or see page 276) 2-3 tablespoons
honey 1 teaspoon
salt

ALLSPICE FRIES
orange kumara or **sweet potato** 600g skin on, scrubbed, cut into 1-2cm-thick wedges
olive oil 1 tablespoon
ground allspice 1 teaspoon
chilli flakes ¼-½ teaspoon (optional)

MANGO SALSA
mango 1 ripe, diced
red onion ½ small, finely diced
spring onion 1, thinly sliced
carrot 1, peeled, shredded or grated
red chilli ½ large, finely chopped (deseed if you want)
black beans ½ x 400g can, drained, rinsed
lemon juice of ½
salt
freshly ground black pepper

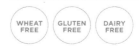

WHEAT FREE • GLUTEN FREE • DAIRY FREE

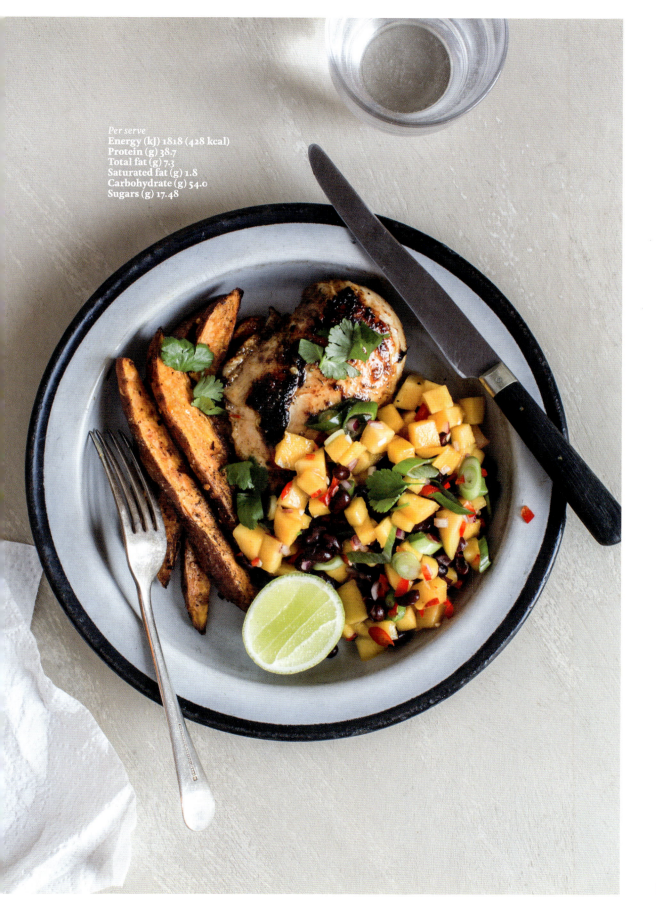

Per serve
Energy (kJ) 1818 (428 kcal)
Protein (g) 38.7
Total fat (g) 7.3
Saturated fat (g) 1.8
Carbohydrate (g) 54.0
Sugars (g) 17.48

TANDOORI ROAST CHICKEN + VEGETABLES WITH RAITA

Everyone will love this quick, tasty Indian-inspired meal. The roasted caramelised vegetables are a delicious accompaniment to the tandoori chicken, and more nutritious than rice.

1. Preheat oven to 200ºC. Line a large oven tray with baking paper. Combine chicken, tandoori paste and olive oil in a bowl and set aside to marinate for at least 15 minutes at room temperature while you prepare the vegetables.

2. Toss carrots, parsnips and red onion with olive oil, honey, cumin and coriander in prepared oven tray. Season well with salt and pepper and roast for 20–25 minutes until soft and starting to caramelise.

3. Season chicken with salt. Heat a drizzle of oil in a large frying pan on medium-high heat and brown chicken for 2–3 minutes, then transfer to oven tray with the vegetables and roast together for a further 10 minutes or until chicken is cooked through.

4. Mix raita ingredients together, seasoning to taste with lemon juice and a little salt.

5. To serve, divide roast vegetables and chicken between plates, spoon over any juices from the oven tray and serve raita on the side.

TIP If you have time, marinate the chicken overnight.

SERVES: 4–6
PREP TIME: 15 MINUTES
COOK TIME: 35 MINUTES

ROAST CHICKEN
chicken thighs 600g, boneless, skinless
tandoori paste (store-bought or see page 279) 2–3 tablespoons
olive oil 2 teaspoons

VEGETABLES
carrots 3 large (about 450g), peeled, cut into 1cm-thick batons
parsnips 2 (about 350g), peeled, cut into 1cm-thick batons
red onion 1 large, cut into 1cm-thick wedges
olive oil 1 tablespoon
liquid honey 2 teaspoons
cumin seeds 1 teaspoon, roughly crushed
coriander seeds 1 teaspoon, roughly crushed
salt
freshly ground black pepper

RAITA
natural unsweetened yoghurt ½ cup
capsicum 1, finely diced
Lebanese cucumber 1, deseeded, diced
tomatoes 2, diced
mint leaves ¼ cup chopped
coriander ¼ cup chopped
lemon juice of ½

WHEAT FREE · GLUTEN FREE · DAIRY FREE

Dairy-free without yoghurt

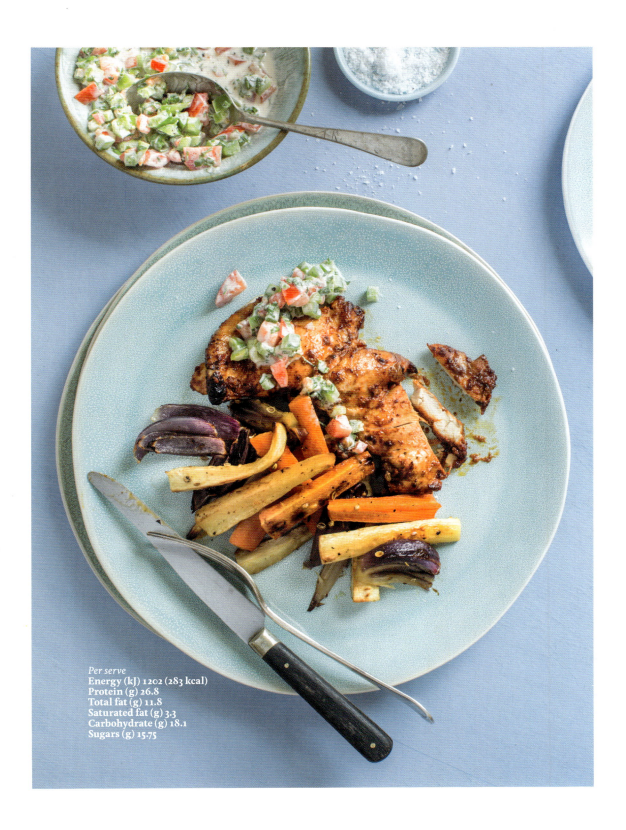

Per serve
Energy (kJ) 1202 (283 kcal)
Protein (g) 26.8
Total fat (g) 11.8
Saturated fat (g) 3.3
Carbohydrate (g) 18.1
Sugars (g) 15.75

DINNER / CHICKEN

177

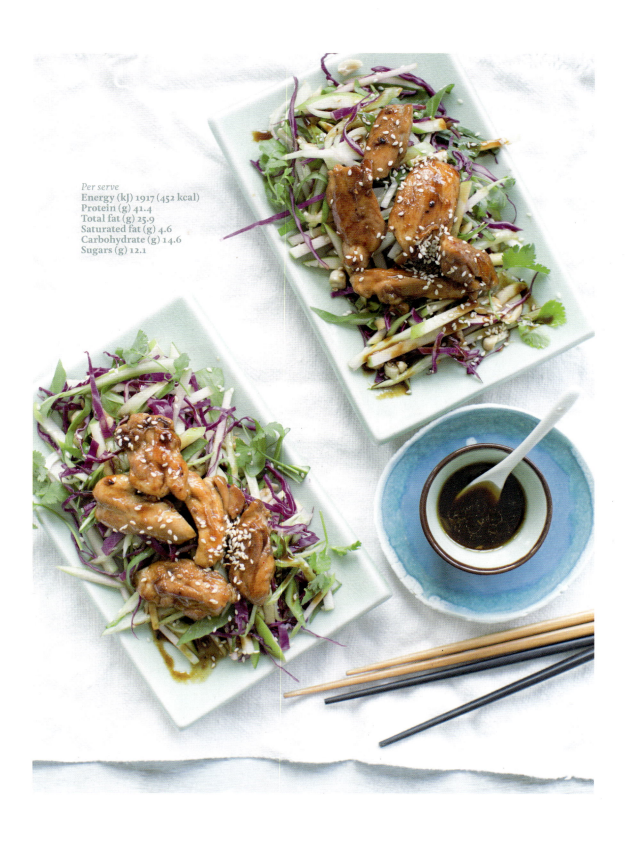

Per serve
Energy (kJ) 1917 (452 kcal)
Protein (g) 41.4
Total fat (g) 25.9
Saturated fat (g) 4.6
Carbohydrate (g) 14.6
Sugars (g) 12.1

TERIYAKI CHICKEN + CRUNCHY BOK CHOY, APPLE + SESAME SLAW

Sweet, sticky teriyaki chicken goes really well with this fresh, crunchy slaw.

1. Mix soy sauce, brown sugar, water and sesame oil together and set aside.

2. Pat chicken dry with paper towels. Heat oil in a wok or large fry pan on high heat. Add chicken to hot pan and stir-fry for about 6-8 minutes or until chicken is browned and just cooked through.

3. Set cooked chicken aside, leaving pan on the heat. Add garlic and ginger to the hot pan and sizzle for 30-60 seconds. Add soy sauce mixture to the hot pan and allow it to bubble away vigorously for about 1 minute, reducing to a thick, sticky glaze. Turn off heat, add back cooked chicken and toss to coat in the glaze.

4. Thinly slice apple (discarding the core), and cut into thin matchsticks. Toss with cabbage, bok choy, peanuts, mint, coriander, and chilli, if using. Mix all dressing ingredients together and toss with salad just before serving.

5. To serve, divide slaw between plates, top with chicken and sauce from the pan, and sprinkle over toasted sesame seeds.

SERVES: 2

PREP TIME: 15 MINUTES

COOK TIME: 10 MINUTES

TERIYAKI CHICKEN

soy sauce 2 tablespoons
brown sugar 2 teaspoons
water 2 tablespoons
sesame oil 1 teaspoon
chicken breast or **thigh meat** 300g boneless skinless, cut into strips
oil 2 teaspoons
garlic 2 cloves, finely chopped
ginger 2cm piece, peeled, grated
toasted sesame seeds 1 teaspoon

APPLE SESAME SLAW

green apple 1 small
purple cabbage ¾-1 cup finely shredded
baby bok choy 2, bottom 2cm of stalk removed, finely sliced
roasted peanuts ¼ cup roughly chopped
mint 2-3 tablespoons chopped
coriander 2-3 tablespoons chopped
red chilli ½ large, finely chopped (optional)

DRESSING

sesame oil 1 teaspoon
soy sauce 2 teaspoons
lime juice 1-2 tablespoons

WHEAT FREE   GLUTEN FREE   DAIRY FREE

Use gluten-free tamari soy sauce

DINNER / CHICKEN

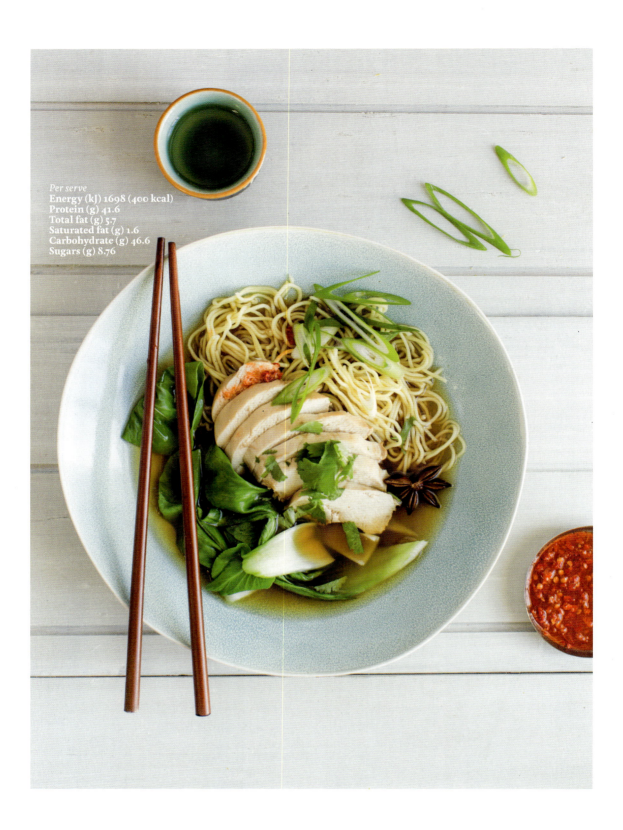

Per serve
Energy (kJ) 1698 (400 kcal)
Protein (g) 41.6
Total fat (g) 5.7
Saturated fat (g) 1.6
Carbohydrate (g) 46.6
Sugars (g) 8.76

ORIENTAL POACHED CHICKEN NOODLE BOWL

This clever method for poaching chicken breast in the stock keeps it moist and cooks it perfectly.

1. Place all stock ingredients in a medium-sized saucepan and stir to combine. Add chicken breasts. There should be enough water to just cover the chicken — if there isn't, top up with a little more water and add a bit more soy sauce. Cover with a tight-fitting lid and bring to a gentle boil. As soon as it comes to the boil, turn off the heat and leave, covered, for 15 minutes. Do not take off the lid during this time (as heat will escape). The residual heat of the stock will cook the chicken through perfectly.

2. Meanwhile, cook noodles and bok choy in a large pot of boiling water for 3-4 minutes until noodles are just cooked. Drain and divide between serving bowls.

3. Remove chicken breast from stock and slice. Strain stock through a sieve, discarding onion and spices, and bring back to a boil. Taste and season with more soy sauce if needed.

4. To serve, ladle hot stock over noodles and vegetables, top with slices of poached chicken, and garnish with spring onion, coriander and chilli.

TIP This recipe can easily be doubled to serve 4 people.

SERVES: 2

PREP TIME: 10 MINUTES

COOK TIME: 20 MINUTES

STOCK + POACHED CHICKEN
ginger 2.5cm piece, peeled, sliced
garlic 2-3 cloves, smashed
red onion 1 small, cut into quarters
whole star anise 4
whole black peppercorns ½ teaspoon
oyster sauce 2 tablespoons
soy sauce 2 tablespoons
rice vinegar or **white or cider vinegar** 2 tablespoons
cold water 2 ½ cups
chicken breasts 300g boneless, skinless

NOODLES + VEGETABLES
dried egg noodles 100g
baby bok choy 6 (350-400g), trimmed

TO SERVE
spring onions 1-2, finely sliced
coriander ¼ cup chopped
chilli paste or sauce 1 tablespoon, or **red chilli** 1 large, finely minced

DAIRY FREE · FREEZES WELL

DINNER / CHICKEN

PAPRIKA CHICKEN WITH APRICOT CAULIFLOWER 'COUSCOUS'

If you love capsicum and paprika, you'll love the flavours in this chicken dish. Cauliflower 'couscous' is so clever — it's entirely made out of cauliflower, so it's gluten-free and bumps up your vege intake, but is light and fluffy.

SERVES: 4
PREP TIME: 10 MINUTES
COOK TIME: 25 MINUTES

PAPRIKA CHICKEN

olive oil 2 tablespoons
red onion 1, thinly sliced
red capsicums 2 large or 3 small, thinly sliced
garlic 2 cloves, chopped
crushed tomatoes 1 x 400g can
chicken thighs 600g boneless skinless, cut into quarters
tomato paste 1½ tablespoons
thyme leaves 1 teaspoon
smoked paprika 1 teaspoon
salt ¾ teaspoon
chilli flakes ½ teaspoon (optional)
lemon juice of 1
salt
freshly ground black pepper

APRICOT CAULIFLOWER 'COUSCOUS'

cauliflower 1 head (750–800g), chopped into florets
dried apricots ½ cup finely chopped
flat-leaf parsley ½ cup finely chopped

1. Heat 1 tablespoon olive oil in a large frying pan over medium heat. Cook red onion and capsicums for about 10 minutes until onion is golden brown and capsicums are slightly charred. If at any time the onions are sticking to the bottom of the pan and burning, just add a tablespoon or two of water or chicken stock. Add garlic and cook for a further 1–2 minutes.

2. Place cooked onion, capsicum and garlic in a food processor with canned tomatoes and blitz together until smooth.

3. Heat remaining olive oil in the pan on high heat. Pat chicken dry with paper towels and season with salt. Brown for about 2 minutes on each side (it does not have to be cooked through). Add puréed tomato capsicum sauce, tomato paste, thyme, smoked paprika, salt and chilli, if using. Simmer uncovered for about 10 minutes until chicken is cooked through and sauce has thickened. Season to taste with lemon juice, salt and pepper.

4. Rinse and dry food processor. To make the 'couscous', blitz cauliflower in the food processor until it resembles the texture of couscous (you may have to do this in batches). Place in a large glass bowl and microwave uncovered for 6–8 minutes. Mix cauliflower 'couscous' with dried apricots and parsley and season to taste with salt and pepper.

5. To serve, divide cauliflower 'couscous' and paprika chicken between plates.

WHEAT FREE · GLUTEN FREE · DAIRY FREE · FREEZES WELL

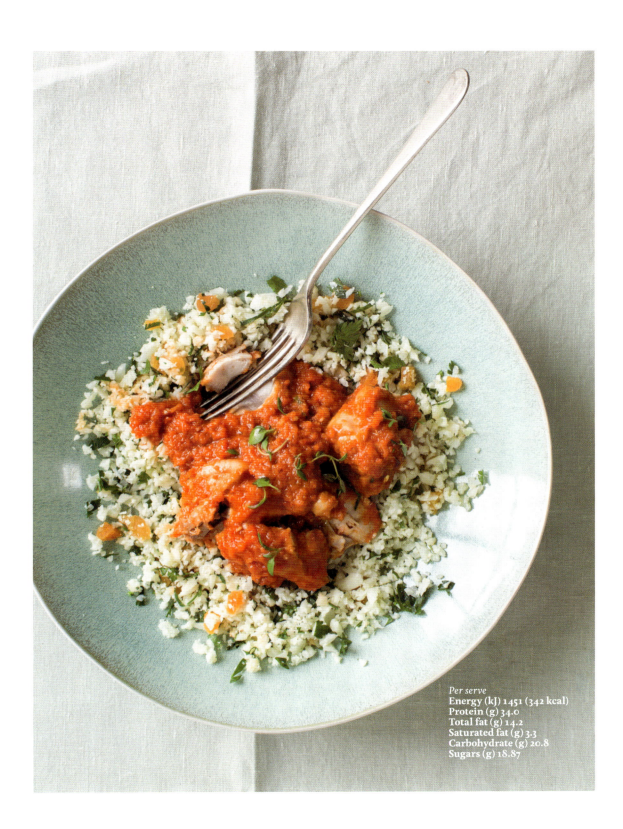

DINNER / CHICKEN

Per serve
Energy (kJ) 1451 (342 kcal)
Protein (g) 34.0
Total fat (g) 14.2
Saturated fat (g) 3.3
Carbohydrate (g) 20.8
Sugars (g) 18.87

CHERMOULA CHICKEN, PUMPKIN + CHERRY TOMATO BAKE WITH CORIANDER + MINT YOGHURT

Chermoula is another great flavour booster to have in your fridge to take a meal from mediocre to amazing. It's full of fresh herbs, lemon, garlic and spices.

SERVES: 4

PREP TIME: 15 MINUTES

COOK TIME: 35-45 MINUTES

CHICKEN, PUMPKIN + TOMATO BAKE

- **chermoula paste** (store-bought or see page 276) ¼ cup
- **chicken thighs** 600g, boneless, skinless
- **olive oil** 1 tablespoon
- **liquid honey** 1 tablespoon
- **butternut** or **pumpkin** 800g skin on, cut into 2cm chunks
- **red onions** 2 medium-sized, cut into 2cm wedges
- **salt**
- **freshly ground black pepper**
- **cherry tomatoes** 1 punnet
- **kale** or **spinach** 3 handfuls, chopped

CORIANDER + MINT YOGHURT

- **natural unsweetened yoghurt** ¾ cup
- **mint leaves** ¼ cup chopped
- **coriander** ¼ cup chopped
- **chermoula paste** 1 tablespoon
- **lemon** juice of ½

Dairy-free without yoghurt

1. Preheat oven to 200°C. Combine chicken with 3 tablespoons of the chermoula paste (reserve remaining 1 tablespoon) and set aside at room temperature to marinate.

2. Toss butternut or pumpkin and red onions together with the honey and olive oil in a large roasting tray lined with baking paper. Season well with salt and pepper and roast for 35-45 minutes or until pumpkin is caramelised. Halfway through cooking time, add whole cherry tomatoes and gently toss through.

3. Heat a drizzle of olive oil in a large frying pan over medium-high heat. Season marinated chicken with salt and brown in the pan (on both sides) for 3-4 minutes. Add to oven tray, on top of roasting pumpkin, to finish cooking for a further 10 minutes or until cooked all the way through.

4. Once chicken is cooked, remove and set aside. Gently toss kale or spinach with roast pumpkin and tomatoes and return to oven for a further 2-3 minutes until wilted.

5. Mix yoghurt with mint, coriander, remaining chermoula paste and lemon juice.

6. To serve, divide vegetables and chicken between plates. Spoon over any juices from the pan and roasting tray, and dollop over coriander mint yoghurt.

TIP You can make chermoula in bulk and store it in the fridge with a very thin layer of oil on top (it will keep for up to a week) or freeze it. It goes well with all sorts of meat and vegetables.

Per serve
Energy (kJ) 1480 (349 kcal)
Protein (g) 33.5
Total fat (g) 13.0
Saturated fat (g) 4.4
Sugars (g) 19.0

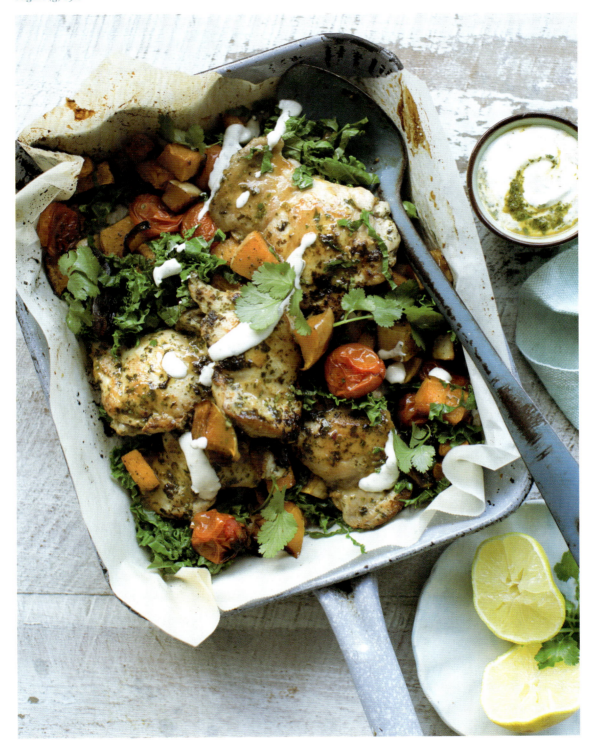

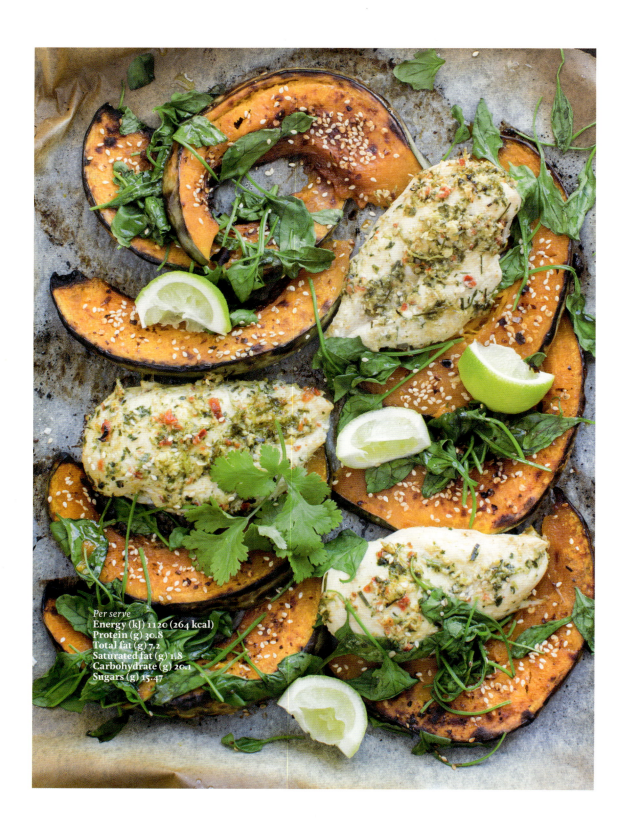

THAI ROAST CHICKEN, PUMPKIN + SPINACH BAKE

Once you've made the spicy, zesty Thai marinade this one-tray meal is a breeze to prepare. I like to leave the skin of the pumpkin on — when roasted it's very tender and there's lots of fibre in it. Make sure the pumpkin is caramelised — it improves the flavour a lot.

1. Preheat oven to 220°C. Line an oven tray with baking paper. Mix all Thai marinade ingredients together, or bash together in a mortar and pestle, until a chunky paste forms.

2. Coat chicken breasts in Thai marinade and set aside to marinate at room temperature. (If you have time, marinate for a few hours or overnight. Toss pumpkin wedges with olive oil and sweet chilli on prepared oven tray and season with salt and pepper. Sprinkle over sesame seeds and chilli flakes, if using. Spread out in a single layer and roast for about 20 minutes or until soft and starting to caramelise. Turn pumpkin over.

3. Place chicken breasts on tray with pumpkin, season with salt and return the tray to the oven to roast for a further 15-20 minutes or until chicken is cooked through and pumpkin is well caramelised. Remove chicken from oven and set aside to rest for 5-10 minutes.

4. Scatter lightly washed baby spinach on top of pumpkin and return tray to the oven for a further 2-3 minutes until the spinach is just wilted.

5. To serve, divide pumpkin and spinach between plates. Slice chicken breasts and place on top. Spoon over any resting juices from the chicken and oven tray. Squeeze over a wedge of lime just before eating.

TIP It is much easier to cut your pumpkin if you pre-cook it a little bit. To do this, I prick the pumpkin skin several times, then microwave it whole for 5-10 minutes on high — this softens the skin and makes it much easier to cut.

SERVES: 4

PREP TIME: 15 MINUTES

COOK TIME: 50 MINUTES

THAI MARINADE

coriander ¼ cup chopped (including stalks)
garlic 1 clove, minced
ginger 2cm piece, peeled, grated
brown sugar 1 teaspoon
red chilli ½, finely chopped (optional)
kaffir lime leaf 2 medium-sized, central stem removed, finely chopped
lime juice of 1

CHICKEN, CARAMELISED PUMPKIN + GREENS

chicken breasts 500g boneless, skinless
pumpkin 800g skin on, cut into 1–2cm-thick wedges
olive oil 1 tablespoon
sweet chilli sauce 1½ tablespoons
salt
freshly ground black pepper
sesame seeds 1½ teaspoons
chilli flakes ½ teaspoon (optional)
baby spinach 4 handfuls
lime 1, cut into wedges

WHEAT FREE GLUTEN FREE DAIRY FREE

DINNER / CHICKEN

THAI CHICKEN MINCE SALAD (LAAB GAI)

I love Thai food, and this dish epitomises the freshness and zestiness that Thai food is all about. Be generous with the fresh herbs — it's what makes the dish. It's great with or without the ground rice powder on top (which is really just there for texture). If you like spicy food, add more chilli.

1. Heat a dry frying pan (with no oil) and toast rice, moving it around the pan frequently, until it is crispy and a deep golden brown. This will take about 5 minutes. Set aside to cool.

2. Heat oil in a large frying pan over medium heat. Sizzle garlic for 30 seconds then add chicken mince, stock and fish sauce. Simmer for 8-10 minutes, breaking up the chicken with a wooden spoon, or until chicken is just cooked through and most of the liquid has evaporated.

3. Mix all dressing ingredients together. Grind toasted rice in a mortar and pestle to a fine powder.

4. Blanch green beans briefly: place in a heatproof bowl, pour over boiling water to cover, wait 20-30 seconds then drain immediately and run under cold water.

5. To serve, toss cooked chicken with beans, spring onion, chilli, carrot, peanuts, lemongrass, kaffir lime leaves, red onion, coriander and mint. Add dressing and rice powder. Arrange cucumber slices around plates and spoon laab gai in the middle.

TIP You might like to serve this with coral lettuce leaves — spoon some mixture in a leaf, wrap and eat.

SERVES: 4

PREP TIME: 15 MINUTES

COOK TIME: 20 MINUTES

jasmine rice ¼ cup
oil 1 teaspoon
garlic 2 cloves, finely minced
chicken mince 500g
chicken stock ½ cup
fish sauce 1 tablespoon

DRESSING

fish sauce 2½ tablespoons
palm or brown sugar 2 teaspoons
limes juice of 2

VEGETABLES + HERBS

green beans 150g, trimmed, finely sliced
spring onions 2, finely chopped
red chilli 1 large, finely chopped
carrot 1, peeled, shredded or grated
roasted peanuts ¼ cup, chopped
lemongrass and **kaffir lime leaves** 1½ tablespoons each very finely chopped
red onion ¼ cup finely diced
coriander ½ cup roughly chopped
mint leaves ½ cup sliced
telegraph cucumber ½, thinly sliced

WHEAT FREE · GLUTEN FREE · DAIRY FREE

Replace butter with oil and omit yoghurt

Per serve
Energy (kJ) 1221 (289 kcal)
Protein (g) 29.7
Total fat (g) 11.7
Saturated fat (g) 2.8
Carbohydrate (g) 16.9
Sugars (g) 5.6

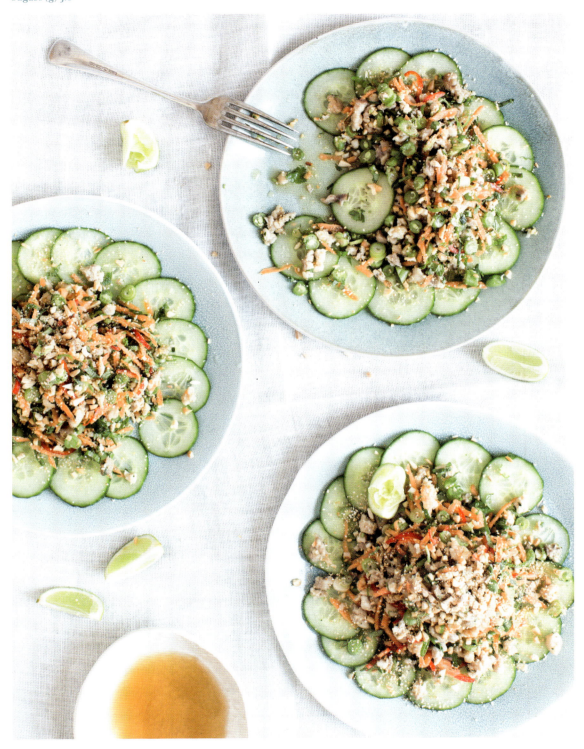

DINNER / CHICKEN

CHICKEN + PINEAPPLE CURRY GARLIC NAAN WRAP

This recipe is inspired by the street food I ate in India. I don't think it's at all traditional, but it's quick and really tasty. I've made a cheat's version of garlic naan that has less than half the calories of standard naan.

1. Preheat oven to 180°C. Heat oil in a wok or large frying pan over medium heat. Cook onion and eggplant for about 8 minutes or until starting to turn golden. If at any time the onion catches on the bottom of the pan, just add 1-2 tablespoons water and stir. Add garlic, ginger, curry powder and curry leaves and continue to cook for a further 1-2 minutes. Add tomatoes, coconut milk and chilli, if using. Simmer for 8-10 minutes until liquid has reduced by half. Stir often to avoid the curry catching and burning.

2. Add chicken and pineapple, cover with a lid, and continue to cook for 5-10 minutes, stirring occasionally, until chicken is cooked through. Stir through spinach until wilted.

3. While the chicken is cooking, make the cheat's garlic naan. Mix melted butter with garlic and turmeric and brush on one side of Lebanese flatbreads. Warm in the oven for 3-4 minutes.

4. To serve, spoon some chicken curry onto each wrap, add a spoonful of yoghurt, garnish with coriander, roll up and eat.

TIP Use fresh ripe or canned pineapple. The chicken curry freezes well, so freeze in individual portions for a quick 'heat and eat' meal. All you'll have to do is make the naan in a couple of minutes.

SERVES: 4
PREP TIME: 15 MINUTES
COOK TIME: 30 MINUTES

CHICKEN CURRY FILLING
oil 1 tablespoon
onion 1, finely chopped
eggplant ½, finely diced
garlic 3 cloves, chopped
ginger 1 tablespoon minced
curry powder 1 tablespoon
curry leaves 1-2 sprigs (about 20 leaves)
crushed tomatoes 1 x 400g can
lite coconut milk ½ x 400g can
red chilli 1, chopped (optional)
chicken breast or thigh 400g boneless, skinless, sliced
pineapple chunks ¾ cup, drained, roughly chopped
spinach 5 cups, washed, chopped

CHEAT'S GARLIC NAAN
butter 2 tablespoons, melted
garlic 2 cloves, minced
ground turmeric ½ teaspoon
Lebanese flatbreads 4 medium-sized

татуSERVE
natural unsweetened yoghurt ½ cup
coriander ½ cup chopped

Replace butter with oil and omit yoghurt

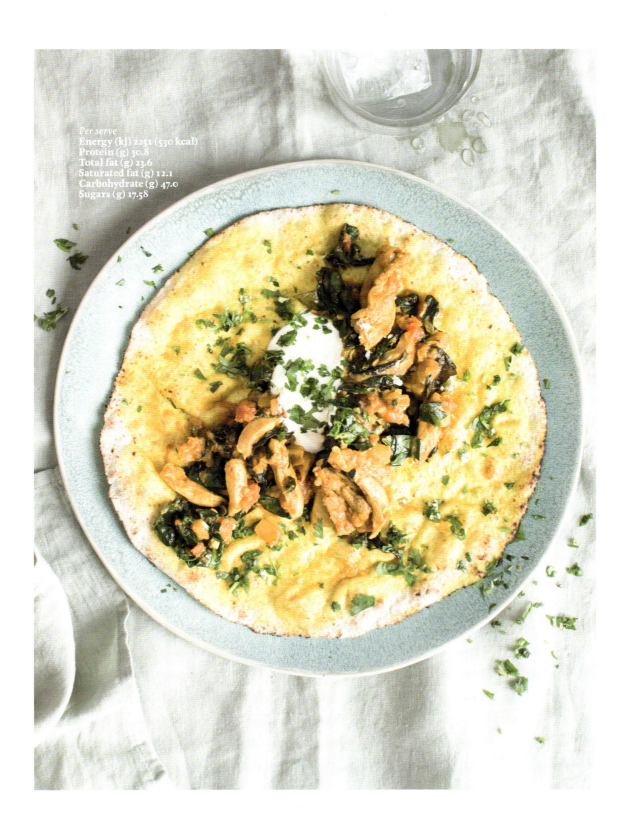

Per serve
Energy (kJ) 2251 (530 kcal)
Protein (g) 30.8
Total fat (g) 23.6
Saturated fat (g) 12.1
Carbohydrate (g) 47.0
Sugars (g) 17.58

DINNER / CHICKEN

191

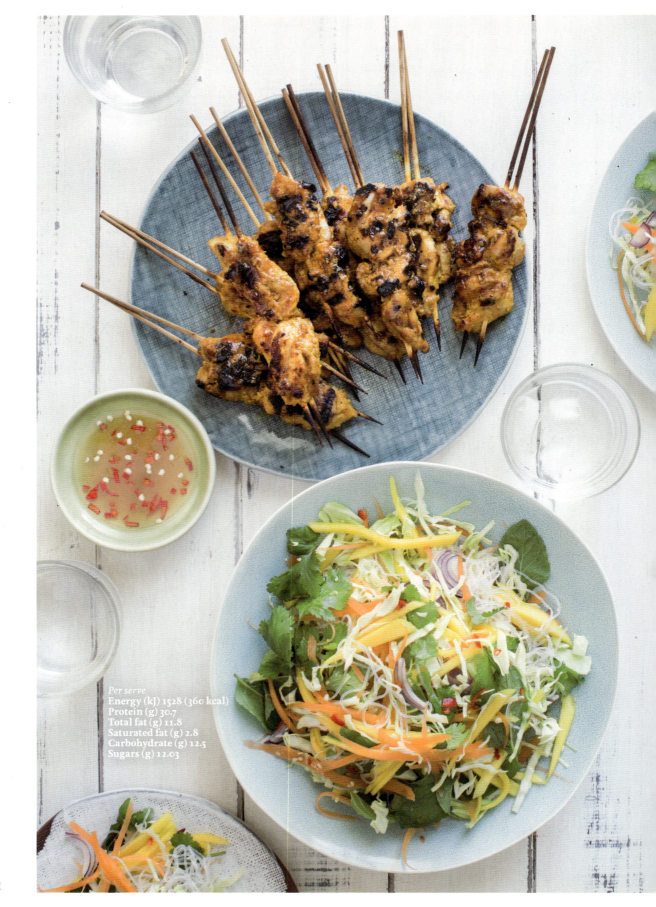

Per serve
Energy (kJ) 1528 (360 kcal)
Protein (g) 30.7
Total fat (g) 11.8
Saturated fat (g) 2.8
Carbohydrate (g) 12.5
Sugars (g) 12.03

LEMONGRASS CHICKEN SKEWERS WITH MANGO SALAD

This is another light, fresh, healthy dish that takes me back to the busy street food alleys in Vietnam. These chicken skewers are great to cook on the barbecue (a little char on them is great), but they can also be cooked in a frying pan or even grilled in the oven.

1. Marinate chicken in the lemongrass paste for 15 minutes at room temperature. (If you have time, marinate for a few hours or overnight in the fridge.)

2. While the chicken is marinating, place vermicelli noodles in a saucepan or a bowl and pour over boiling water to cover. Stir with a fork and leave to stand for 5–10 minutes until noodles are soft. Drain and rinse under cold water to prevent noodles sticking together. Use scissors to snip noodles into shorter lengths.

3. Preheat a barbecue grill or heat a large frying pan over medium-high heat. When ready to cook, thread marinated chicken onto bamboo skewers. Drizzle oil on a plate and lightly roll chicken skewers in the oil to coat. Season chicken with salt. Cook skewers for 2–3 minutes each side or until cooked through.

4. Mix dressing ingredients together. Toss dressing with noodles and salad ingredients. Sprinkle over sesame seeds, if using.

5. To serve, divide noodle salad and lemongrass chicken skewers between plates.

TIP You could use green papaya instead of mango if you can access it.

SERVES: 4

PREP TIME: 30 MINUTES

COOK TIME: 10 MINUTES

CHICKEN SKEWERS + NOODLES

chicken thigh or breast meat 600g boneless, skinless, cut into 3cm strips
lemongrass paste (see page 277) 2–3 tablespoons
mung bean vermicelli noodles (glass noodles) 100g
bamboo skewers 8, soaked in water
oil 1 tablespoon
salt

DRESSING

fish sauce 1½ tablespoons
lime juice 2 tablespoons
liquid honey 1 teaspoon
sesame oil 1 teaspoon
red chilli ½–1 large, finely sliced (optional)

GREEN MANGO SALAD

mango 1 green slightly under-ripe, shredded or cut into thin matchsticks
red onion ½, very finely sliced
carrot 1, peeled, shredded or cut into thin matchsticks
cabbage 2 cups finely shredded
mint leaves ½ cup torn
coriander ½ cup roughly chopped
toasted sesame seeds 1 teaspoon (optional)

WHEAT FREE GLUTEN FREE DAIRY FREE

TERIYAKI SALMON SKEWERS WITH SESAME BROCCOLINI

A super-quick, super-healthy meal of two superfoods: salmon and broccoli. The richness of salmon always works well with this home-made teriyaki sauce. Salmon is best cooked medium (not well done), so it just needs to be seared for 1–2 minutes on each side in a very hot pan.

1. Thread salmon and spring onion pieces onto bamboo skewers. Heat oil in a large non-stick frying pan over medium-high heat. Cook skewers for about 1–2 minutes on each side until salmon is just cooked through and light golden, and spring onion is slightly charred. Use a fish slice to gently press down on the skewers to help them make surface contact with the pan and brown more easily. Set cooked salmon skewers aside. Keep pan on the heat.

2. Mix sugar or honey, soy sauce and cornflour mixture together in a small bowl.

3. Turn down to medium heat and add garlic and ginger to the pan. Fry for 1 minute, then add soy sauce mixture. Bring to a boil, stirring constantly, for 1–2 minutes until sauce has thickened. Turn off the heat. Add salmon skewers back to the pan, gently turning them around to lightly coat in the sauce.

4. Heat sesame oil in a wok or another large pan over medium-high heat. Add broccolini and stir-fry briefly for 1–2 minutes, then add chicken stock and cover with a lid. Steam for 3 minutes until broccolini is bright green and just tender. (I like it to retain a bit of crunch.)

5. To serve, divide broccolini and salmon skewers between plates and sprinkle over sesame seeds. Spoon over any teriyaki sauce left in the pan.

TIP You can use broccoli or any other greens like kale, bok choy or other Asian greens instead of broccolini.

SERVES: 4
PREP TIME: 15 MINUTES
COOK TIME: 10 MINUTES

SALMON SKEWERS
salmon fillet 600g skinless, boneless, cut into 3cm pieces
spring onions 4, cut into 3cm lengths
bamboo skewers 8, soaked in water
peanut or sunflower oil 1 teaspoon

TERIYAKI SAUCE
garlic 2 cloves, minced
ginger 1 tablespoon minced
brown sugar or **liquid honey** 1½ tablespoons
soy sauce 3 tablespoons
cornflour 2 teaspoons mixed with **water** ¼ cup

SESAME BROCCOLINI
sesame oil 2 teaspoons
broccolini 2 bunches (about 400g), ends trimmed, halved
chicken stock ⅓ cup
toasted sesame seeds 2 teaspoons

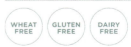

Use gluten-free tamari soy sauce

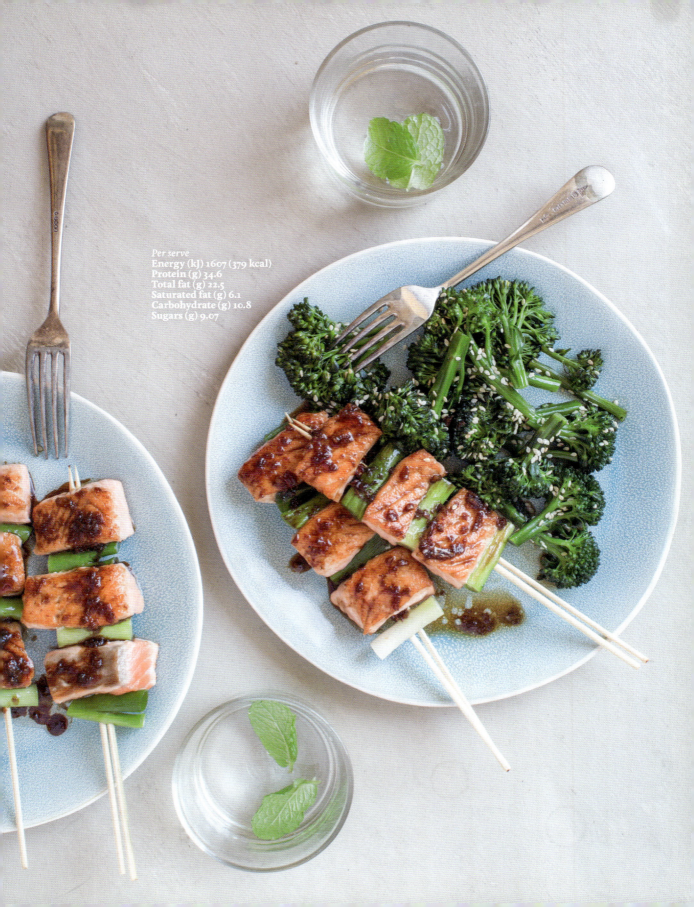

Per serve
Energy (kJ) 1607 (379 kcal)
Protein (g) 34.6
Total fat (g) 22.5
Saturated fat (g) 6.1
Carbohydrate (g) 10.8
Sugars (g) 9.07

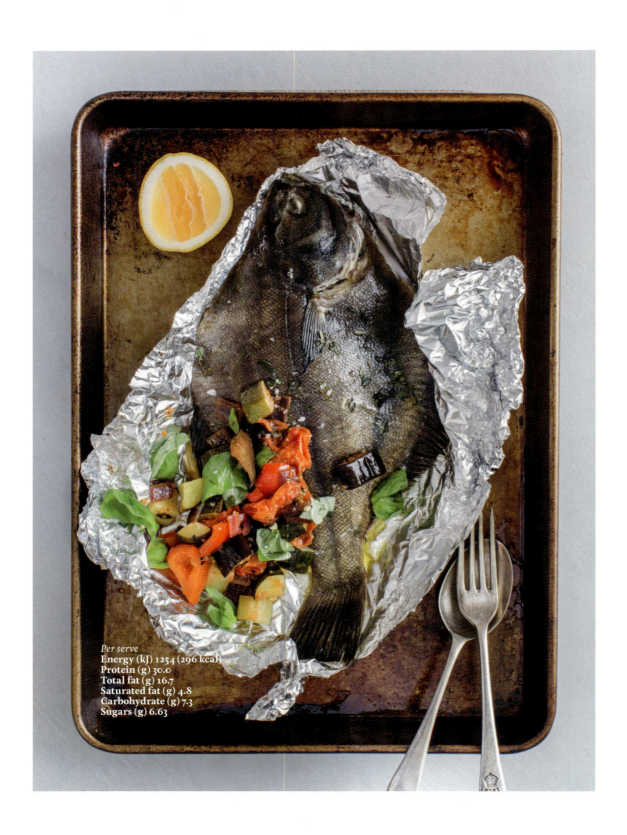

WHOLE FLOUNDER WITH RATATOUILLE

I love having a whole flounder to myself. They're an underrated fish with a lovely delicate, soft white flesh. Delicious served with this colourful summer vegetable ratatouille. If you prefer, use white fish fillets instead (just bake for 7–10 minutes only).

1. Preheat oven to 200°C. Place each flounder on a large rectangle of tinfoil. Squeeze over lemon juice, dot with butter, and sprinkle over thyme leaves. Fold tinfoil up to completely encase the fish and form tight parcels. Bake for 15 minutes until fish is just cooked.

2. Heat 1 tablespoon olive oil in a large frying pan over medium heat. Cook eggplant for about 5 minutes or until soft and cooked through. Add a few tablespoons of chicken stock if it looks like it's drying out at any time. Set aside.

3. Add remaining olive oil and cook red onion for 2–3 minutes until soft, then add garlic and cook for 1 minute further. Add cooked eggplant, tomatoes, capsicum, courgettes, stock or water, vinegar and thyme. Cover and cook over low heat for 10 minutes. Season to taste with salt and pepper and toss with basil leaves and extra virgin olive oil.

4. To serve, place a whole flounder on each plate and top with ratatouille.

SERVES: 4

PREP TIME: 15 MINUTES

COOK TIME: 20 MINUTES

FLOUNDER

whole flounder 4 medium-sized
lemon juice of 1
butter 20g (4 teaspoons), cut into small cubes
thyme leaves 1 teaspoon chopped

RATATOUILLE

olive oil 2 tablespoons
eggplant 1 medium, cut into 2cm dice
red onion ½, cut into 2cm dice
garlic 2 cloves, minced
cherry tomatoes 1 punnet
red capsicum 1, cut into 2cm dice
courgettes 2, cut into 2cm dice
chicken stock or **water** 2–3 tablespoons
white wine vinegar 2 teaspoons
thyme leaves 1–2 teaspoons
salt
freshly ground black pepper
basil leaves 1 handful, torn
extra virgin olive oil 1 tablespoon

WHEAT FREE — GLUTEN FREE

CHERMOULA GRILLED FISH WITH WARM CHICKPEA SALAD

This is one hell of a tasty and healthy meal. You can use any type of fish you like, just adjust the cooking time depending on the thickness and density of your fish fillets. Less dense-fleshed fish (like tarakihi or snapper) may only need a few minutes in the oven.

1. Preheat oven to 200°C. Combine cherry tomatoes, red onion, capsicum, garlic and olive oil in a large roasting dish and season well with salt and pepper. Roast until vegetables are soft, about 20 minutes.

2. Remove from oven and gently toss through chickpeas, olives, capers, lemon zest and chilli flakes, if using. Set aside.

3. Season fish fillets with salt on both sides. Heat olive oil in a frying pan over medium-high heat. Pan-fry fish on one side until just browned, 1–2 minutes. Flip over and transfer to the roasting dish, placing it on top of the chickpeas and vegetables. Spread chermoula paste on fish and return the whole dish to the oven to cook for a further 5–7 minutes, or until fish is just cooked through. Set cooked fish aside and toss herbs through the warm chickpea salad.

4. To serve, divide chickpea salad evenly between plates. Top with a fish fillet and serve with a wedge of lemon to squeeze over just before eating.

SERVES: 4

PREP TIME: 10 MINUTES

COOK TIME: 25 MINUTES

WARM CHICKPEA SALAD

cherry tomatoes 1 punnet

red onion 1 large or 2 medium-sized, cut into wedges

red or yellow capsicum 2, sliced

garlic 3 cloves, minced

olive oil 1½ tablespoons

salt

freshly ground black pepper

chickpeas 2 × 400g cans, drained, rinsed

Kalamata olives ¼ cup, pitted, roughly chopped

capers 2 tablespoons roughly chopped

lemon zest of 1

chilli flakes ½–1 teaspoon (optional)

flat-leaf parsley ½ cup chopped

coriander ½ cup chopped

CHERMOULA FISH

firm white fish fillets (e.g. kingfish, hapuku) 600g

olive oil 2 teaspoons

chermoula paste (store-bought or see page 276) 6 tablespoons

lemon 1, cut into wedges to serve

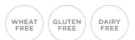

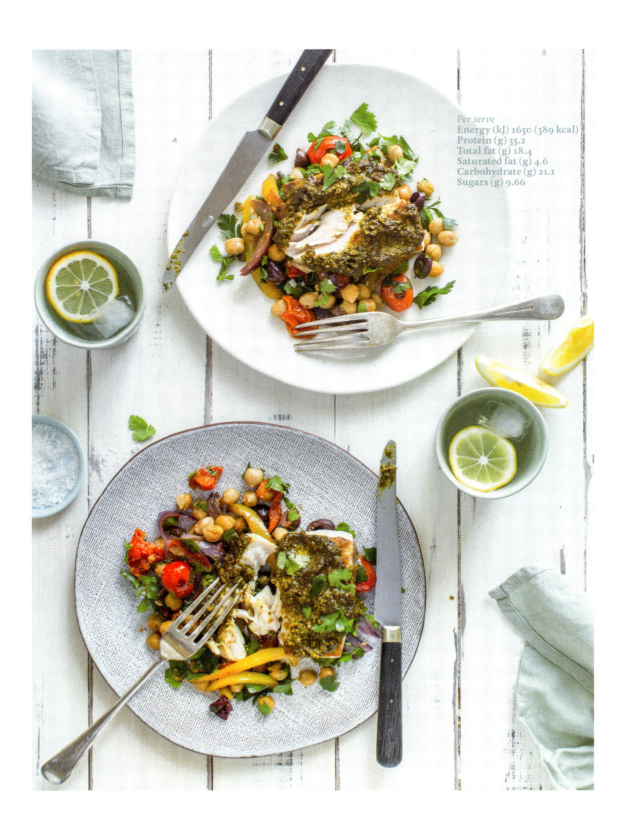

Per serve
Energy (kJ) 1650 (389 kcal)
Protein (g) 35.2
Total fat (g) 18.4
Saturated fat (g) 4.6
Carbohydrate (g) 21.1
Sugars (g) 9.66

DINNER / FISH + SEAFOOD

CREAMY SMOKED SALMON, LEEK + BROCCOLI PASTA

This quick pasta meal is yummy, relaxed comfort food perfect for a Friday night in. Treat yourself and have it with a glass of Chardonnay to make it extra special!

1. Cook pasta in boiling salted water until al dente (just cooked), 10-12 minutes.

2. While the pasta is cooking, melt butter in a large frying pan over medium heat. Cook leek for 3-4 minutes until soft. Add garlic and cook for 1 minute further. Stir in lemon zest and juice, crème fraîche or sour cream, chicken stock and capers. Simmer for a few minutes until sauce has slightly thickened. Turn off the heat.

3. Drop broccoli into the saucepan to briefly cook with the pasta for 1 minute. Drain pasta and broccoli and add to the sauce, along with salmon. Toss pasta and broccoli with sauce and salmon and season to taste with salt and pepper.

4. To serve, divide pasta and sauce between serving bowls and garnish with basil or parsley. Squeeze over a little more lemon juice.

SERVES: 4

PREP TIME: 10 MINUTES

COOK TIME: 10 MINUTES

dried linguine, spaghetti or **fettuccine** 280g
butter 1 tablespoon
leek 1½ cups finely sliced
garlic 2 cloves, minced
lemon finely grated zest and juice of 1
crème fraîche or **sour cream** 150g
chicken stock ¾ cup
capers 1 tablespoon, chopped
broccoli 2 cups chopped florets
hot smoked salmon 200g, flaked
salt
freshly ground black pepper
basil leaves or **flat-leaf parsley** ¼ cup chopped
lemon 1 to serve

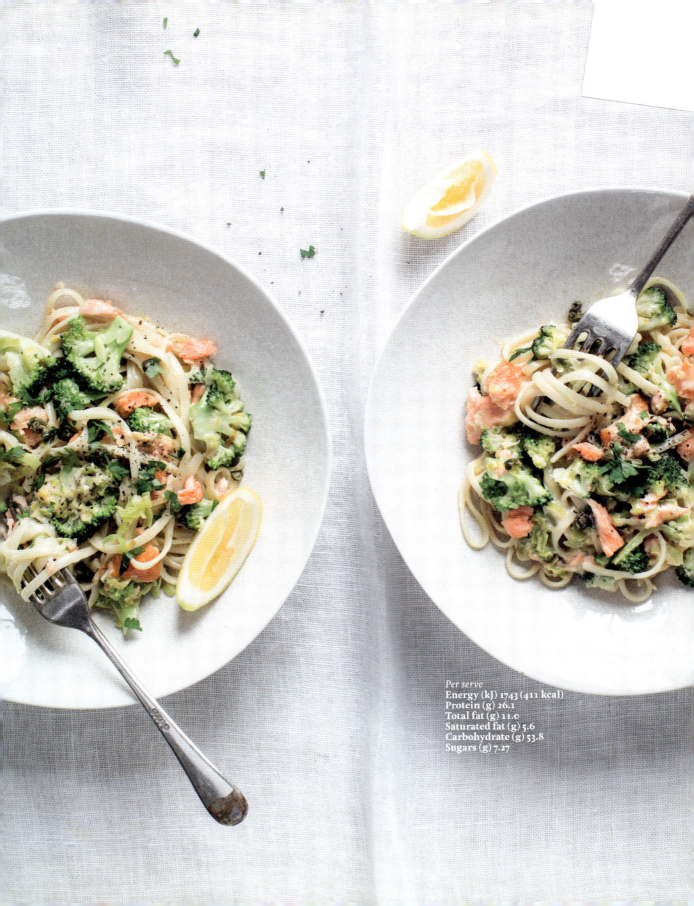

Per serve
Energy (kJ) 1743 (411 kcal)
Protein (g) 26.1
Total fat (g) 11.0
Saturated fat (g) 5.6
Carbohydrate (g) 53.8
Sugars (g) 7.27

COCONUT, CHILLI + CORIANDER STEAMED FISH WITH SOBA NOODLES

This dish is a fusion of Asian and Pacific flavours. The fish is steamed in its own juices and a delicious coconut, soy and chilli sauce.

1. Preheat oven to 220°C. Lay 4 large rectangles of tinfoil about 40cm long on the bench and place a fish fillet in the centre of each. Mix garlic, ginger, chilli, if using, soy sauce, sesame oil and coconut cream together. Spoon mixture over each fish fillet, dividing equally. Wrap up tinfoil to encase fish. Place parcels on an oven tray and bake for about 8 minutes or until fish is just cooked through.

2. Add noodles to a saucepan of boiling water and cook until al dente (just cooked), 4-5 minutes. Do not overcook. Drain and rinse under cold water to prevent noodles sticking together.

3. Heat oil in a wok or large frying pan. Stir-fry garlic and vegetables for 2-3 minutes. Add drained noodles to vegetables. Toss everything together to heat through.

4. To serve, divide noodles and vegetables between plates. Unwrap fish parcels and place a fish fillet on top. Pour over juices from the tinfoil parcels and garnish with coriander.

SERVES: 4

PREP TIME: 10 MINUTES

COOK TIME: 10 MINUTES

STEAMED FISH

white fish (e.g. tarakihi, snapper, gurnard, blue cod) 4 x 150g fillets
garlic 1 large clove, finely chopped
ginger 2.5cm piece, peeled, cut into thin matchsticks
red chilli ½-1 large, finely chopped (optional)
soy sauce 2 tablespoons
sesame oil 2 teaspoons
coconut cream ¼ cup

NOODLES + VEGETABLES

dried soba or thin rice stick noodles 250g
oil 1 tablespoon
garlic 1 clove, chopped
Chinese vegetables (e.g. bok choy, gai lan, choy sum, broccolini) 2 large bunches, trimmed, chopped
coriander ¼ cup chopped

Use gluten-free rice stick noodles and tamari soy sauce

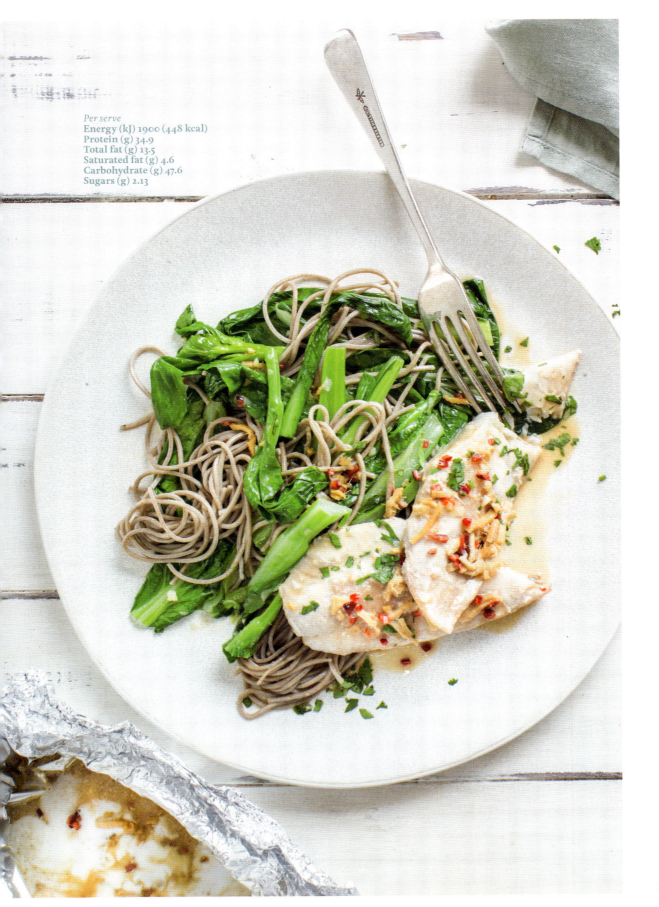

Per serve
Energy (kJ) 1900 (448 kcal)
Protein (g) 34.9
Total fat (g) 13.5
Saturated fat (g) 4.6
Carbohydrate (g) 47.6
Sugars (g) 2.13

DINNER / FISH + SEAFOOD

203

MEDITERRANEAN BAKED FISH WITH HERBY SPINACH + POTATOES

Another really quick, no-fuss, simple meal that has loads of flavour from the sundried tomato, olive and pinenut topping.

1. Preheat oven to 200°C. Line an oven tray with baking paper. Cut any larger potatoes in half or into quarters so they are all roughly the same size. Cook potatoes in a pot of boiling salted water until tender, 10-12 minutes.

2. Place olives, sundried tomatoes, shallot, parsley, lemon zest and pinenuts in a pile on your chopping board. Use a large sharp knife to chop and combine everything together for the topping — doing it this way gives a nice rustic texture and helps combine the flavours perfectly.

3. Place fish fillets on prepared tray and season with salt and pepper. Spoon topping on fish and gently press down with the back of a spoon so the topping sticks. Drizzle with a little olive oil and bake for 8-10 minutes (depending on the thickness of your fish) until the fish is just cooked through.

4. Meanwhile, drain potatoes and return back to the pan with extra virgin olive oil. Gently crush potatoes with a fork, then fold through remaining ingredients. Season to taste with salt and pepper.

5. To serve, divide fish and herby spinach and potatoes between plates. Serve with a wedge of lemon to squeeze over just before eating.

TIP Use kumara, sweet potato or pumpkin instead of potato if you prefer.

SERVES: 4

PREP TIME: 10 MINUTES

COOK TIME: 15 MINUTES

HERBY SPINACH + POTATOES
baby potatoes 400g
extra virgin olive oil 1½ tablespoons
baby spinach 3 handfuls
spring onion 1, finely sliced
mixed fresh herbs (e.g. chives, flat-leaf parsley and a little dill) ½ cup chopped
capers 1 tablespoon, chopped

BAKED FISH
green olives ¼ cup, pitted
sundried tomatoes ¼ cup roughly chopped
shallot 1 small, chopped
flat-leaf parsley ⅓ cup roughly chopped
lemon zest of 1
pinenuts 2 tablespoons
white fish fillets (e.g. tarakihi, snapper, gurnard, hoki) 600g skinless
salt
freshly ground black pepper

TO SERVE
lemon 1, cut into wedges to serve

WHEAT FREE   GLUTEN FREE   DAIRY FREE

Per serve
Energy (kJ) 1232 (290 kcal)
Protein (g) 27.9
Total fat (g) 11.0
Saturated fat (g) 1.8
Carbohydrate (g) 21.3
Sugars (g) 5.20

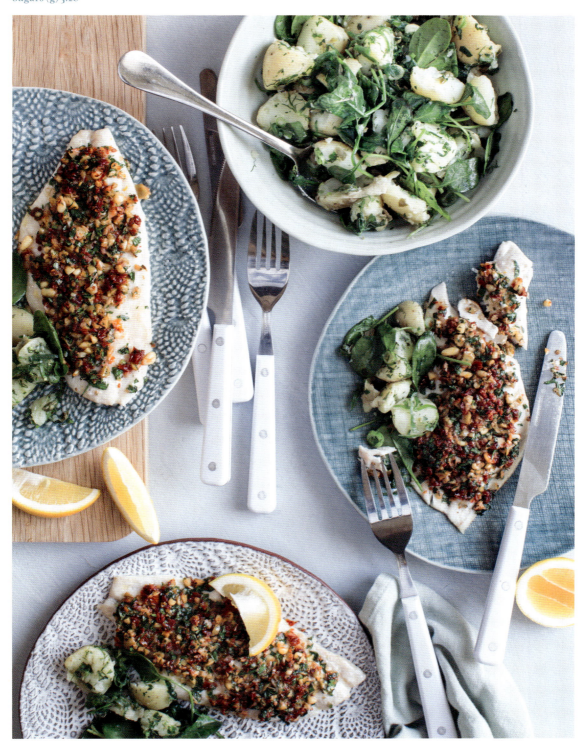

DINNER / FISH + SEAFOOD

205

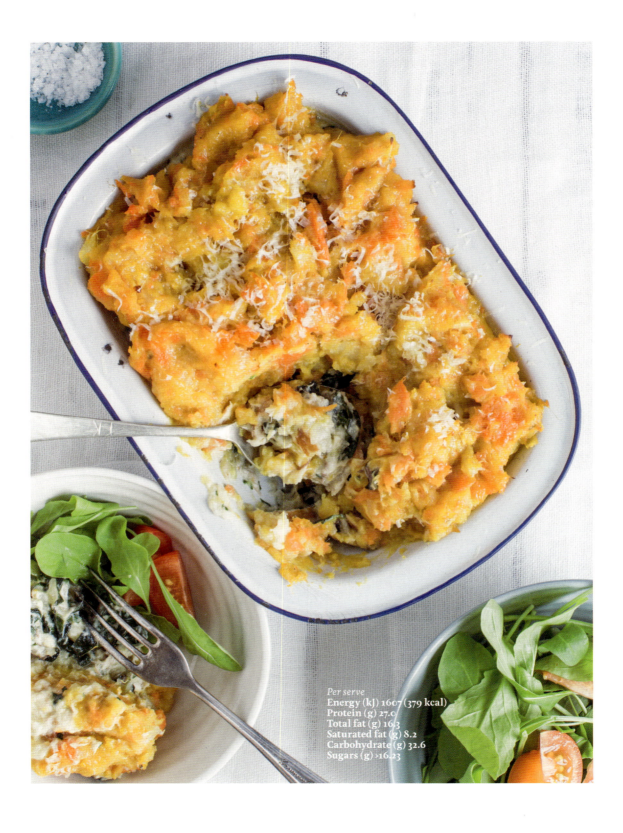

Per serve
Energy (kJ) 1607 (379 kcal)
Protein (g) 27.0
Total fat (g) 16.3
Saturated fat (g) 8.2
Carbohydrate (g) 32.6
Sugars (g) >16.23

ROOT VEG TOPPED SMOKED FISH + SILVERBEET PIE

To make this dish more interesting and nutritious, I've replaced the standard potato mash topping with a mash of parsnip, carrots and kumara, and folded silverbeet or spinach through the creamy smoked fish filling.

1. Preheat oven to 200°C. Cook root vegetables in boiling salted water until soft, about 12 minutes. Drain well and return to pot. Place back over low heat for a few minutes to evaporate excess moisture. Mash with butter and milk. Season to taste with salt and pepper.

2. Heat oil in a frying pan over medium heat and sauté onion and leek until soft, about 4 minutes. Add butter and when melted add flour and stir continuously with a wooden spoon for 1 minute to cook the flour. Add milk gradually, stirring continuously to avoid any lumps forming. Simmer, stirring continuously, until thickened, 3-4 minutes. Mix in mustard, parmesan, capers (if using) and parsley.

3. Steam damp silverbeet or spinach in the microwave until just wilted, about 2 minutes. Squeeze out excess water by wringing in a tea towel.

4. Fold smoked fish and silverbeet into cheese sauce. Season to taste with salt and pepper — you may not need much salt as smoked fish can be quite salty. Spoon into a baking dish and top with mashed root vegetables and a sprinkle of parmesan. Cook in the oven for 10-15 minutes until the top is golden.

5. To serve, spoon some fish pie onto each plate. Serve with salad on the side.

TIP This freezes well so would make a great 'heat and eat' dinner.

SERVES: 5

PREP TIME: 15 MINUTES

COOK TIME: 25 MINUTES

VEGETABLE TOPPING

parsnips 250g (about 1 medium-sized), peeled, chopped
carrots 250g (about 2 medium-sized), peeled, chopped
kumara, sweet potato or **potato** 300g, peeled, chopped
butter 2 tablespoons
milk 1-2 tablespoons
salt
freshly ground black pepper

ONION + CHEESE SAUCE

olive oil 1 tablespoon
onion 1, diced
leek 1 medium, chopped
butter 2 tablespoons
plain flour 2 tablespoons
milk 2 cups
Dijon mustard 1 teaspoon
parmesan 30g (¾ cup), grated
capers 1½ tablespoons, chopped
flat-leaf parsley ¼ cup chopped

TO ASSEMBLE

silverbeet or **spinach** 3 cups
good-quality smoked fish (e.g. kahawai) 400g, flaked
parmesan ¼ cup grated

TO SERVE

leafy green salad (see page 277)

DINNER / FISH + SEAFOOD

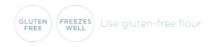
GLUTEN FREE   FREEZES WELL   Use gluten-free flour

207

OVEN-BAKED FISH WITH CAPERS, DILL + PARSLEY, WEDGES + AÏOLI

A deliciously simple fish and chips dinner with the three things that go best with fish: herbs, lemon and capers.

1. Preheat oven to 200°C. Line an oven tray and a baking dish with baking paper. Toss potatoes with olive oil in oven tray and season with salt and pepper. Bake for about 40 minutes until golden and crispy.

2. Place parsley, capers, dill and lemon zest on a chopping board and finely chop everything together, mixing all ingredients well.

3. Place fish fillets in prepared baking dish. Season with salt and pepper. Dot with butter and scatter over herb mixture. Squeeze over lemon juice. Bake for 6-8 minutes or until fish is just cooked through.

4. Mix all aïoli ingredients together.

5. To serve, divide fish and chips between plates and serve with a dollop of aïoli, and salad and tomato on the side.

SERVES: 4

PREP TIME: 15 MINUTES

COOK TIME: 50 MINUTES

WEDGES
Agria potatoes 600g, cut into 1-2cm thick wedges
olive oil 1 tablespoon
salt
freshly ground black pepper

FISH
flat-leaf parsley ½ cup roughly chopped
capers 2-3 teaspoons, chopped
dill 3 tablespoons roughly chopped
lemon zest and juice of 1
white fish fillets (e.g. tarakihi, snapper, gurnard, hoki) 600g skinless
butter 1½ tablespoons, chopped

AÏOLI
good-quality mayonnaise 2 tablespoons
natural unsweetened thick Greek yoghurt 2 tablespoons
garlic 1 small clove, minced
smoked paprika ¼ teaspoon
cayenne pepper pinch of (optional)

TO SERVE
leafy green salad (see page 277) 4 servings
tomatoes 2 sliced

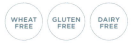

Dairy-free without yoghurt + use olive oil instead of butter

Per serve
Energy (kJ) 1709 (403 kcal)
Protein (g) 33.9
Total fat (g) 19.4
Saturated fat (g) 6.6
Carbohydrate (g) 24.7
Sugars (g) 1.94

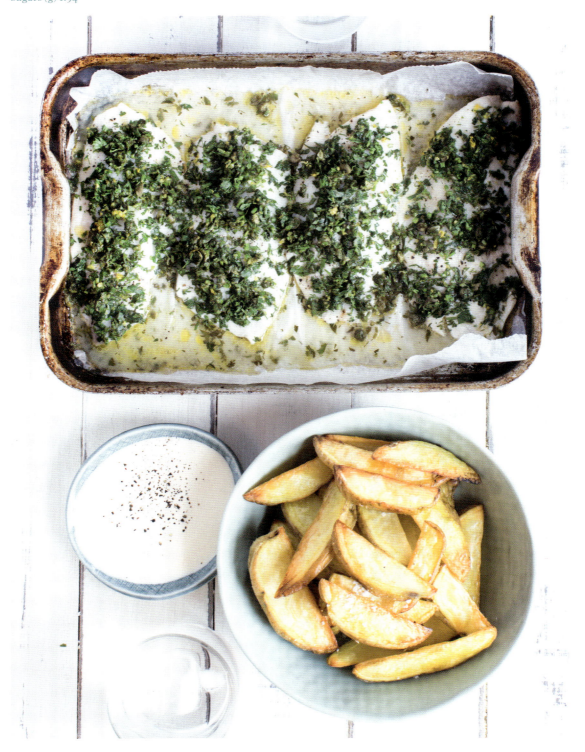

DINNER / FISH + SEAFOOD

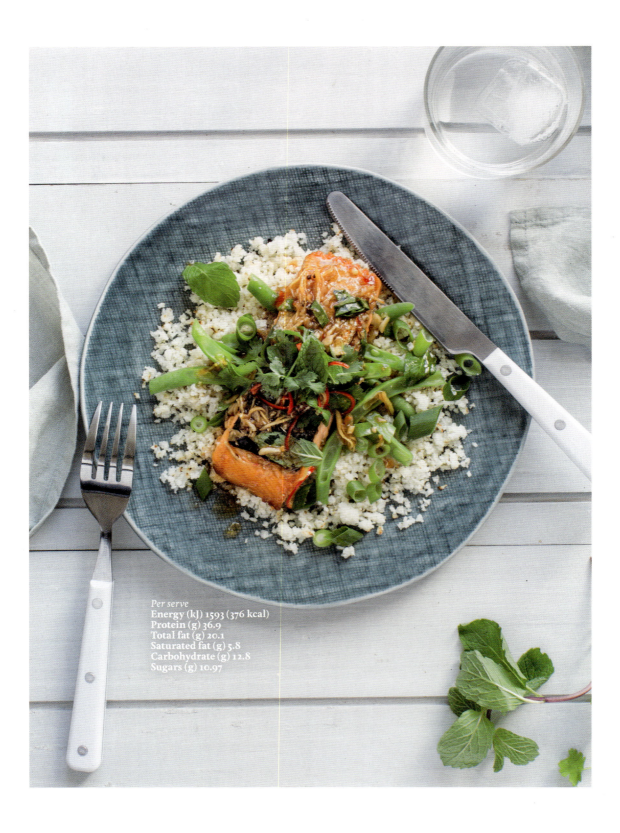

Per serve
Energy (kJ) 1593 (376 kcal)
Protein (g) 36.9
Total fat (g) 20.1
Saturated fat (g) 5.8
Carbohydrate (g) 12.8
Sugars (g) 10.97

STICKY CHILLI SALMON WITH BEANS, ASIAN HERBS + CAULIFLOWER 'RICE'

You'll love this way of doing salmon. The sweet, sticky chilli sauce also goes really well with chicken too if you want to change it up.

1. Place cauliflower in a food processor and blitz to a crumbly texture that resembles breadcrumbs or rice. You may have to do this in a couple of batches to avoid overcrowding the food processor. Place in a large bowl and microwave on high, uncovered, for a few minutes (this lightly steams the cauliflower and evaporates excess moisture to make it fluffy). Season with salt and pepper.

2. Pat salmon dry with paper towels. Heat oil in a large frying pan over medium-high heat. Pan-fry salmon, skin side down, for 3-4 minutes until skin is golden and crispy, then flip over and cook on the other side for a further 2 minutes or until salmon is just cooked through (salmon is best cooked medium, so try not to overcook it). Set salmon aside. Keep pan on the heat.

3. Add ginger and lemongrass to the pan and stir-fry for 1 minute, then add chilli, fish sauce, vinegar, sweet chilli sauce and water. Allow the sauce to bubble for 1-2 minutes until sticky and reduced. Turn off the heat.

4. Briefly cook beans in boiling water for 1-2 minutes until bright green and just tender.

5. To serve, divide hot cauliflower rice, beans and salmon between plates and spoon over sticky chilli sauce. Garnish with plenty of fresh mint and coriander, and a lime wedge to squeeze over just before eating.

SERVES: 4

PREP TIME: 10 MINUTES

COOK TIME: 15 MINUTES

CAULIFLOWER RICE

cauliflower 1 head (750–800g), chopped into florets
salt

SALMON

salmon fillet 600g skin on, cut into 4 portions
oil 1 teaspoon

STICKY CHILLI SAUCE

ginger 3cm piece, peeled, cut into thin matchsticks
lemongrass 1 stalk, tough outer leaves removed, finely chopped
red chilli 1 large, finely sliced (deseed if you want)
fish sauce 3 tablespoons
rice or white wine vinegar 3 tablespoons
sweet chilli sauce 3 tablespoons
water 2 tablespoons

TO SERVE

green beans 400g, trimmed
mint and coriander leaves 1 cup total
lime 1, cut into wedges

WHEAT FREE • GLUTEN FREE • DAIRY FREE

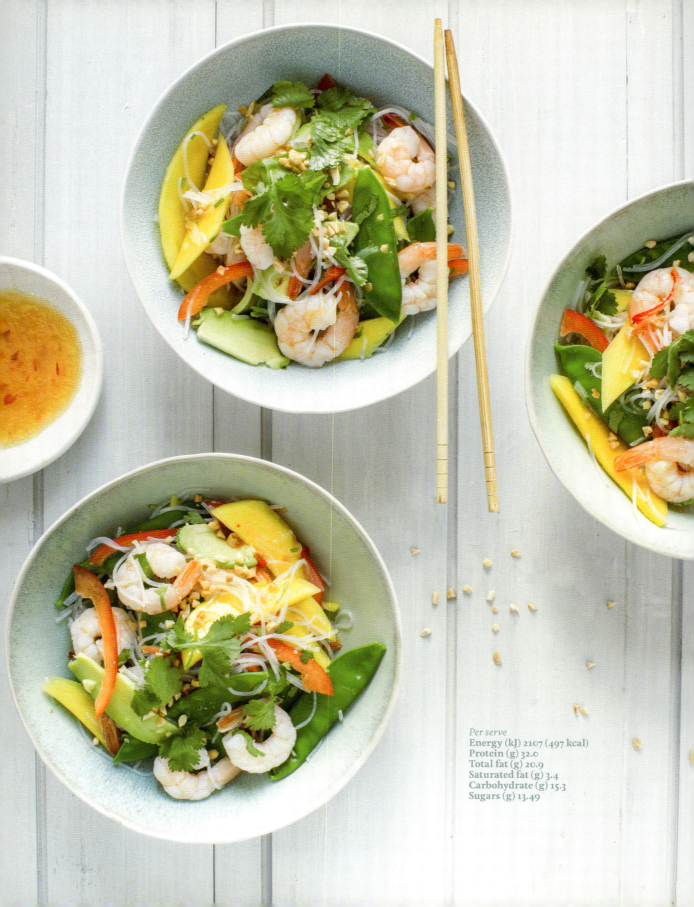

Per serve
Energy (kJ) 2107 (497 kcal)
Protein (g) 32.0
Total fat (g) 20.9
Saturated fat (g) 3.4
Carbohydrate (g) 15.3
Sugars (g) 13.49

PRAWN, AVOCADO + MANGO GLASS NOODLE SALAD

Prawns, mango and avocado are sublime together, especially if you throw in chilli, citrus, basil, coriander and roasted peanuts. Simply delicious. Stir-fried chicken or shredded meat from pre-cooked chicken can be used instead of prawns, too.

1. Place noodles in a pot or heatproof bowl and cover with boiling water. Stir with a fork and leave to stand for about 5 minutes until soft, then drain and run under cold water to prevent noodles sticking together. Use scissors to snip noodles into shorter lengths (which makes them easier to eat).

2. Pat prawns dry with paper towels and season with salt. Heat oil in a wok or large frying pan over high heat. Add prawns and stir-fry for 2–3 minutes until prawns are almost cooked. Add garlic and cook for 1 minute further. Squeeze in lemon juice and turn off the heat.

3. Pour boiling water over snow peas to cover and leave for 1–2 minutes until bright green. Refresh in iced water — this helps them stay crunchy.

4. To serve, toss noodles, prawns, snow peas, avocado, mango, capsicum, chilli, if using, basil and coriander with sweet chilli dressing. Divide between bowls and garnish with peanuts and more fresh herbs.

SERVES: 4

PREP TIME: 15 MINUTES

COOK TIME: 10 MINUTES

dried mung bean vermicelli noodles (glass noodles) 150g
frozen raw prawns 500g, defrosted, shelled with tails left on
salt
oil 1 teaspoon
garlic 2 cloves, minced
lemon juice of 1
snow peas 200g
avocado 1 ripe, sliced
mango 1 slightly under-ripe, thinly sliced
red capsicum 1, thinly sliced
red chilli 1, finely chopped (optional)
basil leaves ½ cup roughly torn + extra for serving
coriander ½ cup chopped + extra for serving
sweet chilli dressing (see page 279) ½ cup
roasted peanuts ¼ cup, roughly chopped

WHEAT FREE · GLUTEN FREE · DAIRY FREE

DINNER / FISH + SEAFOOD

PRAWN LAKSA

I love a good laksa — it's Asian comfort food. Use a store-bought laksa paste (there are lots of good-quality ones available now) to fast-track this meal, or use the recipe on page 277 to make your own — which you can also freeze to use in other meals.

1. Heat oil in a medium-sized saucepan over medium heat. Fry laksa paste along with a few tablespoons coconut milk until very fragrant, 2-3 minutes. Add tomatoes and cook for 1-2 minutes, then add remaining coconut milk and stock and bring to a gentle boil.

2. Meanwhile, place noodles in a bowl and cover with boiling water. Stir with a fork and leave to stand for 5 minutes until soft. Drain and rinse under cold water to help prevent noodles from sticking together. Use scissors to snip in a few places to shorten the strands. Divide noodles between serving bowls.

3. Add prawns and beans to laksa broth and continue to simmer for about 2 minutes until prawns are just cooked through. Season broth to taste with a little salt or soy sauce if needed.

4. To serve, ladle hot laksa broth and contents over noodles in serving bowls. Top with bean sprouts, spring onions, carrot, chilli and coriander. Serve with a wedge of lime to squeeze over just before eating.

TIP Look for a good-quality laksa paste that is free of MSG, such as Asian Home Gourmet.

SERVES: 4
PREP TIME: 15 MINUTES
COOK TIME: 10 MINUTES

oil 1 tablespoon
laksa paste ¼ cup (store-bought or see page 277)
lite coconut milk 1 x 400g can
vine-ripened tomatoes 2-3, chopped or **canned crushed tomatoes** ¾ cup
chicken or fish stock 4 cups
dried mung bean vermicelli noodles (glass noodles) 280g
frozen raw prawns 500g, defrosted, shelled with tails left on
green beans 200g, trimmed, sliced
salt or **soy sauce** to taste

TO SERVE

mung bean sprouts 4 small handfuls
spring onions 2-3, finely sliced
carrot 1 large, peeled, shredded or cut into thin matchsticks
red chilli 1 large, deseeded, finely sliced
coriander ½ cup chopped
lime 1, cut into wedges

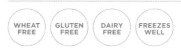

Use salt instead of soy sauce

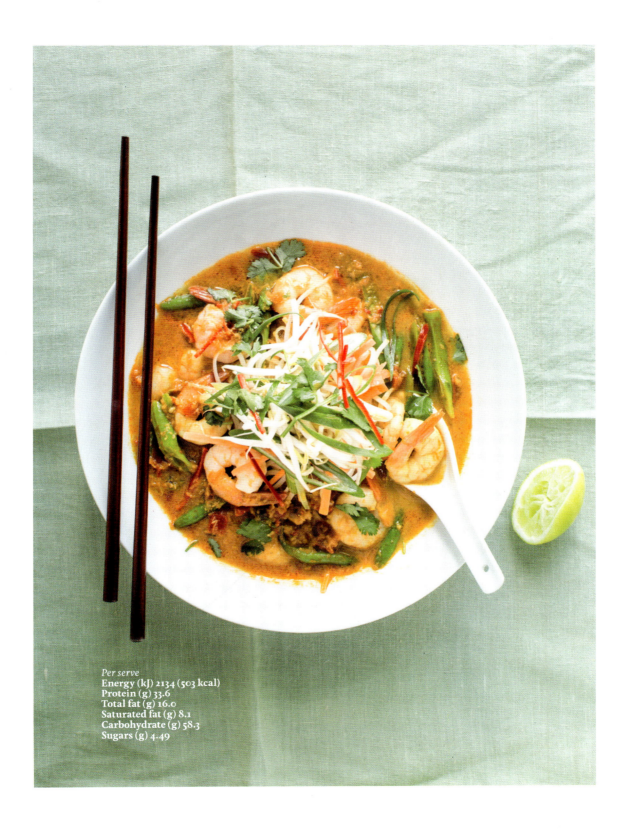

Per serve
Energy (kJ) 2134 (503 kcal)
Protein (g) 33.6
Total fat (g) 16.0
Saturated fat (g) 8.1
Carbohydrate (g) 58.3
Sugars (g) 4.49

DINNER / FISH + SEAFOOD

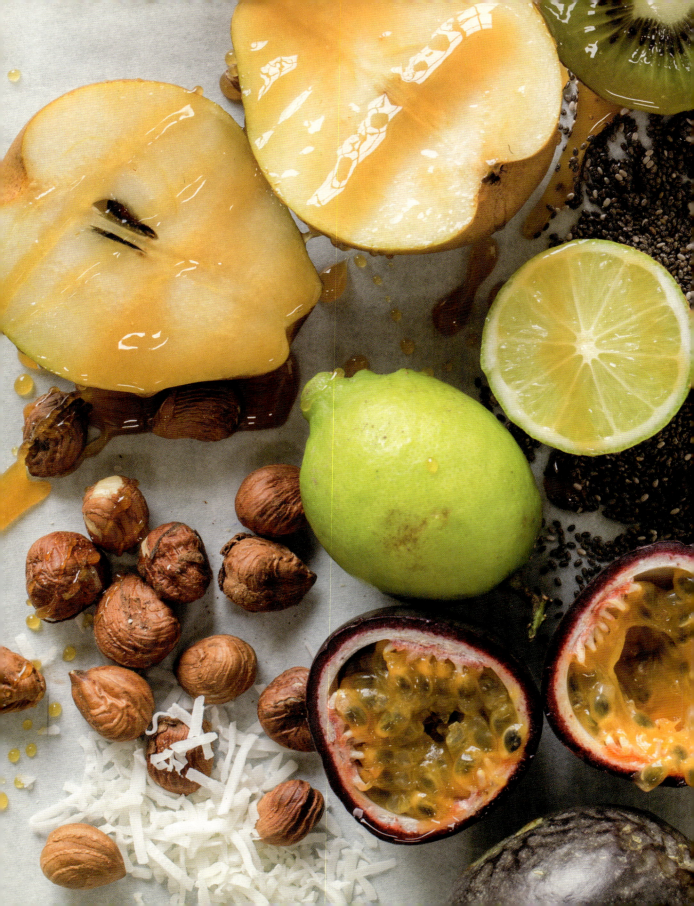

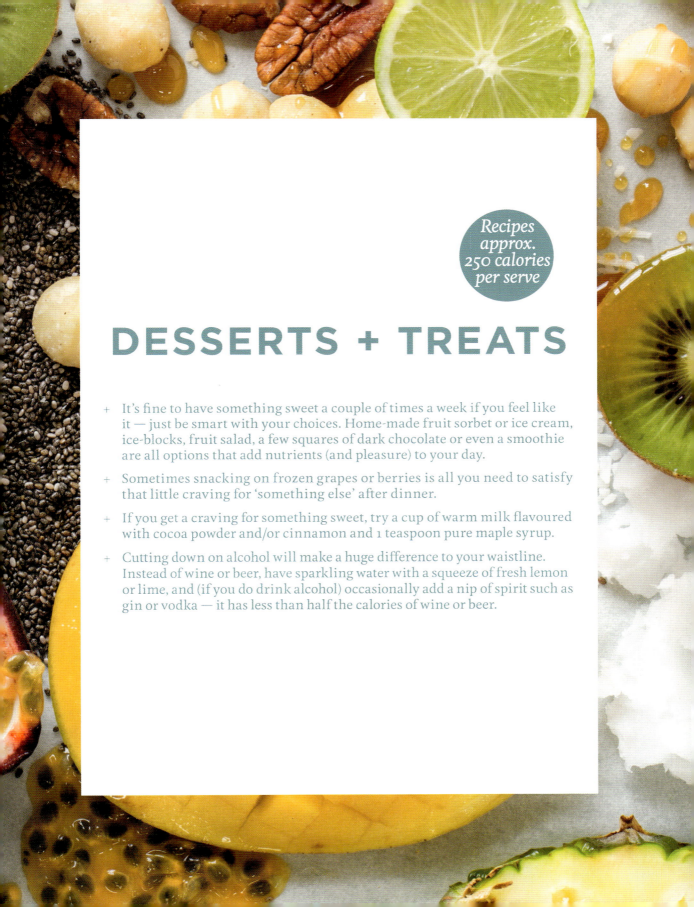

Recipes approx. 250 calories per serve

DESSERTS + TREATS

+ It's fine to have something sweet a couple of times a week if you feel like it — just be smart with your choices. Home-made fruit sorbet or ice cream, ice-blocks, fruit salad, a few squares of dark chocolate or even a smoothie are all options that add nutrients (and pleasure) to your day.

+ Sometimes snacking on frozen grapes or berries is all you need to satisfy that little craving for 'something else' after dinner.

+ If you get a craving for something sweet, try a cup of warm milk flavoured with cocoa powder and/or cinnamon and 1 teaspoon pure maple syrup.

+ Cutting down on alcohol will make a huge difference to your waistline. Instead of wine or beer, have sparkling water with a squeeze of fresh lemon or lime, and (if you do drink alcohol) occasionally add a nip of spirit such as gin or vodka — it has less than half the calories of wine or beer.

MELON WITH MINT + TAMARIND, CHILLI + GINGER SYRUP

Cold slices of refreshing melon, drizzled with a sweet and sour syrup with hints of ginger and chilli, makes a beautifully simple dessert.

1. Put all tamarind syrup ingredients in a small saucepan over a high heat and bring to the boil. Stir to break up tamarind pulp. Continue boiling until reduced by half, about 12 minutes. Strain and discard any seeds, pulp, ginger and chilli. You should have about ¾ cup syrup. Chill syrup in the freezer for 10-15 minutes until cold, thick and syrupy.

2. Cut melon into 8 slices and arrange on a serving plate. Sprinkle over mint and drizzle over tamarind syrup. Serve with lime wedges to squeeze over just before eating.

TIP The syrup keeps in the fridge for a couple of weeks and is great topped up with cold soda water and a squeeze of lime in a tall glass for a refreshing drink. Tamarind is a fruit with sweet and sour flavours similar to prunes. You can find it in Asian grocery stores or sometimes in the international section of the supermarket.

SERVES: 4

PREP TIME: 10 MINUTES

COOK TIME: 12 MINUTES

TAMARIND SYRUP

tamarind pulp 3 tablespoons
water 1½ cups
coconut sugar or **honey** 4-5 tablespoons
ginger 2cm piece, peeled, thinly sliced
red chilli (seeds in) ½ large, sliced

TO SERVE

melon (e.g. rockmelon, honeydew or small watermelon) ½
mint leaves 4-5, finely chopped
lime 1, cut into wedges

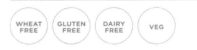

Per serve
Energy (kJ) 469 (110 kcal)
Protein (g) 1.4
Total fat (g) 0.3
Saturated fat (g) 0.0
Carbohydrate (g) 26.3
Sugars (g) 25.93

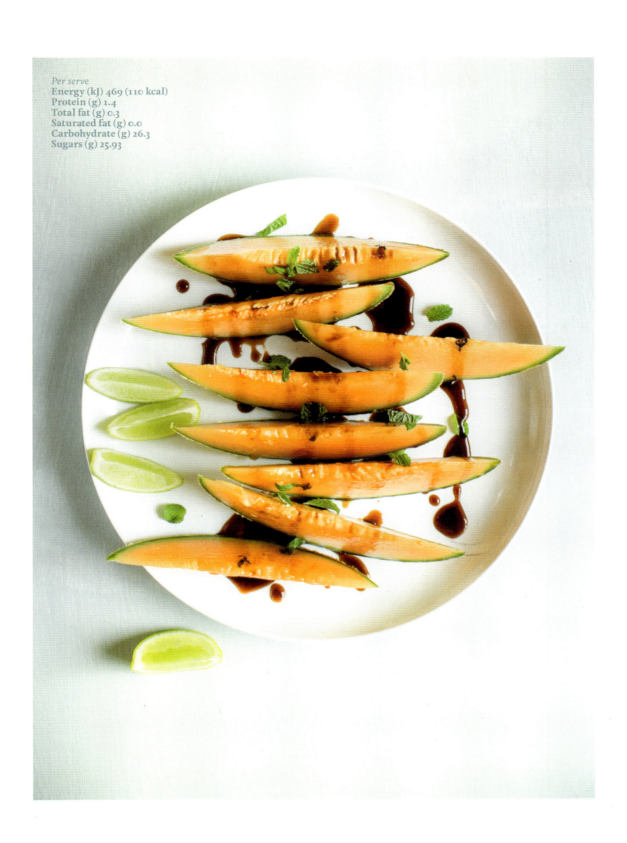

DESSERTS + TREATS

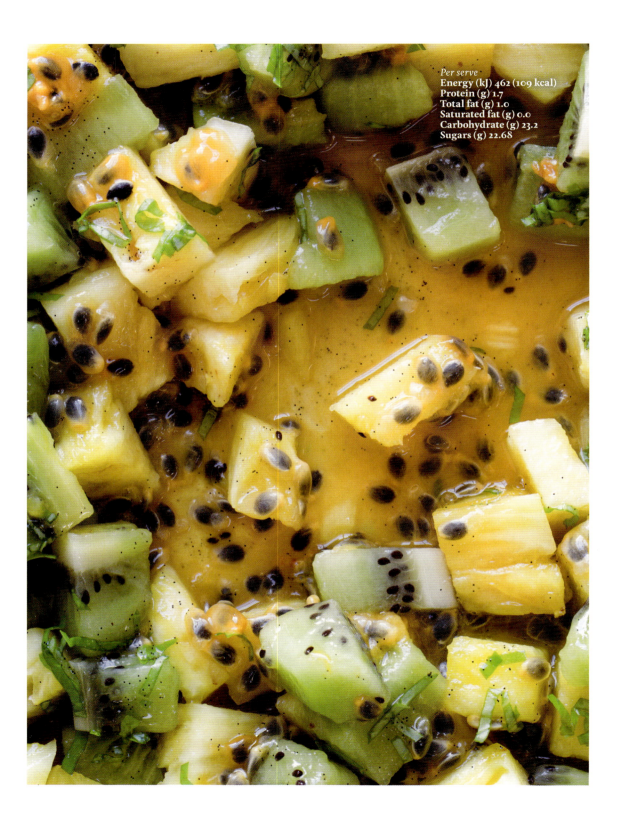

PINEAPPLE, KIWIFRUIT + PASSIONFRUIT SALAD WITH VANILLA SYRUP + BASIL

How do you make an ordinary fruit salad sensational? Add some vanilla and chopped fresh mint and basil! If you have rose or orange blossom water on hand, you could also add a few drops.

1. Mix pineapple, kiwifruit, passionfruit pulp and mint or basil together in a large serving bowl.
2. Gently heat all syrup ingredients together in a small saucepan on the stovetop, or in a small bowl in the microwave for 30-60 seconds.
3. To serve, pour syrup over the fruit salad and divide between bowls.

SERVES: 4

PREP TIME: 10 MINUTES

COOK TIME: 1 MINUTE

pineapple ½ fresh ripe, cored, diced
kiwifruit 4 ripe green, peeled, diced
passionfruit 4 ripe, scooped-out flesh
mint or basil leaves 1-2 tablespoons finely chopped

SYRUP

liquid honey 1 tablespoon or **agave nectar** 2 tablespoons
water 1 tablespoon
vanilla bean paste or **vanilla extract or essence** ¼ teaspoon
lime juice of 1

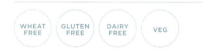

WHEAT FREE | GLUTEN FREE | DAIRY FREE | VEG

DESSERTS + TREATS

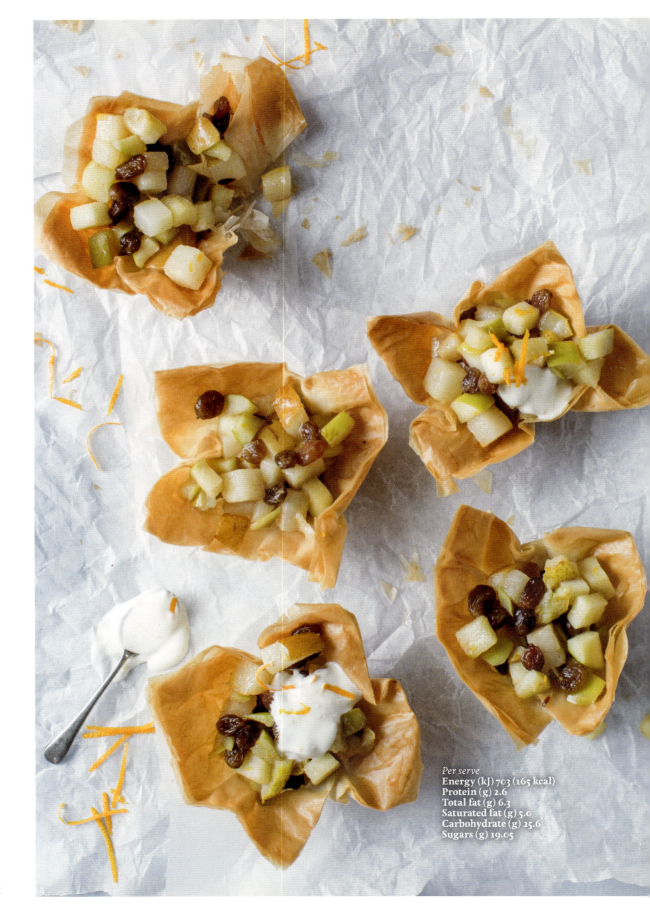

Per serve
Energy (kJ) 703 (165 kcal)
Protein (g) 2.6
Total fat (g) 6.3
Saturated fat (g) 5.0
Carbohydrate (g) 25.6
Sugars (g) 19.05

APPLE, PEAR + SULTANA FILO BASKETS

These gorgeous little open filo pies are so delicious, easy to make, and a much healthier version of traditional apple pie. Adding the rosemary sprig adds a subtle, fragrant flavour, but is optional.

1. Preheat oven to 180°C. Lightly grease 6 moulds in a 12-mould muffin tray. Combine sultanas or raisins and hot water and set aside for about 10 minutes to plump up.

2. While the sultanas are soaking, make the filo baskets. Mix melted coconut oil or butter and cinnamon together, then lightly brush a sheet of filo with the mixture and top with another sheet of filo. Repeat until all the pastry has been used.

3. Cut the layered pastry into 6 small rectangles. Push pastry rectangles into the 6 greased moulds of the muffin tray to create basket shapes and bake for 10-12 minutes or until filo is golden and crisp.

4. While the filo baskets are cooking, make the filling. Heat butter or coconut oil in a frying over medium-high heat. Cook apple, pear, cinnamon, rosemary sprig, if using, and lemon zest for 6-8 minutes until fruit is starting to soften (but still holds its shape). Remove rosemary sprig, add drained sultanas or raisins and honey and toss with the fruit.

5. Mix yoghurt with grated orange zest, if using.

6. To serve, place a filo basket on each plate and spoon in some fruit filling. Serve with a dollop of yoghurt.

TIP In summer I like to use stone fruit like apricots and nectarines instead of apples and pears.

SERVES: 6

PREP TIME: 20 MINUTES

COOK TIME: 10-12 MINUTES

FILLING

sultanas or **raisins** ⅓ cup
hot water 2 tablespoons
butter or **coconut oil** 1½ tablespoons
apples 2, peeled, cored, cut into 1cm dice
pears 2, peeled, cored, cut into 1cm dice
ground cinnamon ½ teaspoon
rosemary 1 small sprig (optional)
lemon zest of 1
honey 1½ tablespoons

FILO BASKETS

coconut oil or **butter** 1 tablespoon, melted
ground cinnamon ¼ teaspoon
filo pastry 5 sheets

TO SERVE

natural sweetened or unsweetened yoghurt ½ cup
orange zest of ½ (optional)

DAIRY FREE | VEG

Dairy-free with coconut oil + serve with coconut yoghurt

DESSERTS + TREATS

LEMONGRASS, GINGER + HONEY POACHED PEARS

Simple, elegant poached pears are one of my favourite desserts. You can poach them in any flavours you like (e.g. cinnamon, star anise, orange, lemon, wine, etc.). Here I've given them a fragrant Asian-inspired twist with lemongrass. They're simple to make and delicious with yoghurt, or some crème fraîche, mascarpone or ice cream.

1. Peel pears, leaving the stalk intact. Cut a thin slice off the bottom of each pear so that they will stand upright when served.

2. Use a vegetable peeler to peel the lemon skin, trying not to get too much of the white pith. Slice lemon peel into thin strips and place in a medium-sized saucepan. Add lemongrass along with ginger, honey and water. Stir to mix everything together.

3. Place pears on their sides in the liquid, cover and bring to a gentle boil. Reduce heat and simmer gently, partially covered, for 1–1½ hours or until pears are soft and an amber colour, and the liquid has reduced by about two-thirds to a syrup. Turn the pears gently during cooking, to make sure they cook evenly.

4. Serve pears warm or cold, with a little syrup drizzled over and a dollop of yoghurt.

TIP The poached pears last in the fridge, stored in their syrup, for up to a week, so you can make them in advance if you are having a dinner party.

SERVES: 6

PREP TIME: 5–10 MINUTES

COOK TIME: 1–1½ HOURS

pears (e.g. Beurre Bosc) 6 medium-sized firm, ripe
lemon 1 smooth-skinned
lemongrass 2 stalks, bruised with the back of a knife, roughly chopped
ginger 2.5cm piece, peeled, thinly sliced
liquid honey 4 tablespoons
water 3 cups

TO SERVE

natural unsweetened yoghurt 2 tablespoons per serving

(WHEAT FREE) (GLUTEN FREE) (DAIRY FREE) (VEG)

Dairy-free with coconut yoghurt

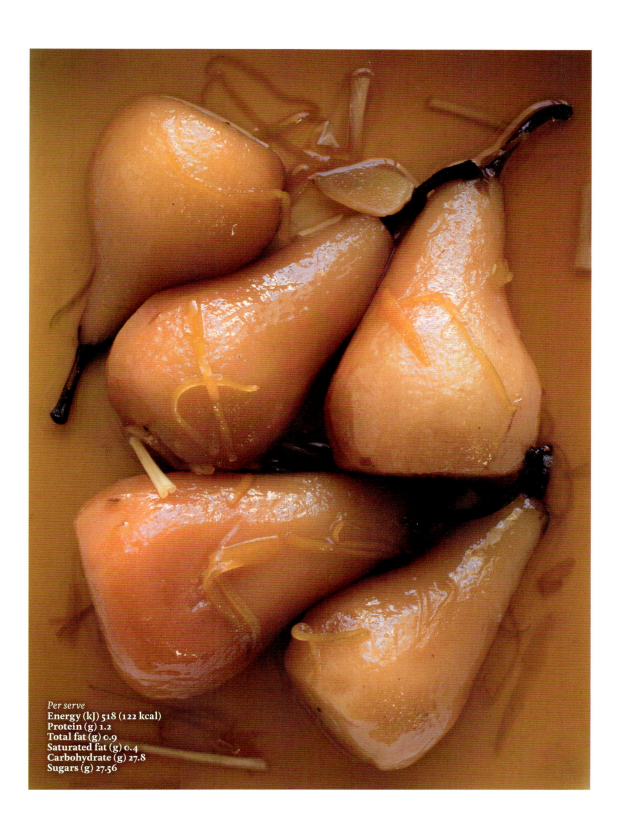

Per serve
Energy (kJ) 518 (122 kcal)
Protein (g) 1.2
Total fat (g) 0.9
Saturated fat (g) 0.4
Carbohydrate (g) 27.8
Sugars (g) 27.56

DESSERTS + TREATS

GRILLED CINNAMON BANANAS WITH MAPLE CARAMELISED PECANS + YOGHURT

This quick, yummy dessert serves as a great way to hit the spot if you still feel like a little something after dinner. They're ready in less than 15 minutes, and you feel like you're eating a decadent treat.

1. Preheat grill to 200°C or to high. Line an oven tray with baking paper for easy clean up. Trim the stems of the bananas, then cut them in half lengthways. Arrange cut side up on prepared oven tray. Sprinkle over cinnamon and drizzle with maple syrup. Place under grill for 10-12 minutes until bananas are starting to bubble and turn golden brown.

2. Toast pecans in a dry frying pan (no oil required) for about 2 minutes over medium heat (be careful they don't burn). Turn off the heat and add maple syrup — it will start to bubble and caramelise — and stir to coat the nuts.

3. To serve, place two grilled banana halves on each plate and scatter over caramelised pecans. Serve with a dollop of yoghurt on the side.

TIP You can use apple syrup instead of maple syrup if you prefer.

SERVES: 4

PREP TIME: 5 MINUTES

COOK TIME: 10-12 MINUTES

BANANAS
bananas 4 ripe
ground cinnamon 1 teaspoon
pure maple syrup 2 tablespoons

CARAMELISED PECANS
pecans ¼ cup, chopped
pure maple syrup 2 tablespoons

TO SERVE
natural unsweetened yoghurt
1 tablespoon per serving

WHEAT FREE · GLUTEN FREE · DAIRY FREE · VEG

Dairy-free with coconut yoghurt

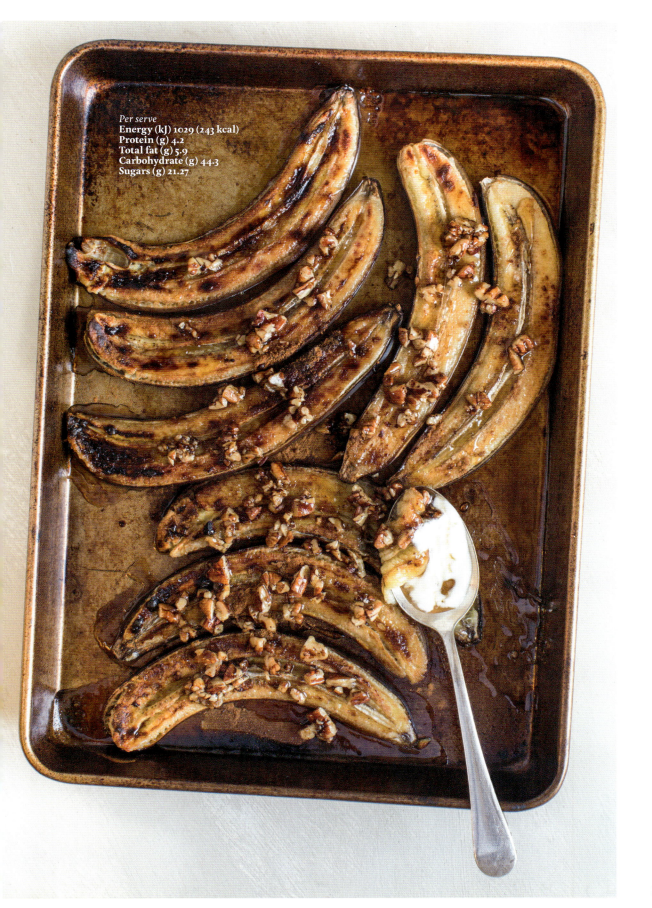

Per serve
Energy (kJ) 1029 (243 kcal)
Protein (g) 4.2
Total fat (g) 5.9
Carbohydrate (g) 44.3
Sugars (g) 21.27

DESSERTS + TREATS

227

Per serve
Energy (kJ) 414 (97 kcal)
Protein (g) 4.4
Fat (g) 4.6
Saturated fat (g) 2.8
Carbohydrate (g) 9.5
Sugar (g) 9.4

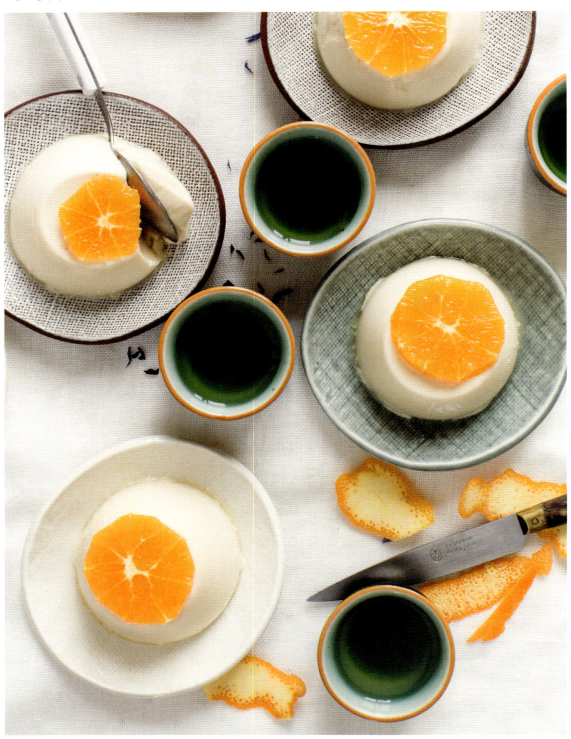

HONEY MILK JELLIES

My mum used to make these as a healthy dessert when we were kids. I love their wobbliness and creamy texture. If you're a fan of it, add some almond essence. Serve with fresh or canned fruit such as berries, peaches or oranges.

1. If using moulds, lightly grease them with a little neutral flavoured or nut oil (e.g. grapeseed or almond oil), melted butter or coconut oil. If you are using glasses or tea cups, you don't need to grease them. Mix gelatine with cold water and set aside for a few minutes to swell — it will form one big lump.

2. Place milk and honey in a saucepan over a gentle heat and warm until honey has dissolved.

3. Whisk gelatine into hot milk and honey until the gelatine is fully dissolved and there are absolutely no specks or lumps. Allow to cool completely, then whisk in yoghurt. Transfer to a jug for easy pouring.

4. Pour mixture into moulds or cups, dividing equally. Place in the fridge to set for at least 4 hours or overnight.

5. To serve, briefly dip moulds into a bowl of warm water for a few seconds, then run a knife around the inside of the moulds to pop the 'seal'. Carefully invert each jelly onto a plate and serve with fruit. If using glasses or tea cups, garnish with fruit on top and serve in the cups.

SERVES: 6

PREP TIME: 5 MINUTES

SETTING TIME: AT LEAST 4 HOURS

small moulds, glasses or **tea cups** 6
gelatine powder 2 teaspoons
cold water 2 tablespoons
almond or cow's milk 1½ cups
honey 2 tablespoons
natural unsweetened thick Greek yoghurt 1 cup

TO SERVE

oranges (or other fresh fruit) 2, peeled, sliced

WHEAT FREE · GLUTEN FREE

DESSERTS + TREATS

Per serve
Energy (kJ) 403 (95 kcal)
Protein (g) 1.1
Fat (g) 6.4
Saturated fat (g) 0.9
Carbohydrate (g) 8.3
Sugar (g) 8.1

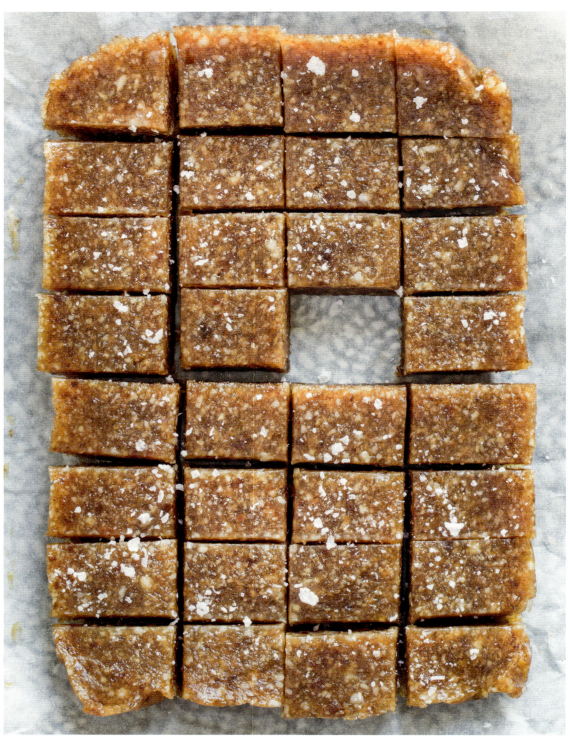

SALTED CARAMEL FUDGE

This salted caramel fudge is to die for! I seriously couldn't believe how good it tasted when I first experimented making this recipe. It is simply medjool dates, vanilla and macadamias blended up to create a thick, sticky fudge that tastes better than the real (unhealthy, sugar-laden) thing. This contains only natural sugars and healthy fats but, even still, make sure you only have 1 or 2 pieces and savour them.

1. Line a 20cm square or rectangular dish with baking paper. Place dates, macadamias, vanilla and salt in a food processor and blitz until smooth and well combined. Drizzle in milk with the motor running. At first it may seem like the mixture isn't coming together, but then it suddenly will in one big sticky lump.

2. Spoon into prepared dish. Use the back of a wet spoon to press down and spread the mixture evenly. The wet spoon will help you to deal with the sticky mixture. Sprinkle with flaky sea salt, if using. Set in the freezer for at least 3 hours or until firm.

3. Use a hot knife (run under hot water) to cut fudge into 32 pieces once set. Best stored in and eaten from the freezer.

MAKES: 32 SMALL PIECES (2 PIECES PER SERVING)

PREP TIME: 5 MINUTES

SETTING TIME: 3 HOURS

medjool dates 1 cup (about 10–12 dates), pitted
macadamia nuts 1 cup
vanilla bean paste or **vanilla extract or essence** 1 teaspoon
salt ¼ teaspoon
milk (e.g. cow's, almond, rice, oat) 2 teaspoons
flaky sea salt good pinch of (optional)

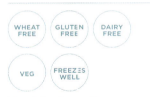

Use dairy-free milk

DESSERTS + TREATS

CHIA PUDDING WITH FRUIT SALSA

Chia puddings make a quick, nutritious dessert. Top with any fruit you like.

1. Place chia seeds in a bowl and whisk in water, milk, maple syrup or honey and vanilla. Briskly whisk the ingredients together for about 5 minutes until mixture has thickened slightly.

2. Divide mixture between 2 serving glasses and leave in the fridge to chill for a few hours or overnight — the puddings should have a gel-like texture, like not-quite-set jelly. You may need to whisk the mixture a few times with a fork while the puddings are chilling to stop the seeds from clumping and sinking to the bottom.

3. Mix all fruit salsa ingredients together.

4. To serve, spoon fruit salsa on top of chia puddings.

TIP The trick to avoiding the chia seeds clumping together and going gluggy is to briskly whisk them continuously for a good 5 minutes before placing in the fridge to set. This movement 'activates' the seeds, releasing their gelatinous texture.

SERVES: 2

PREP TIME: 5 MINUTES

SETTING TIME: 3–4 HOURS

chia seeds 3 tablespoons
water ½ cup
milk (e.g. cow's, almond, soy, rice) ½ cup
pure maple syrup or **liquid honey** 1½ tablespoons
vanilla bean paste or **vanilla extract or essence** 1 teaspoon

FRUIT SALSA

mango ½ (about 250g) ripe, finely diced
green kiwifruit 1 small ripe, peeled, finely diced
liquid honey 1 teaspoon
mint leaves 3–4, finely sliced (optional)

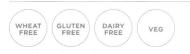

Use dairy-free milk

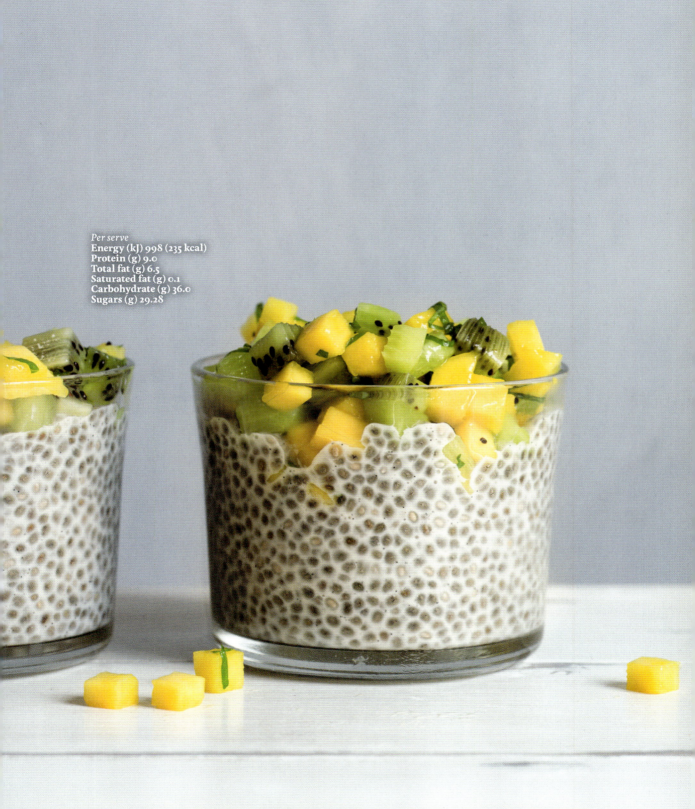

Per serve
Energy (kJ) 998 (235 kcal)
Protein (g) 9.0
Total fat (g) 6.5
Saturated fat (g) 0.1
Carbohydrate (g) 36.0
Sugars (g) 29.28

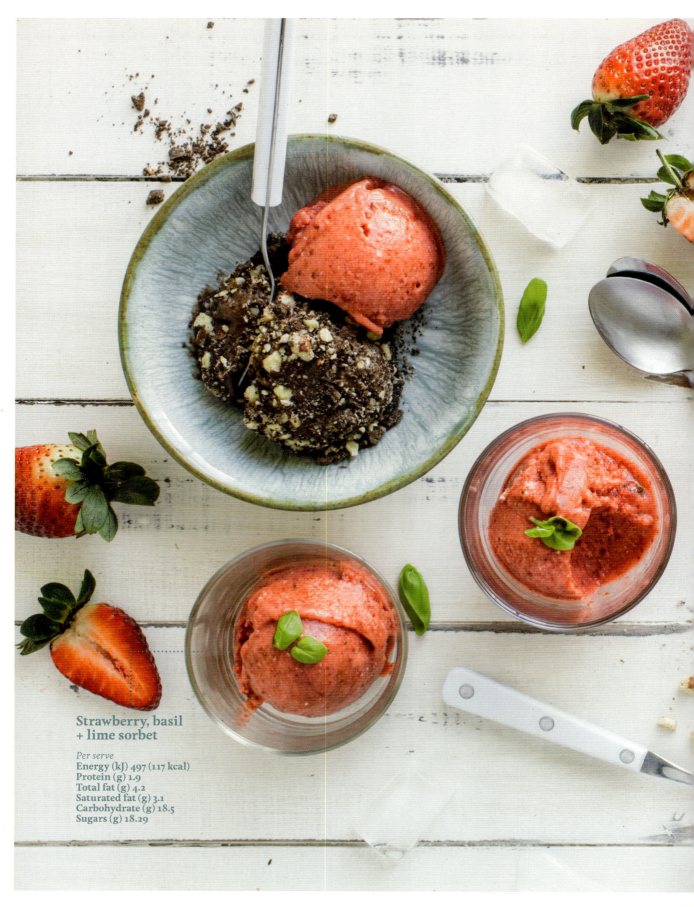

Strawberry, basil + lime sorbet

Per serve
Energy (kJ) 497 (117 kcal)
Protein (g) 1.9
Total fat (g) 4.2
Saturated fat (g) 3.1
Carbohydrate (g) 18.5
Sugars (g) 18.29

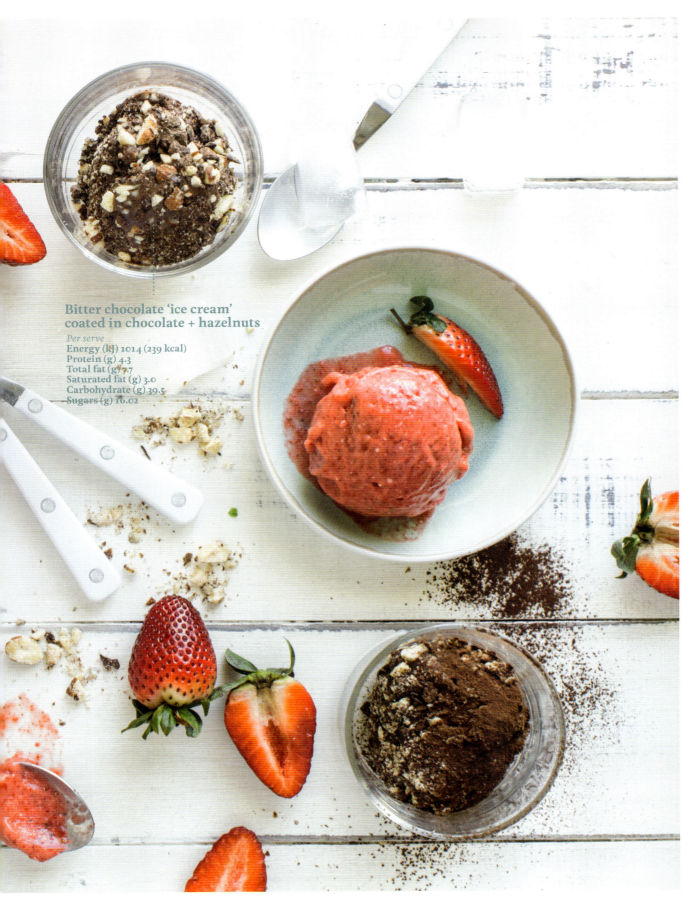

Bitter chocolate 'ice cream' coated in chocolate + hazelnuts

Per serve
Energy (kJ) 1014 (239 kcal)
Protein (g) 4.3
Total fat (g) 7.7
Saturated fat (g) 3.0
Carbohydrate (g) 39.5
Sugars (g) 16.02

STRAWBERRY, BASIL + LIME SORBET

It's hard to think of a more refreshing and delicious treat than this sorbet. And yes, basil goes amazingly well with strawberries, but you can use mint if you prefer.

1. Place serving bowls in the freezer to chill. Place frozen berries, honey or apple syrup, lime juice and zest, and basil or mint in a food processor and blitz until crumbly. Keep the motor running and pour in cream. Keep blending until it turns into a smooth sorbet consistency — it will form one big lump. Serve immediately or place in the freezer for up to 4 hours, until ready to serve.

2. To serve, place 2 scoops of sorbet into each chilled serving bowl.

TIP You can use frozen mixed berries instead of just strawberries to make this sorbet. This sorbet is best served within 4 hours of freezing — any longer than that and it can go a bit 'icy'.

SERVES: 4

MAKES: 8 SCOOPS

PREP TIME: 10 MINUTES

FREEZING TIME: UP TO 4 HOURS

frozen strawberries or other berries 4 cups (500g)

liquid honey or **apple syrup** 1½ tablespoons

lime zest and juice of 1

basil or mint leaves 10

coconut cream or **cream** 3 tablespoons

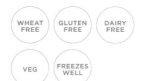

Dairy-free with coconut cream

BITTER CHOCOLATE 'ICE CREAM' COATED IN CHOCOLATE + HAZELNUTS

You'll be amazed at how the texture of this 'ice cream', using frozen bananas as the base — which have an amazing ability to whip up to a fluffy, creamy consistency — is just like the real thing. I've added cocoa to turn it into a decadent (but healthy) chocolate ice cream, and then coated it in hazelnuts and dark chocolate — yum!

1. Place serving bowls in the freezer to chill. Very finely chop nuts and chocolate together. Alternatively, you can blitz them in the food processor until finely chopped and slightly crumbly. Set aside. This is your coating.

2. Place frozen bananas, maple syrup, cocoa or cacao powder and cream in the food processor and blitz to a smooth ice-cream consistency — it will form one big lump. Serve immediately or place in freezer for up to 4 hours until ready to serve.

3. Place scoops of chocolate ice cream in the hazelnut chocolate mixture. Use two spoons to roll them around gently to coat them well in the mixture.

4. To serve, place 2 scoops ice cream into each chilled serving bowl.

SERVES: 4

MAKES: 8 SCOOPS

PREP TIME: 10 MINUTES

FREEZING TIME: UP TO 4 HOURS

hazelnuts (or other nuts, e.g. almonds) 3 tablespoons
good-quality dark eating chocolate 3 tablespoons
frozen bananas 4, peeled, chopped
pure maple syrup 2 tablespoons
good-quality dark cocoa powder or **raw cacao powder** ¼ cup
coconut cream or **cream** 1 tablespoon

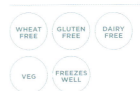

Dairy-free with coconut cream + dairy-free dark chocolate

CHOCOLATE BERRY FUDGE BROWNIES

This brownie contains a secret ingredient that makes it so much healthier than other brownies (as well as gluten free). You'll never believe it, but black beans make a great substitute to flour in baking — the end result is a moist, fudgy chocolate brownie (that you could never tell contained beans). You'll have to make it to believe it!

1. Preheat oven to 150°C. Lightly grease and line a 18-20cm square cake or slice tin with baking paper. If using frozen berries, make sure you drain as much liquid off them as possible before scattering over the brownie mixture.

2. Place coconut oil or butter, honey, agave or maple syrup and dark chocolate in a medium-sized saucepan and gently heat on medium, stirring frequently, until chocolate is melted. Allow to cool slightly.

3. Transfer to a food processor with beans, baking powder and eggs and blitz until smooth and well combined, scraping down the sides of the food processor with a spatula a few times.

4. Spoon mixture into prepared tin. Scatter berries over and bake for 20-25 minutes until brownie is mostly set around the edges, but still slightly soft and fudgy in the middle. (Twenty minutes if you prefer it more fudgy, 25 minutes if you prefer it slightly firmer — I go in between!)

5. Place in the fridge for about 10 minutes to allow it to set slightly. Cut into 16 pieces with a large sharp knife. Delicious eaten warm or cold, and stores well in the freezer or in an airtight container in the fridge for up to a week.

TIP If you don't have a food processor, you can make this in a blender.

MAKES: 16 PIECES

PREP TIME: 10 MINUTES

COOK TIME: 25 MINUTES

fresh or frozen berries (e.g. blueberries, raspberries, boysenberries) 1 cup, defrost if frozen

coconut oil or **butter** ¼ cup melted

liquid honey, pure maple syrup or **agave nectar** 4 tablespoons

good-quality dark eating chocolate (at least 70% cocoa solids) 100g

canned black beans or kidney beans 1 x 400g can, drained, rinsed

baking powder 1 teaspoon

free-range eggs 2

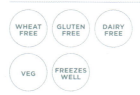

Dairy-free with coconut oil + use dairy-free dark chocolate

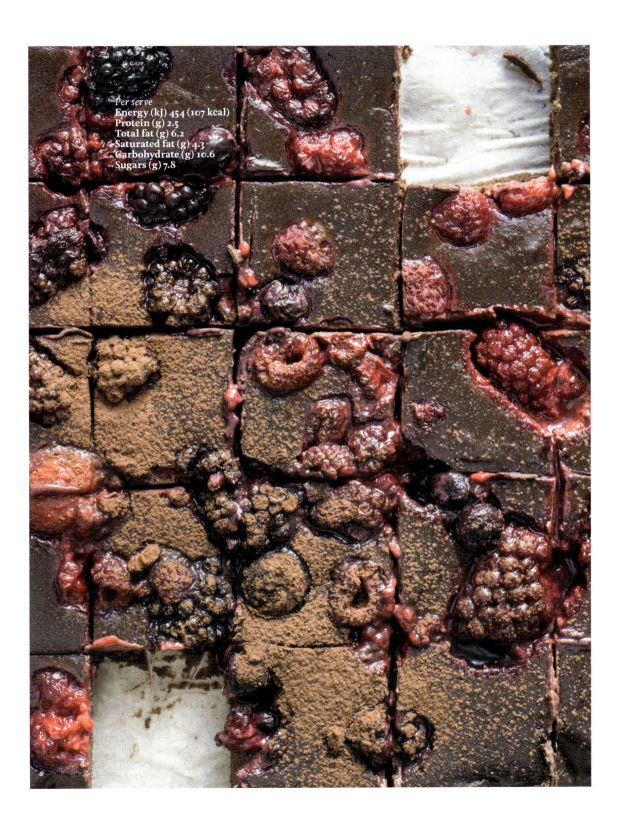

Per serve
Energy (kJ) 454 (107 kcal)
Protein (g) 2.5
Total fat (g) 6.2
Saturated fat (g) 4.3
Carbohydrate (g) 10.6
Sugars (g) 7.8

DESSERTS + TREATS

239

APPLE, BLACKBERRY + DATE NUT CRUMBLE

This crumble topping, sweetened with dates instead of sugar, is amazing. As well as rolled oats, I've added nuts for extra flavour and texture. Everyone will love this dessert, and the fact that it's healthy is a bonus!

1. Preheat oven to 180°C. Heat butter or coconut oil in a frying pan over medium heat. Cook apples and cinnamon for 8-10 minutes until apples are soft (but still loosely holding their shape). Toss warm apples with blackberries and honey and spoon into a medium-sized pie or baking dish.

2. Place nuts, oats, dates, butter or coconut oil and salt in a food processor and blitz until well combined and a crumbly texture.

3. Sprinkle crumble over fruit and bake for about 20 minutes until golden.

4. Serve warm with a dollop of yoghurt.

TIP If you don't have a food processor, very finely chop the nuts and dates and mix well with oats, butter/coconut oil and salt to make the crumble topping.

SERVES: 5

PREP TIME: 10 MINUTES

COOK TIME: 30 MINUTES

FILLING
butter or **coconut oil** 1 tablespoon
apples (e.g. Granny Smith or Braeburn) 4 (about 700-800g), cored, diced
ground cinnamon ¾ teaspoon
fresh, frozen or canned blackberries 1 cup, frozen (defrosted) or canned (drained)
liquid honey 1 teaspoon

CRUMBLE TOPPING
almonds or **hazelnuts** ⅓ cup
rolled oats ¾ cup
dates ⅓ cup, pitted
butter or **coconut oil** 2 tablespoons
salt pinch of

TO SERVE
natural unsweetened yoghurt 1 tablespoon per serving

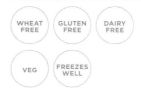

Dairy-free with coconut oil + serve with coconut yoghurt

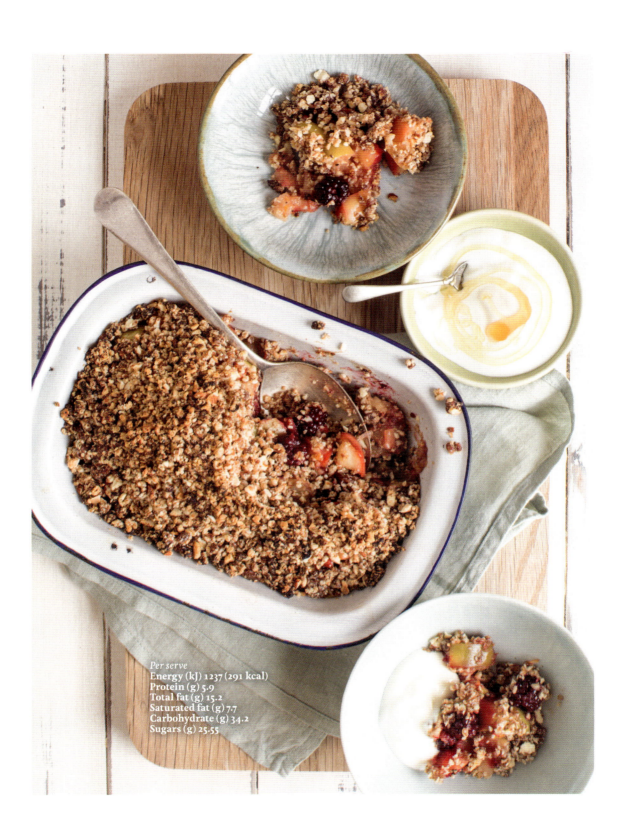

Per serve
Energy (kJ) 1237 (291 kcal)
Protein (g) 5.9
Total fat (g) 15.2
Saturated fat (g) 7.7
Carbohydrate (g) 34.2
Sugars (g) 25.55

DESSERTS + TREATS

241

BAKED CUSTARD

This is a childhood favourite that my mum used to make — a nutritious dessert made with just eggs, milk and honey, baked into a smooth, creamy custard.

1. Preheat oven to 180°C. Bring a full kettle of water to the boil. Use a fork to whisk eggs, egg yolk and vanilla together in a large bowl until well combined. Do not use a whisk as this will froth the eggs up too much.

2. Place milk and honey in a small saucepan and gently heat until it almost comes to the boil, however do not let the mixture boil. Stir well to make sure all the honey has dissolved. Transfer to a pouring jug and allow to cool in the fridge for a few minutes until it is lukewarm — if the mixture is too hot you risk scrambling the eggs.

3. Gradually pour lukewarm milk and honey into the egg mixture while continuously whisking with a fork. Transfer to a jug for easy pouring.

4. Pour into 6 small or medium-sized ramekins or tea cups, dividing equally. Place in a casserole dish or roasting pan with high sides. Grate over a little fresh nutmeg. Pour enough boiling water into the dish or pan to come halfway up the sides of the ramekins or tea cups.

5. Carefully place in oven and cook for 25–30 minutes or until the custards are just set but still have a slight wobble in the middle. Serve hot or cold.

SERVES: 6

PREP TIME: 10 MINUTES

COOK TIME: 25–30 MINUTES

free-range eggs 3
free-range egg yolk 1
vanilla bean paste or **vanilla extract or essence** 1 teaspoon
full-fat milk 2¼ cups
honey 4 tablespoons
whole nutmeg freshly grated

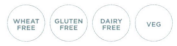

Use dairy-free milk

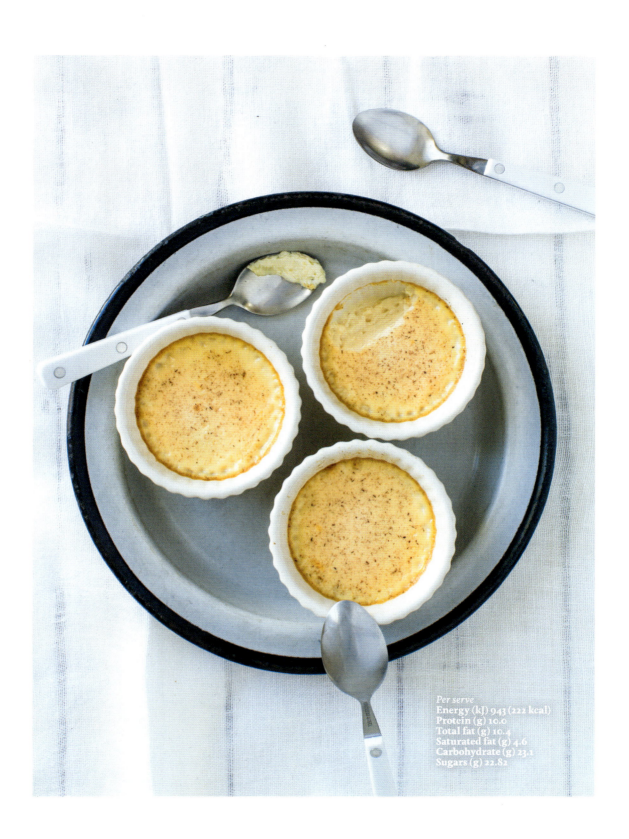

DESSERTS + TREATS

Per serve
Energy (kJ) 943 (222 kcal)
Protein (g) 10.0
Total fat (g) 10.4
Saturated fat (g) 4.6
Carbohydrate (g) 23.1
Sugars (g) 22.82

LEMON COCONUT SLICE

If you love lemon, you will LOVE this slice — it's super lemony, with just the perfect amount of sweetness (not too much) to balance it out. Amazingly, it's only made with nutritious whole ingredients and no refined sugar.

1. Line a 18-20cm square cake tin with baking paper. Place all base ingredients in a food processor and blitz until well combined and crumbly, and the mixture holds together easily when pinched between your fingers.

2. Use the back of a wet spoon to firmly and evenly press the base mixture into prepared tin. The base layer will be quite thin.

3. Place all topping ingredients in the food processor and blitz to a smooth and creamy consistency (this will take at least a few minutes), scraping down the sides a few times with a spatula.

4. Spread topping mixture evenly over the base. Place in the freezer to set for at least 2 hours.

5. Use a large sharp knife to cut the slice into 20 pieces. Best stored in and eaten from the freezer.

TIP This slice keeps best in the freezer. If you don't have a food processor, you can make the base in a blender, however for the topping use ⅔ cup thick coconut cream blended with the lemon zest and maple syrup/honey (you can also add the pulp of 2 passionfruit to make it a lemon passionfruit slice). Set it in the freezer until the topping is solid.

MAKES: 20 PIECES

PREP TIME: 10 MINUTES

SETTING TIME: 2-3 HOURS

BASE

lemons zest of 2
thread or desiccated coconut ½ cup
fine rolled oats ¾ cup
medjool dates 10, pitted
salt pinch of
coconut oil or **butter** 1 tablespoon, melted

TOPPING

macadamia nuts ¾ cup
thread or desiccated coconut ¾ cup
lemons zest of 2
lemon juice ¼-⅓ cup
pure maple syrup, liquid honey or **agave nectar** 2-3 tablespoons

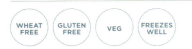

For wheat-free use ground almonds instead of rolled oats

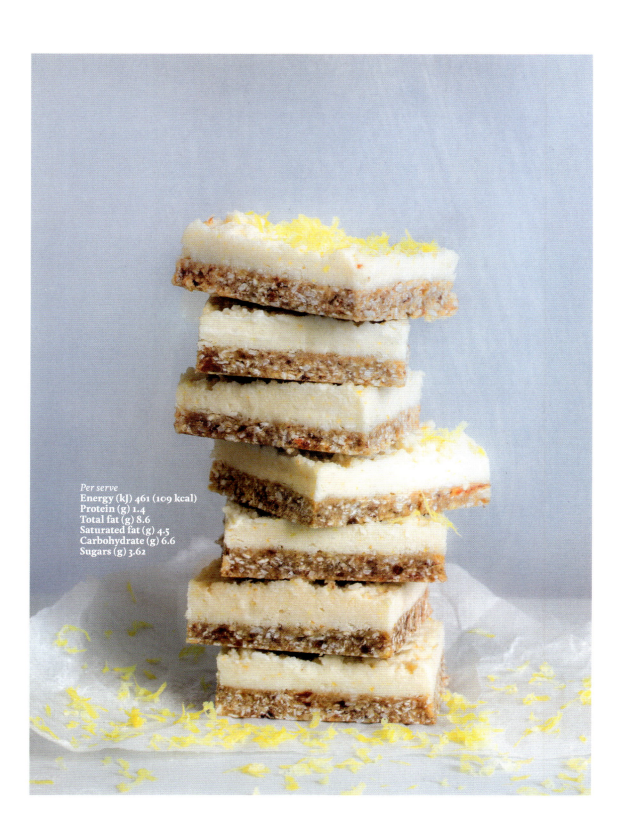

Per serve
Energy (kJ) 461 (109 kcal)
Protein (g) 1.4
Total fat (g) 8.6
Saturated fat (g) 4.5
Carbohydrate (g) 6.6
Sugars (g) 3.62

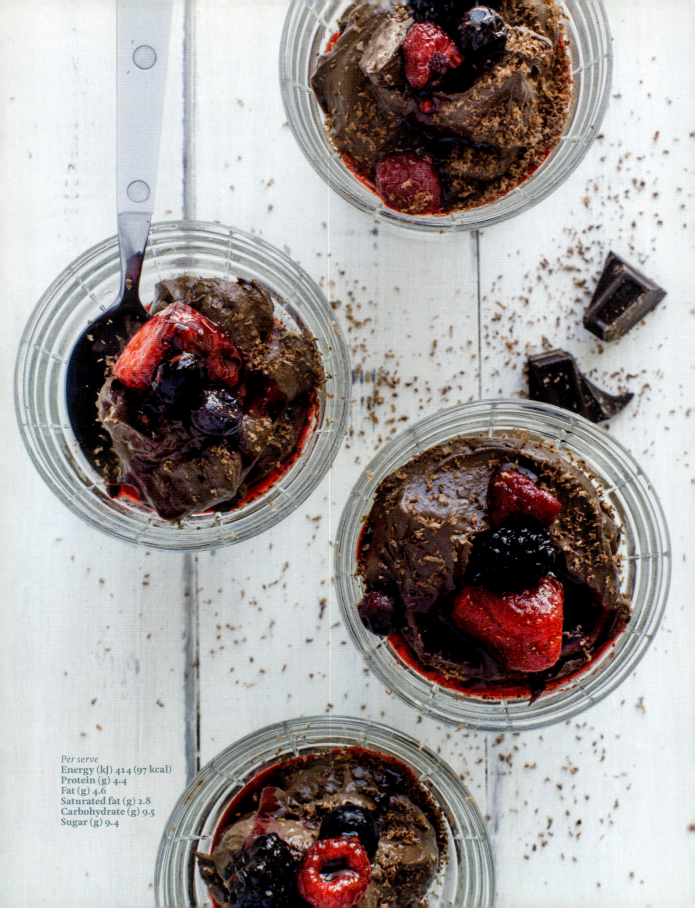

Per serve
Energy (kJ) 414 (97 kcal)
Protein (g) 4.4
Fat (g) 4.6
Saturated fat (g) 2.8
Carbohydrate (g) 9.5
Sugar (g) 9.4

INSTANT CHOCOLATE AVOCADO MOUSSE

Who would have thought that you could make a creamy, decadent healthy chocolate mousse? Well, by using avocado, you can! Thousands of people have made this recipe and told me they can't believe how delicious it is.

1. Melt chocolate in a double boiler or in a glass bowl set above a saucepan of simmering water (make sure the water does not touch the bottom of the bowl or the chocolate could overheat or become grainy). Stir a few times until melted.

2. Place avocado, milk and melted chocolate in a food processor and blend together until smooth. Keep adding a little more liquid until the mousse is very smooth and light. Blend in honey, maple syrup or agave to taste.

3. Spoon into serving glasses and serve immediately. Garnish with berries.

TIP Use the best quality chocolate you can afford — the better the quality, the better the flavour of the mousse.

SERVES: 6

PREP TIME: 10 MINUTES

- **good-quality dark eating chocolate** (at least 70% cocoa solids) 150g, broken into pieces
- **avocados** 2 ripe small to medium-sized or 1½ large
- **milk** (e.g. cow's, almond, rice, oat) ⅓–½ cup
- **liquid honey, pure maple syrup** or **agave nectar** 1–2 tablespoons to taste

TO SERVE

- **fresh or frozen berries** ¼ cup per serving, defrost if frozen

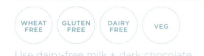

Use dairy-free milk + dark chocolate

DESSERTS + TREATS

Per serve
Energy (kJ) 1261 (297 kcal)
Protein (g) 4.0
Total fat (g) 21.3
Saturated fat (g) 13.2
Carbohydrate (g) 23.3
Sugars (g) 11.4

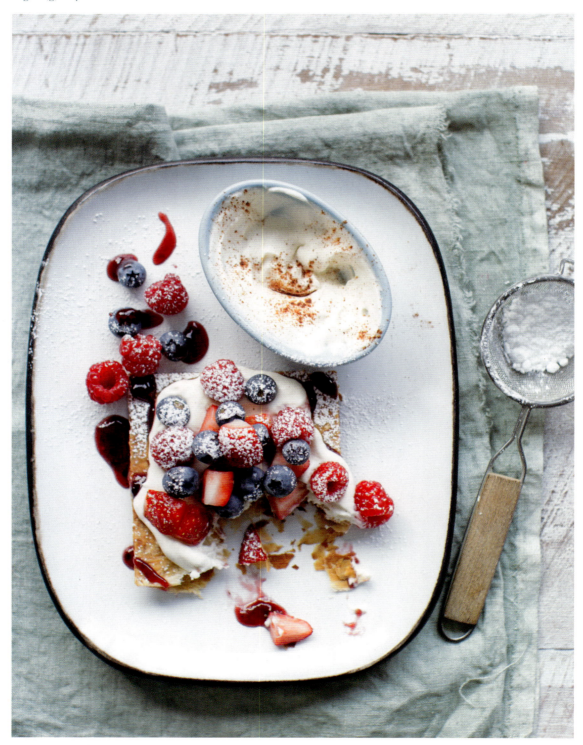

BERRY + CINNAMON CREAM YOGHURT MILLE-FEUILLE

This simple, pretty dessert is what I make for guests if I am short on time. It's loved by everyone.

1. Preheat oven to 180°C. Line a baking tray with baking paper and place sheet of pastry on top. Place another sheet of baking paper on top of pastry and then another baking tray on top (this will help to keep the pastry flat). Bake for about 8-10 minutes, then flip the trays over and turn them around so the front is now the back. Continue to cook for a further 5-10 minutes or until the pastry is crisp and golden. Check on the pastry halfway through cooking to make sure it's not burning (as some ovens and oven trays get hotter than others). Remove pastry from the trays and allow to cool completely.

2. Lightly whip cream, then fold through yoghurt and cinnamon.

3. Briefly melt jam in the microwave or in a small pot on the stovetop to loosen.

4. Use a large sharp knife to cut the cooked pastry into quarters so you have four squares. To assemble, place one pastry square on a serving plate. Drizzle over melted jam and spread with one quarter of the yoghurt cream and top with one quarter of the berries. Grate over a little dark chocolate if desired. Repeat with remaining ingredients. Dust with icing sugar and serve immediately.

SERVES: 4

PREP TIME: 10 MINUTES

COOK TIME: 30 MINUTES

flaky puff pastry 1 square sheet (just thawed)
cream ½ cup
natural yoghurt ½ cup
ground cinnamon ½ teaspoon
berry jam 3 tablespoons
fresh or frozen berries (e.g. blueberries, boysenberries, raspberries or strawberries) 2 cups, defrosted
good-quality dark eating chocolate (at least 70% cocoa solids) for grating
icing sugar 1 tablespoon

VEG

DESSERTS + TREATS

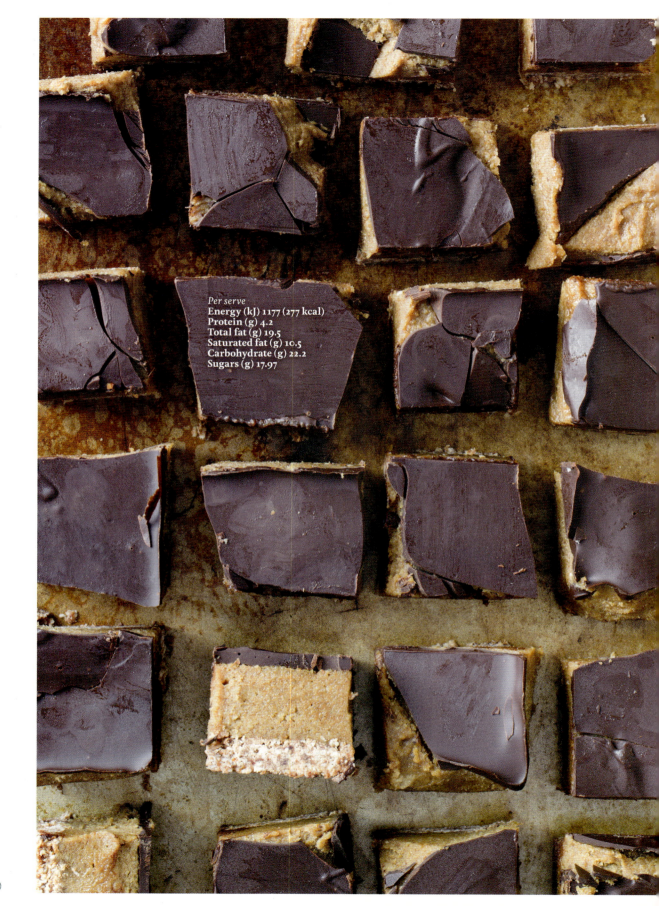

DATE + CASHEW CARAMEL CHOCOLATE SLICE

I love caramel slice, so I created this recipe in an attempt to make something just as delicious but using much more wholesome ingredients. I was stoked with the end result, as were over half a million people that downloaded this recipe from my blog. It's become a favourite all around the world since, with many cafés even making and selling it! It contains no refined sugar, and can be gluten and dairy free.

MAKES: 25 PIECES

PREP TIME: 15 MINUTES

COOK TIME: 30 MINUTES

SETTING TIME: 4 HOURS

BASE

fine rolled oats ¾ cup
desiccated coconut ¾ cup
good-quality dark cocoa or raw cacao powder 1 tablespoon
medjool dates 6, pitted
raw natural almonds ½ cup
salt pinch of
coconut oil or **butter** 6 tablespoons, melted

FILLING

dried pitted dates 1 x 400g packet
boiling water ¾ cup
raw natural cashew nuts 2 cups, soaked (see page 32)
pure maple syrup ¼ cup
coconut oil ½ cup, melted
vanilla extract or essence 1 teaspoon

CHOCOLATE TOPPING

good-quality dark eating chocolate (at least 70% cocoa solids) 100–120g
coconut oil 1 tablespoon

1. Lightly grease and line the bottom and sides of a 20cm square baking tin. Place oats, coconut, cocoa, dates, almonds and salt in a food processor and blitz to a fine, crumbly texture. Drizzle in melted coconut oil or butter and pulse until well combined and the mixture holds together when pressed between your fingers. Press mixture firmly into the prepared tin using the back of a wet spoon or spatula.

2. Place dried dates and water in a medium-sized saucepan and boil, stirring frequently, until the dates are very soft and mushed up, and all the water has evaporated. Place dates in the food processor along with soaked cashew nuts, maple syrup, coconut oil and vanilla. Blitz for a few minutes until smooth.

3. Spread caramel evenly over the base in the tin. Place in the freezer for at least 4 hours or until quite firm.

4. Once the caramel has set, melt chocolate in the top of a double boiler or in a glass bowl set above a small saucepan of simmering water. Mix in oil — this softens the chocolate a little, so it doesn't set too hard. Pour melted chocolate over the filling and spread out evenly. Place in the fridge for 20 minutes until the chocolate is firm.

5. Cut into 25 pieces using a sharp knife dipped in hot water in between each cut. It can be easier to cut it upside down. Keep in an airtight container in the fridge for a few weeks, or longer in the freezer.

TIP If you don't have a food processor, you can make this in a blender by roughly chopping the dates and blending with the almonds, then mixing with remaining base ingredients. To make the topping in a blender, blend cashew nuts, maple syrup, coconut oil and vanilla until smooth, then mix well with dates.

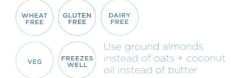

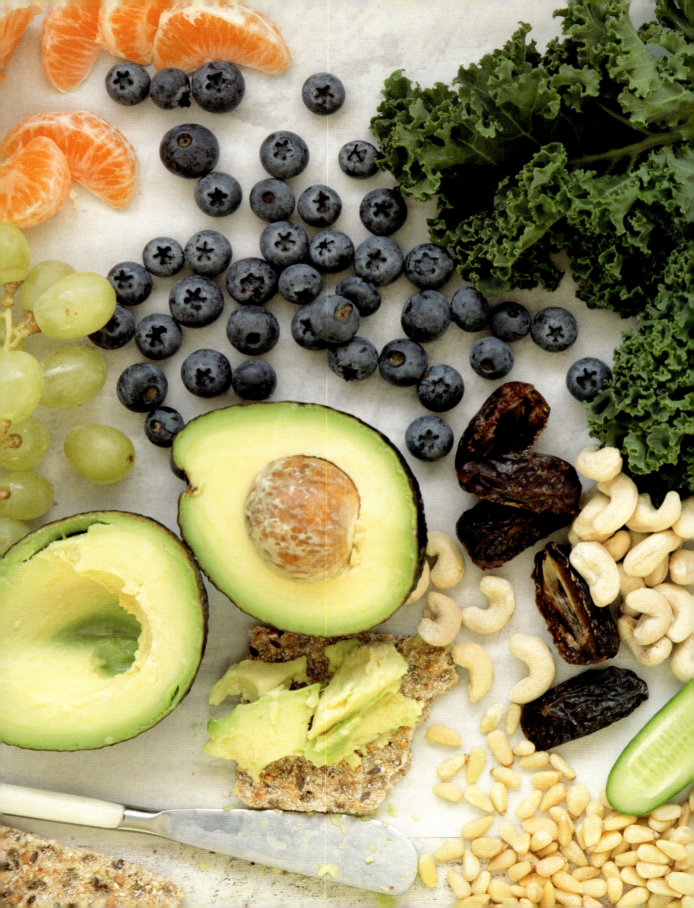

Recipes approx. 100 calories per serve

HEALTHY SNACKS

+ Sometimes you'll need a snack to get you from one meal to the next, or if you're doing more exercise. Pick from any of these options or have a smoothie (from the breakfast section) — they also make great snacks that add nutrients to your day.

+ Do some healthy baking every few weeks and freeze muffins and cookies (to keep them fresh) for healthy snacks.

+ With all your meals, even if it's just a snack, serve your portion (e.g. a bliss ball or a cookie) on a little plate and put the rest away, out of sight, to avoid over-eating.

+ Free morning teas at work can be a trap for many people — don't eat just because it's there and it's free; stop for a few seconds and think 'do I really want this, and would I still eat it if I had to pay for it?' Have a cup of herbal tea in your hands instead.

+ Other quick snack ideas include ½ apple with 1 tablespoon nut butter, or ½ cup yoghurt with a sprinkle of cinnamon and a handful of fresh or frozen berries.

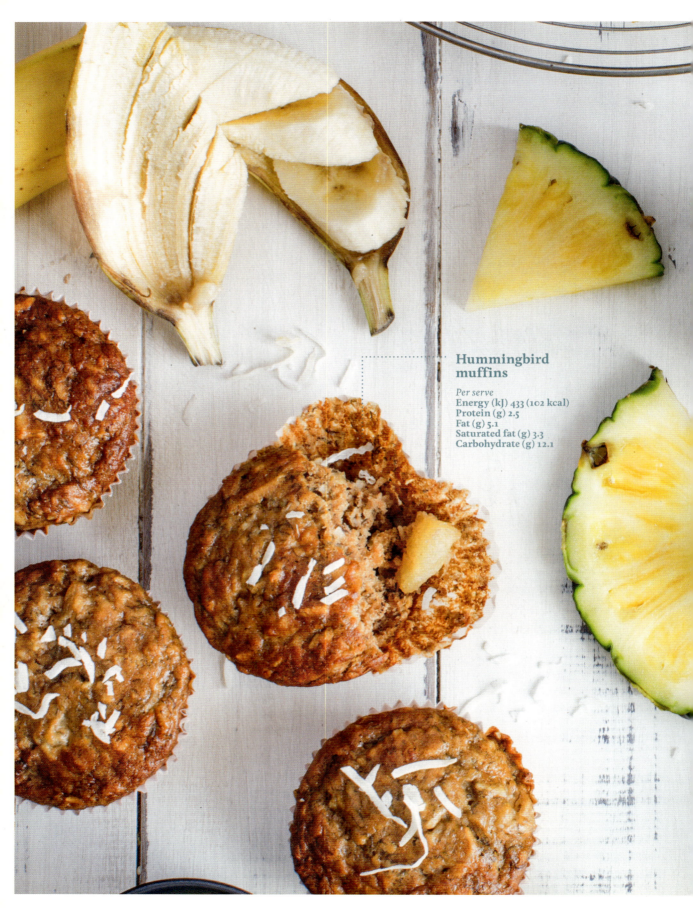

Hummingbird muffins

Per serve
Energy (kJ) 433 (102 kcal)
Protein (g) 2.5
Fat (g) 5.1
Saturated fat (g) 3.3
Carbohydrate (g) 12.1

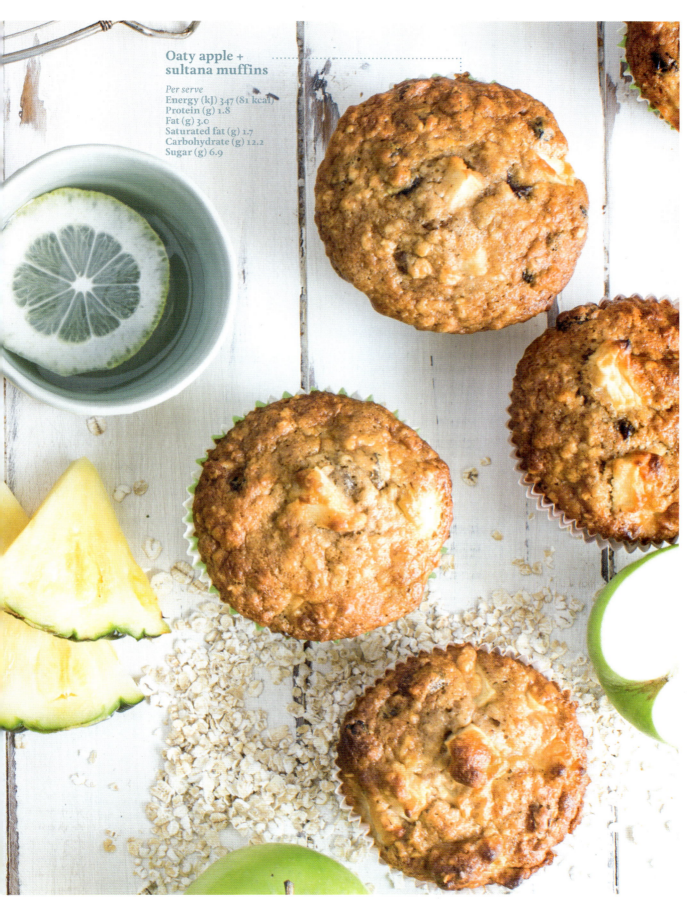

Oaty apple + sultana muffins

Per serve
Energy (kJ) 347 (81 kcal)
Protein (g) 1.8
Fat (g) 3.0
Saturated fat (g) 1.7
Carbohydrate (g) 12.2
Sugar (g) 6.9

HUMMINGBIRD MUFFINS

Based on the famous hummingbird cake, these healthy, high-fibre muffins are flavoured with coconut, lime, pineapple and banana. I've also added in some grated carrot for extra goodness.

1. Preheat oven to 180°C fanbake. Line a 12-mould muffin tray with paper cases. Sift flour and cinnamon into a large mixing bowl.

2. In a large bowl, mix baking soda mixture, eggs, mashed banana, grated carrot, melted butter or coconut oil, honey, vanilla, pineapple, zest and coconut together.

3. Add flour to wet mixture and fold together with a large metal spoon until just combined — be careful not to over-mix to avoid the muffins becoming tough.

4. Spoon mixture into paper cases and bake for 15-18 minutes or until muffins have risen and the tops are lightly browned. Leave muffins in the tray for about 5 minutes to cool slightly before removing to a wire rack.

5. Eat warm or allow to cool completely before storing. These muffins will keep in an airtight container in the fridge for a few days or in the freezer. Briefly warm up frozen muffins in the microwave for about 30 seconds before eating.

TIP These muffins freeze really well. Try one for a breakfast on the go. To make baking soda mixture warm 2 tablespoons milk in a small bowl in the microwave for 15-20 seconds, then stir in baking soda and it will froth up.

MAKES: 12 SMALL MUFFINS
PREP TIME: 10 MINUTES
COOK TIME: 20-25 MINUTES

spelt, wholemeal or gluten-free flour ⅔ cup
ground cinnamon 1 teaspoon
baking soda 1½ teaspoons mixed with 2 tablespoons warm **milk**
free-range eggs 2, beaten
bananas 1 cup mashed (about 2 large)
carrot ⅔ cup grated
butter or **coconut oil** ¼ cup melted
honey ¼ cup
vanilla bean paste or **vanilla extract** or **essence** 1 teaspoon
pineapple chunks ⅔ cup, drained, chopped
lemon zest of 1 or **limes** zest of 2
desiccated coconut ⅓ cup

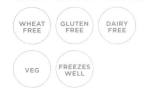

Use gluten-free flour + coconut oil

OATY APPLE + SULTANA MUFFINS

These muffins are made with fresh apple, cinnamon, sultanas, yoghurt and oats. Even though they're a very high-fibre muffin, they're light and fluffy in texture.

1. Preheat oven to 180°C fanbake. Line a 12-mould muffin tray with paper cases. Sift flour, baking powder, and cinnamon into a bowl, then mix in remaining dry ingredients.

2. In a large mixing bowl, beat together eggs, baking soda mixture, maple syrup or honey, vanilla, yoghurt and melted butter or oil with a whisk until smooth and well combined. Stir in diced apple.

3. Add dry mixture to wet mixture and fold together using a large metal spoon until just combined — be careful not to over-mix to avoid the muffins becoming tough.

4. Spoon mixture into paper cases, filling up to the top. Bake for 15-18 minutes or until muffins have risen and are golden brown. Leave muffins in the tray for about 5 minutes to cool slightly before removing to a wire rack.

5. Eat warm or allow to cool completely before storing. These muffins will keep in an airtight container in the fridge for a few days or in the freezer. Briefly warm up frozen muffins in the microwave for about 30 seconds before eating.

TIP These muffins freeze really well. Try one for a breakfast on the go. To make baking soda mixture, warm 1 tablespoon milk in a small bowl in the microwave for 10-15 seconds, then stir in baking soda and it will froth up.

MAKES: 12 SMALL MUFFINS
PREP TIME: 15 MINUTES
COOK TIME: 20-25 MINUTES

DRY MIXTURE
spelt, wholemeal or gluten-free flour ⅔ cup
baking powder 2 teaspoons
ground cinnamon 1 teaspoon
fine rolled oats ⅔ cup
lemon zest of 1
sultanas or **currants** ½ cup

WET MIXTURE
free-range eggs 1 large
baking soda 1 teaspoon mixed with 1 tablespoon warm **milk**
pure maple syrup or **liquid honey** ¼ cup
vanilla extract or essence ½ teaspoon
natural unsweetened thick Greek yoghurt ½ cup
butter or **coconut oil** ¼ cup melted
apples (e.g. Braeburn or Granny Smith) 1⅓ cups (about 2 small) peeled, diced

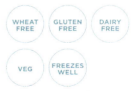

Use gluten-free flour + coconut yoghurt + oil

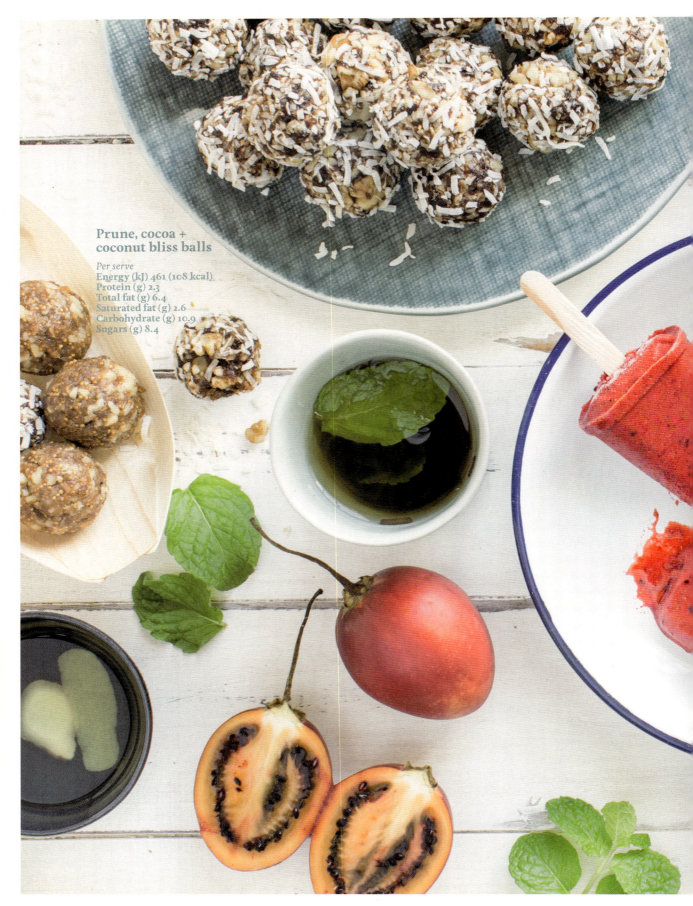

Prune, cocoa + coconut bliss balls

Per serve
Energy (kJ) 461 (108 kcal)
Protein (g) 2.3
Total fat (g) 6.4
Saturated fat (g) 2.6
Carbohydrate (g) 10.9
Sugars (g) 8.4

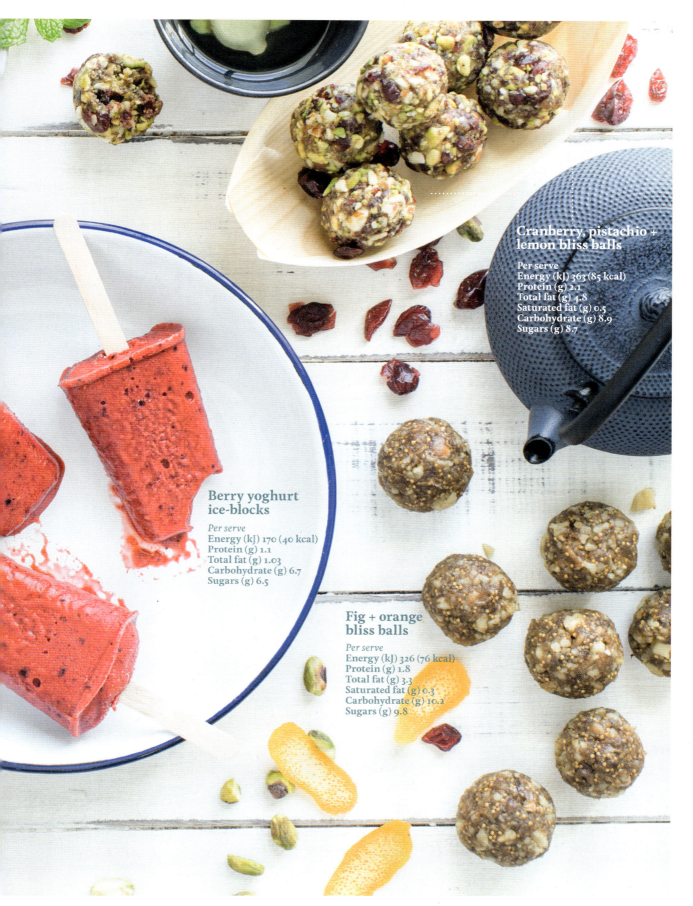

Cranberry, pistachio + lemon bliss balls

Per serve
Energy (kJ) 363 (85 kcal)
Protein (g) 2.1
Total fat (g) 4.8
Saturated fat (g) 0.5
Carbohydrate (g) 8.9
Sugars (g) 8.7

Berry yoghurt ice-blocks

Per serve
Energy (kJ) 170 (40 kcal)
Protein (g) 1.1
Total fat (g) 1.03
Carbohydrate (g) 6.7
Sugars (g) 6.5

Fig + orange bliss balls

Per serve
Energy (kJ) 326 (76 kcal)
Protein (g) 1.8
Total fat (g) 3.3
Saturated fat (g) 0.3
Carbohydrate (g) 10.2
Sugars (g) 9.8

BERRY YOGHURT ICE-BLOCKS

So simple to make, these taste amazing — just blend up yoghurt, berries and honey and freeze. The perfect refreshing healthy snack or treat!

1. Place all ingredients except moulds and sticks in a blender or food processor and blend until smooth.

2. Pour mixture into ice-block moulds, pop in a wooden stick and place in the freezer for at least 8 hours or overnight, until frozen hard.

3. To unmould ice-blocks, dip moulds into warm water for a few seconds to loosen — they should come out easily.

MAKES: 8–10 SMALL ICE-BLOCKS

PREP TIME: 5 MINUTES

FREEZING TIME: 8 HOURS

fresh or frozen boysenberries (or other berries e.g. strawberries, raspberries) 500g, defrost if frozen
natural unsweetened thick Greek yoghurt ½ cup
liquid honey 2 tablespoons
vanilla extract or essence 1 teaspoon
ice-block moulds 8–10 × 65ml (¼ cup)
wooden sticks 8–10

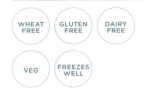

Dairy-free with coconut yoghurt

BLISS BALLS

Bliss balls are handy little snacks full of goodness. You can get creative with different flavours, here are just a few suggested combinations.

CRANBERRY, PISTACHIO + LEMON

MAKES: 12   **PREP TIME:** 10 MINUTES

Place 4 pitted **medjool dates**, ½ cup **dried cranberries** or **cherries**, ½ cup **raw natural almonds** or **macadamias** or ¼ cup **pistachio nuts**, a pinch of **salt**, the zest of 1 **lemon** and juice of half a lemon in a food processor and blitz until well combined and the mixture holds together when you pinch it between your fingers. Roll heaped tablespoonfuls of mixture into balls and serve. Keep in an airtight container in the pantry for up to 1½ weeks. Alternatively, you can freeze the bliss balls.

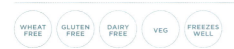

PRUNE, COCOA + COCONUT

MAKES: 12   **PREP TIME:** 10 MINUTES

Place 200g **pitted prunes**, 6 pitted **medjool dates**, ½ cup **thread coconut**, ½ cup **raw natural macadamias** or **almonds**, 2 tablespoons **good-quality dark cacao or cocoa powder** and ½ teaspoon **vanilla extract or essence** in a food processor and blitz until well combined and the mixture holds together when you pinch it between your fingers. Roll heaped tablespoonfuls of mixture into balls and serve. Keep in an airtight container in the pantry for up to 1½ weeks. Alternatively, you can freeze the bliss balls.

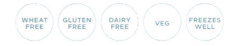

FIG + ORANGE

MAKES: 12   **PREP TIME:** 10 MINUTES

Place 6 pitted **medjool dates**, 3 **dried figs** (use the plumper, more juicy dried figs not the hard, very dry ones), ½ cup **raw natural cashews** or **almonds**, ½ cup **desiccated coconut**, zest of 1 **orange**, a pinch of **salt** and 2 tablespoons **orange or lemon juice** in a food processor and blitz until well combined and the mixture holds together when you pinch it between your fingers.

Roll heaped tablespoonfuls of mixture into balls and serve. Keep in an airtight container in the pantry for up to 1½ weeks. Alternatively, you can freeze the bliss balls.

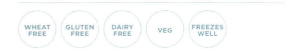

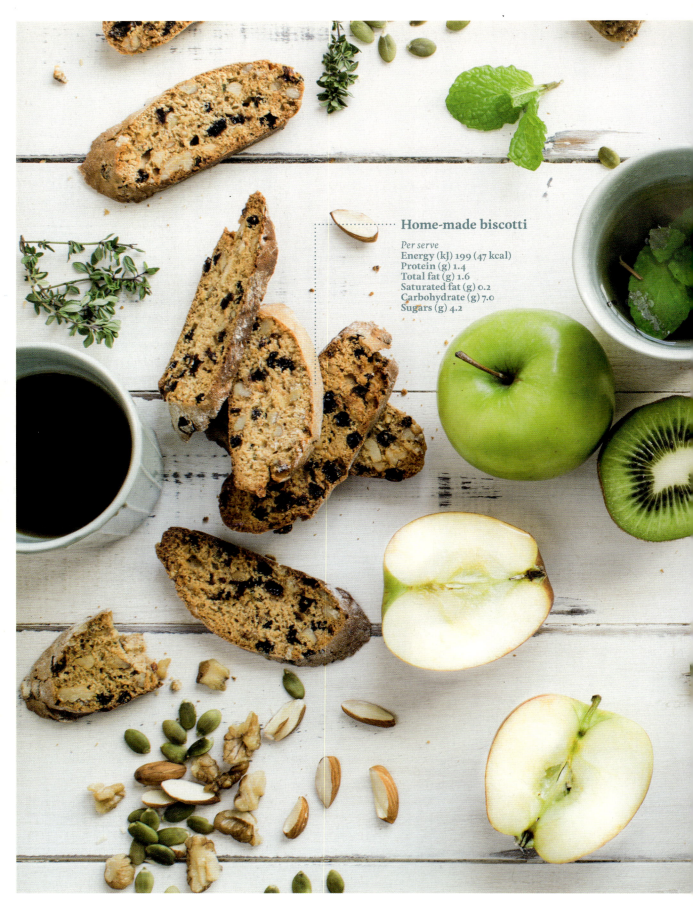

Home-made biscotti

Per serve
Energy (kJ) 199 (47 kcal)
Protein (g) 1.4
Total fat (g) 1.6
Saturated fat (g) 0.2
Carbohydrate (g) 7.0
Sugars (g) 4.2

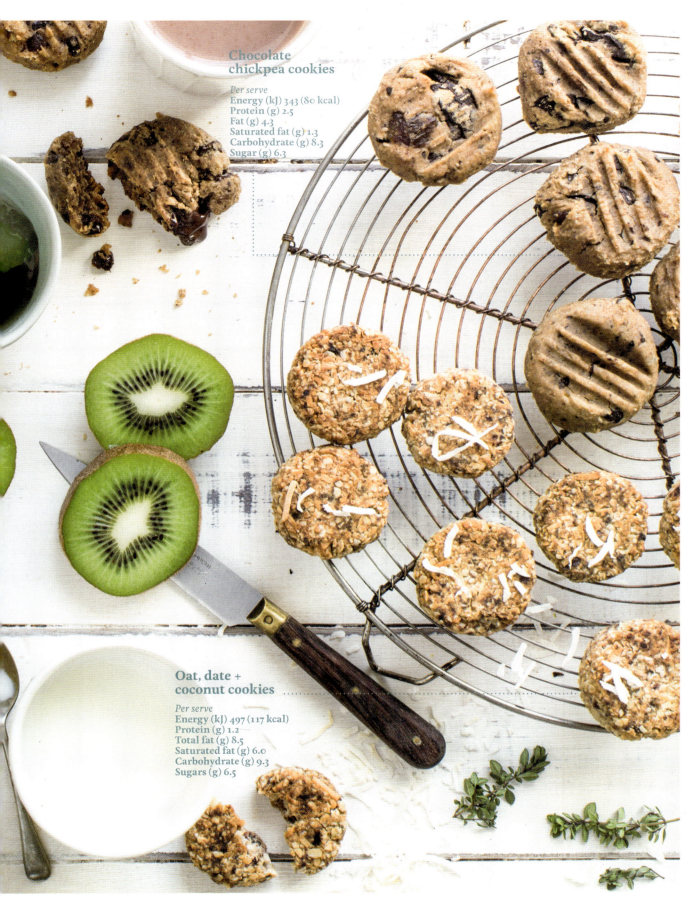

Chocolate chickpea cookies

Per serve
Energy (kJ) 343 (80 kcal)
Protein (g) 2.5
Fat (g) 4.3
Saturated fat (g) 1.3
Carbohydrate (g) 8.3
Sugar (g) 6.3

Oat, date + coconut cookies

Per serve
Energy (kJ) 497 (117 kcal)
Protein (g) 1.2
Total fat (g) 8.5
Saturated fat (g) 6.0
Carbohydrate (g) 9.3
Sugars (g) 6.5

HOME-MADE BISCOTTI

You can easily make your own biscotti (that taste much better than anything bought from a café) to have as a treat with a coffee or hot chocolate.

1. Preheat oven to 190°C. Line a baking tray with baking paper. Sift flour, baking powder and mixed spice into a mixing bowl, then mix in dried fruit and nuts.

2. Beat egg, almond or vanilla essence, honey, lemon or orange zest and rosemary or thyme, if using, until well combined.

3. Make a well in the centre of the dry ingredients and pour in the beaten egg mixture. Mix together until combined — be careful not to overmix. Add a little more flour if the mixture seems too sticky to roll.

4. Divide dough in half and roll into logs, about 3cm in diameter, on a lightly floured surface. Place logs on prepared tray and bake for 20 minutes. Remove from oven and allow to cool slightly.

5. Lower oven temperature to 160°C. Use a serrated bread knife to cut the logs into thin slices, about 0.5cm thick, on the diagonal. Lay individual biscotti on 2 baking trays and return to the oven to dry out for 20-30 minutes. Leave to cool completely.

TIP Biscotti will keep, stored in an airtight container, for a couple of months. Make sure they have completely cooled before storing them, or they risk going soft.

MAKES: 25-30 (2 BISCOTTI PER SERVE)

PREP TIME: 10 MINUTES

COOK TIME: 30-35 MINUTES

spelt, wholemeal or gluten-free flour 1 cup
baking powder 1 teaspoon
ground mixed spice or **Chinese five spice** or **cinnamon** 1 teaspoon
currants or **chopped dried dates or apricots** ½ cup
walnuts (or other nuts e.g. almonds, brazil nuts, hazelnuts) ½ cup finely chopped
free-range egg 1 small
almond or vanilla essence 1 teaspoon
honey ¼ cup
lemon or **orange** zest of ½
rosemary or **thyme leaves** ½ –1 teaspoon finely chopped (optional)

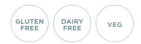

Use gluten-free flour

OAT, DATE + COCONUT COOKIES

These cute little cookies remind me of Anzac biscuits, except they've got no refined sugar in them.

1. Preheat oven to 180°C. Line a baking tray with baking paper. Place all ingredients in a food processor and blitz until just combined — the mixture should stick together well when pinched between your fingers. Do not over-blend.

2. Roll heaped tablespoonfuls of dough into balls and place on prepared tray, evenly spaced about 3cm apart. Flatten slightly with the back of a fork.

3. Bake for 8-10 minutes until light golden. Remove from oven and allow to cool slightly. Transfer carefully with a fish slice to a wire rack to cool completely — they will be quite delicate.

4. Keep in an airtight container in the pantry for up to a week, or freeze.

MAKES: 20
PREP TIME: 10 MINUTES
COOK TIME: 8-10 MINUTES

medjool dates 1 cup, pitted
fine rolled oats or **ground almonds** 1 cup
desiccated or thread coconut 1 cup
butter or **coconut oil** ½ cup, softened
vanilla or almond essence 1 teaspoon; or **lemon** zest of 1; or **ground mixed spice, cinnamon** or **ginger** 1 teaspoon (optional)

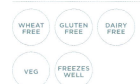

For wheat-free use ground almonds + for dairy-free use coconut oil

HEALTHY SNACKS

CHOCOLATE CHICKPEA COOKIES

You might be surprised that chickpeas make a great gluten-free (and more nutritious) alternative to wheat flour in baking, as they provide the same substance and floury texture. I've used them in these chocolate nut-butter cookies to boost their nutrition.

1. Preheat oven to 170°C. Line a baking tray with baking paper. Pat chickpeas dry with paper towels. Place in a food processor with nut butter, vanilla, brown sugar, baking powder, ground almonds, and butter or coconut oil. Blitz until all ingredients are well combined and have formed a cookie-dough consistency.

2. Add dark chocolate and pulse briefly to distribute the chocolate throughout the cookie dough.

3. Roll heaped tablespoonfuls of cookie dough into balls — wet hands help deal with the sticky dough — and place on prepared baking tray about 3cm apart (they won't spread much). Flatten slightly with the back of a wet fork.

4. Bake for 20-25 minutes until lightly golden. Remove from oven and leave cookies to cool slightly. Use a fish slice to transfer them carefully to a wire rack to cool completely — they will be quite delicate.

5. These cookies are lovely eaten warm, but also keep in an airtight container in the pantry for up to a week, or frozen for several weeks. Warm a frozen cookie (or two!) for about 10 seconds in the microwave — the chocolate will melt and go gooey.

TIP These cookies are best eaten after microwaving for about 10 seconds — the chocolate will melt slightly and they'll be at the perfect temperature. Yummy with a small glass of milk!

MAKES: 16

PREP TIME: 10 MINUTES

COOK TIME: 12-15 MINUTES

chickpeas 1 x 400g can, drained, rinsed
nut butter (e.g. almond, cashew or peanut) ½ cup
vanilla essence 1 teaspoon
brown sugar ½ cup
baking powder 1 teaspoon
ground almonds 2 tablespoons
butter or **coconut oil** 1 tablespoon melted
good-quality dark eating chocolate (at least 70% cocoa solids) 70g (about ½ cup), finely chopped

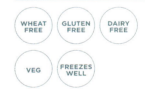

Use dairy-free dark chocolate

AVOCADO, TOMATO, OLIVE + BASIL RYVITA

It's no secret that avocados are one of nature's super foods. They're chocka-full of vitamins and minerals, and their protein and mono-unsaturated fat content means they help keep you fuller for longer. The combination of avocado, basil, tomato and olives makes a healthy, tasty snack.

1. Combine tomatoes, salt, olives, if using, and lemon juice.
2. Spread each Ryvita or Cruskit cracker with a little avocado and top with tomato mixture. Grind over black pepper and garnish with basil leaves.

SERVES: 2 AS A SNACK

PREP TIME: 5 MINUTES

vine-ripened tomatoes 2–3 small, diced
salt pinch of
Kalamata olives 1–2 tablespoons chopped (optional)
lemon juice squeeze of
Ryvita or Cruskit crackers 4
avocado ¼ ripe
freshly ground black pepper
basil leaves 6–8

HEALTHY SNACKS

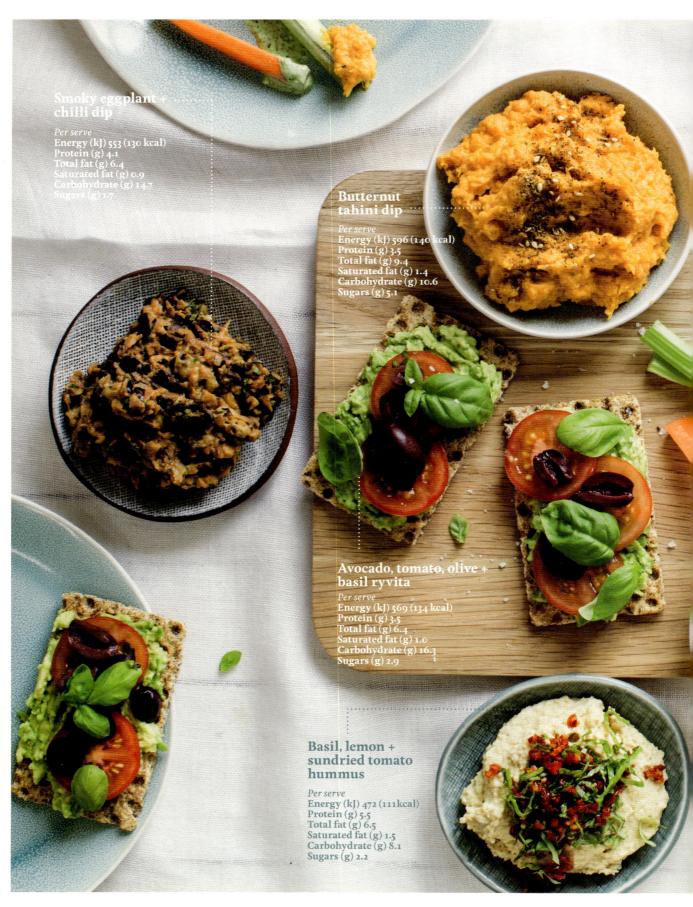

Smoky eggplant + chilli dip

Per serve
Energy (kJ) 553 (130 kcal)
Protein (g) 4.1
Total fat (g) 6.4
Saturated fat (g) 0.9
Carbohydrate (g) 14.7
Sugars (g) 1.7

Butternut tahini dip

Per serve
Energy (kJ) 596 (140 kcal)
Protein (g) 3.5
Total fat (g) 9.4
Saturated fat (g) 1.4
Carbohydrate (g) 10.6
Sugars (g) 5.1

Avocado, tomato, olive + basil ryvita

Per serve
Energy (kJ) 569 (134 kcal)
Protein (g) 3.5
Total fat (g) 6.4
Saturated fat (g) 1.0
Carbohydrate (g) 16.3
Sugars (g) 2.9

Basil, lemon + sundried tomato hummus

Per serve
Energy (kJ) 472 (111 kcal)
Protein (g) 5.5
Total fat (g) 6.5
Saturated fat (g) 1.5
Carbohydrate (g) 8.1
Sugars (g) 2.2

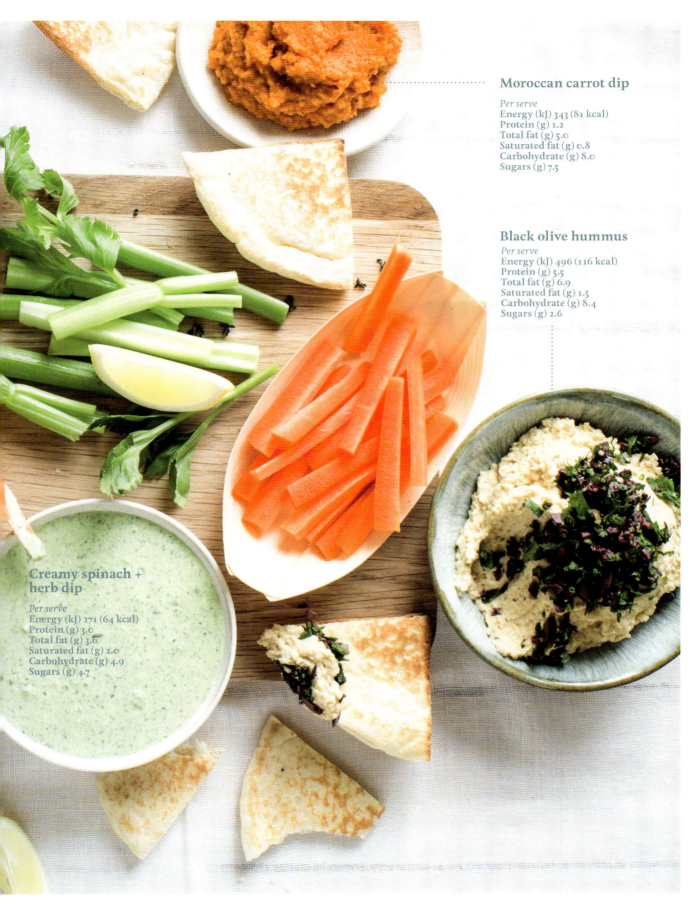

Moroccan carrot dip

Per serve
Energy (kJ) 343 (81 kcal)
Protein (g) 1.2
Total fat (g) 5.0
Saturated fat (g) 0.8
Carbohydrate (g) 8.0
Sugars (g) 7.5

Black olive hummus

Per serve
Energy (kJ) 496 (116 kcal)
Protein (g) 5.5
Total fat (g) 6.9
Saturated fat (g) 1.5
Carbohydrate (g) 8.4
Sugars (g) 2.6

Creamy spinach + herb dip

Per serve
Energy (kJ) 271 (64 kcal)
Protein (g) 3.0
Total fat (g) 3.6
Saturated fat (g) 2.0
Carbohydrate (g) 4.9
Sugars (g) 4.7

DIPS

I love having tasty dips as a snack to fill the gap until the next meal. Serve these with toasted pita bread or vegetable crudités for a gluten-free option.

BASIC HUMMUS

SERVES: 4 AS A SNACK

PREP TIME: 10 MINUTES

Place 1 x 400g can rinsed, drained **chickpeas**, 2 cloves crushed **garlic**, 3 tablespoons **tahini**, 1–2 tablespoons **lemon juice** and a good pinch of **salt** in a food processor and blitz until well combined. With the motor running, drizzle in 4–5 tablespoons **iced water** and continue blending to a nice smooth consistency. Season to taste with **salt** and **freshly ground black pepper**.

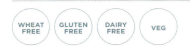

BLACK OLIVE HUMMUS

SERVES: 4 AS A SNACK

PREP TIME: 10 MINUTES

Mix 2 tablespoons pitted, chopped **Kalamata olives** and 1 tablespoon finely chopped **flat-leaf parsley** together and spoon on top of 1 quantity **basic hummus**.

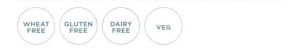

BASIL, LEMON + SUNDRIED TOMATO HUMMUS

SERVES: 4 AS A SNACK

PREP TIME: 10 MINUTES

Mix 2 tablespoons chopped **basil**, zest of ½ **lemon** and 1 tablespoon finely chopped **sundried tomatoes** together and spoon on top of 1 quantity **basic hummus**.

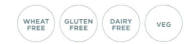

CREAMY SPINACH + HERB DIP

SERVES: 6 AS A SNACK

PREP TIME: 10 MINUTES

Place 125g **lite cream cheese**, 3–4 handfuls **baby spinach**, 1 small clove crushed **garlic**, zest of 1 **lemon**, 2–3 tablespoons chopped **mixed fresh herbs** (e.g. parsley or basil) and 2–3 teaspoons **lemon juice** in a food processor and blitz until well combined. Season to taste with **salt** and **freshly ground black pepper**.

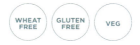

MOROCCAN CARROT DIP

1. Preheat oven to 200°C. Line an oven tray with baking paper. Toss carrots with spices, ginger, honey and olive oil in prepared tray and season well with salt. Roast for about 30 minutes or until carrots are soft and caramelised.

2. Transfer roasted carrots and any juices to a food processor. Add lemon juice and garlic and blitz a few times until well combined — you can leave the texture slightly chunky if you like, or keep blending until it is smoother. Add 1-2 tablespoons or more of water to achieve your desired consistency. Season to taste with salt and pepper.

3. To serve, garnish with chopped parsley or coriander and extra virgin olive oil. Serve with crudités or toasted pita bread.

SERVES: 4 AS A SNACK
PREP TIME: 10 MINUTES
COOK TIME: 30 MINUTES

carrots 3 (about 300g), peeled, sliced 1cm thick
ground cumin 1 teaspoon
ground coriander ½ teaspoon
ground cinnamon ¼ teaspoon
ginger 1 tablespoon minced
liquid honey 1 tablespoon
olive oil 1 tablespoon
salt
lemon juice of ½
garlic 1 small clove, chopped
freshly ground black pepper

TO SERVE

flat-leaf parsley or **coriander** 2 tablespoons chopped
extra virgin olive oil 1 teaspoon
vegetable crudités 1 cup or **lightly toasted pita bread** ½ small per serving

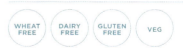

For wheat-free serve with vegetable crudités

HEALTHY SNACKS

SMOKY EGGPLANT + CHILLI DIP

1. Preheat oven to 220°C. Line an oven tray with baking paper. Toss eggplant, olive oil and paprika in prepared tray. Season well with salt and bake for about 20 minutes or until eggplant is very soft and starting to caramelise.

2. Finely chop roast eggplant and mix in a bowl with garlic, lemon zest and juice, cayenne pepper or chilli and tahini. Season to taste with salt. Alternatively, blitz all ingredients together in a food processor if you prefer a smoother texture.

3. To serve, garnish with parsley or coriander. Serve with toasted pita breads.

SERVES: 6 AS A SNACK
PREP TIME: 10 MINUTES
COOK TIME: 20 MINUTES

eggplants 2 medium-sized, cut into 2–3cm cubes
olive oil 2 tablespoons
smoked paprika 1 teaspoon
salt
garlic 1 small clove, minced
lemon zest and juice of 1
cayenne pepper or **ground chilli** pinch of
tahini 2 teaspoons

TO SERVE

flat-leaf parsley or **coriander** 1–2 tablespoons chopped
vegetable crudités 1 cup or **lightly toasted pita bread** ½ small per serving

WHEAT FREE · GLUTEN FREE · DAIRY FREE · VEG

For gluten-free serve with vegetable crudités

BUTTERNUT TAHINI DIP

SERVES: 4 AS A SNACK
PREP TIME: 10 MINUTES
COOK TIME: 25-30 MINUTES

1. Preheat oven to 200°C. Line an oven tray with baking paper. Toss butternut with olive oil and cumin in prepared tray. Season with salt and pepper and roast for 25-30 minutes until soft and caramelised.

2. Crush butternut with a fork or masher and mix with garlic, lemon juice, yoghurt, tahini and coriander. Alternatively, place ingredients in a food processor and blitz until smooth. Season to taste with more salt and pepper if needed. Garnish with dukkah, za'atar or sesame seeds, if using.

butternut 400g, peeled, deseeded, cut into 1-2cm chunks
olive oil 1 tablespoon
ground cumin 1½ teaspoons
salt
freshly ground black pepper
garlic 1 small clove, minced
lemon juice of 1
natural unsweetened thick Greek yoghurt 2 tablespoons
tahini 2 tablespoons
coriander ¼ cup chopped
dukkah, za'atar or **black and white sesame seeds** 1 teaspoon, to garnish (optional)

WHEAT FREE · GLUTEN FREE · DAIRY FREE · VEG

Dairy-free with coconut yoghurt

KALE CHIPS

Kale chips make a delicious, crunchy, salty snack — just like deep-fried potato chips, but considerably better for you!

1. Preheat oven to 120°C. Line an oven tray with baking paper. Tear kale leaves into roughly 3-4cm bite-sized pieces and pat dry with paper towels. Toss kale well with olive oil, chilli flakes, if using, and sesame seeds in prepared tray. Season with just a pinch of flaky salt — be careful not to over-salt.

2. Arrange in a single layer on the tray and bake for 30-40 minutes until crispy. The kale will go a dark green colour with a little brown around the edges. You don't want the chips to burn or they will taste bitter, so watch carefully and take them out as soon as the chips are done.

3. Serve in a bowl for a tasty, salty, crispy snack.

TIP Make sure you use curly kale, as other varieties of kale do not work as well and tend not to crisp up, or burn. Feel free to play around with different flavours — a pinch of curry powder, cumin or smoked paprika are all good!

SERVES: 2 AS A SNACK
PREP TIME: 5 MINUTES
COOK TIME: 30-40 MINUTES

curly kale 150g, tough stems removed
olive oil 1 tablespoon
chilli flakes pinch of (optional)
sesame seeds 1 teaspoon
flaky sea salt pinch of

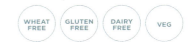

WHEAT FREE | GLUTEN FREE | DAIRY FREE | VEG

Per serve
Energy (kJ) 331 (78 kcal)
Protein (g) 1.6
Total fat (g) 7.7
Saturated fat (g) 1.3
Carbohydrate (g) 0.7
Sugars (g) 0.7

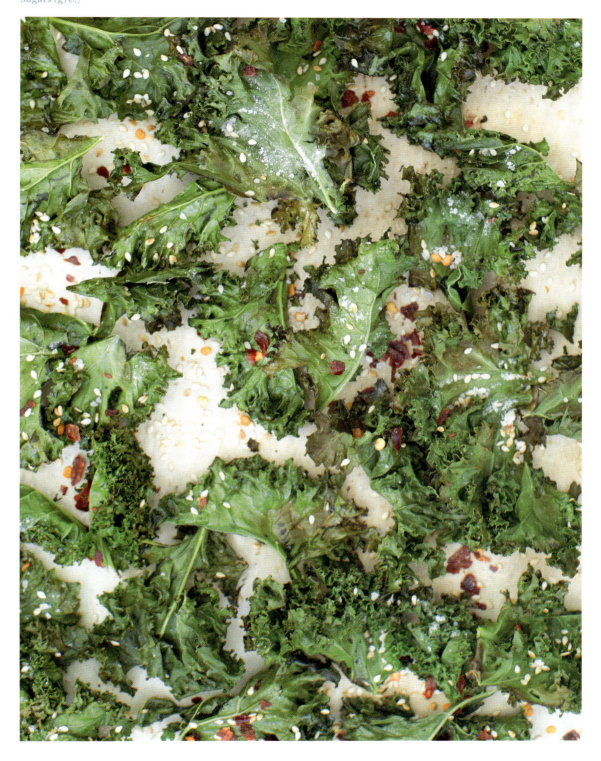

HEALTHY SNACKS

ESSENTIALS

CARAMELISED ONIONS

MAKES: ¾ CUP   PREP TIME: 10 MINUTES

Heat 1 tablespoon **olive oil** in a medium frying pan over medium heat. Cook 2 **onions**, thinly sliced, for about 6-8 minutes, until soft and browned. Stir occasionally. If at any time the onions are sticking to the bottom of the pan and burning, just add a tablespoon of water, stir, and continue cooking (they should lift from the bottom of the pan). Be patient and get the onions nice and caramelised, then add 1 teaspoon **brown sugar** and 1 tablespoon **balsamic vinegar**, and continue cooking for about 2 more minutes.

CHERMOULA PASTE

MAKES: ½ CUP   PREP TIME: 10 MINUTES

Place 2 cups (40-50g) roughly chopped **coriander** (leaves and stalks), ½ cup roughly chopped **parsley**, 8 cloves **garlic**, zest and juice of 2 lemons, 2 tablespoons **white vinegar**, 2 tablespoons **ground cumin**, 3 teaspoons **ground coriander**, 4 teaspoons **smoked paprika**, 2 large **red chillies**, ½ cup **olive oil** and 1 teaspoon **salt** in a small food processor and blitz until well combined. Alternatively, very finely chop herbs and garlic and mix with all other ingredients.

JAMAICAN JERK PASTE

MAKES: ½ CUP   PREP TIME: 10 MINUTES

Place 2 **spring onions**, chopped, 3 tablespoons **thyme leaves**, 2.5cm piece of **ginger**, peeled and chopped, 4 cloves **garlic**, chopped, 1 tablespoon **ground allspice**, 2 tablespoons **brown sugar**, juice of 2 **limes**, 1 tablespoon **tomato paste**, 1 tablespoon **soy sauce**, ¼ cup **olive oil**, 2 large **red chillies** and 1 teaspoon **salt** in a small food processor and blitz until well combined.

HARISSA PASTE

MAKES: ½ CUP   PREP TIME: 10 MINUTES

Place 3 cloves **garlic**, chopped, 1-2 large **red chilies**, chopped, 1½ tablespoons crushed **cumin seeds**, 1 tablespoons crushed **coriander seeds**, ¼ cup **olive oil**, 2 tablespoons **tomato paste**, 1 teaspoon **brown sugar**, juice of ½ **lemon** and 1 teaspoon **salt** in a small food processor and blitz until well combined.

KASUNDI (INDIAN SPICED TOMATO CHUTNEY)

MAKES: 1 CUP   PREP TIME: 10 MINUTES

Heat 2 tablespoons **oil** in a medium frying pan over medium heat. Cook 1 **onion**, diced, for a few minutes until soft. Add 1½ teaspoons crushed **cumin seeds** or **ground cumin**, 1 teaspoon crushed **coriander seeds** or **ground coriander**, ½–1 teaspoon **ground chilli** or **chilli flakes**, and 1 teaspoon crushed **fennel seeds** (optional) and continue cooking for a further 2 minutes. Add 1 x 400g can **crushed tomatoes**, 2 teaspoons **sugar** and 2 teaspoons **vinegar**. Simmer for 10–15 minutes until reduced to a thick chutney-like consistency. Season to taste with **salt** and **pepper**.

LEAFY GREEN SALAD

PREP TIME: 5 MINUTES

Per serving: Toss a large handful of **green salad leaves** (e.g. rocket, mesclun, lettuce, mizuna, watercress, baby spinach, or a mixture) with ½ teaspoon **extra virgin olive oil**, squeeze of **lemon** and pinch of **salt** just before serving.

LAKSA PASTE

MAKES: ⅔ CUP   PREP TIME: 10 MINUTES

Place 5 small, peeled **shallots**, 3 cloves **garlic**, 2.5cm piece **ginger**, peeled and chopped, 2 large stalks **lemongrass**, finely chopped, 1 large **red chilli**, chopped, ¼ cup **raw cashew nuts**, 1 tablespoon **dried shrimp paste** (belachan), 1 teaspoon **ground turmeric**, 1 teaspoon **ground cumin**, 2 teaspoons **ground coriander**, 1 teaspoon **ground chilli** and 1½ teaspoons **salt** in a small food processor and blend until a smooth paste forms. Alternatively, you can bash and grind the ingredients together in a large mortar and pestle. Heat 1 tablespoon **oil** in a medium frying pan over medium heat and cook laksa paste for 3–4 minutes until fragrant and thickened. Add 1–2 tablespoons **coconut milk** during cooking to loosen the paste, if you need to.

LEMONGRASS PASTE

MAKES: ½ CUP   PREP TIME: 10 MINUTES

Place 3 stalks **lemongrass** (tough outer layer removed), 2 tablespoons **oil**, 2½ tablespoons **fish sauce**, 2 teaspoons each **ground turmeric**, **brown sugar** and minced **red chilli** and 2 cloves **garlic** in the bowl of a small food processor and blitz until a paste forms. Alternatively, pound all ingredients together in a mortar and pestle.

PIZZA SAUCE

MAKES: 1 CUP   PREP TIME: 15 MINUTES

Heat 2 tablespoons **olive oil** in a medium frying pan over medium heat. Cook 1 **onion**, diced, and 2 cloves **garlic**, finely chopped, for 3-4 minutes until soft. Stir in 3-4 tablespoons **tomato paste** and 1 x 400g can **crushed tomatoes**. Simmer uncovered, stirring occasionally, until sauce is thick and jam-like. Season to taste with salt and pepper.

PINEAPPLE + COCONUT SALSA

MAKES: 1 CUP   PREP TIME: 15 MINUTES

Heat 1 teaspoon **oil** in a small frying pan over medium heat. Cook 10-15 **fresh curry leaves** for 1-2 minutes until fragrant, then add 2 tablespoons **thread coconut** and continue to fry for 1 minute further until coconut is golden brown. Combine curry leaves and coconut with 1 cup finely diced **fresh** or **canned pineapple**, 1 large **red chilli**, diced, 1 **spring onion**, diced, ½ cup chopped **coriander** and juice of 1 **lime** and season to taste with **salt**.

QUICK BEETROOT RELISH

MAKES: 1 CUP   PREP TIME: 15 MINUTES

Heat 1 tablespoon **olive oil** in a frying pan over medium heat. Cook ½ small red **onion**, sliced, for 2-3 minutes until soft and just starting to caramelise. Add 2 cups coarsely grated **beetroot** (about 1 medium-sized beetroot), 1 teaspoon grated **ginger**, 1 tablespoon **balsamic vinegar** and 2 teaspoons **liquid honey** and continue cooking, stirring frequently, for 3-4 minutes.

SALSA VERDE

MAKES: ½ CUP   PREP TIME: 10 MINUTES

Place ½ cup roughly chopped **flat-leaf parsley**, 1½ tablespoons **thyme leaves**, 1 small clove **garlic**, chopped, 2 teaspoons **capers** and 2 **anchovy fillets** (optional) in a pile on a chopping board and finely chop everything together. Place in a bowl and mix in 1 teaspoon **Dijon mustard**, 2 tablespoons **lemon juice** and 2 tablespoons **extra virgin olive oil**. Season to taste with **salt** and **pepper**.

SWEET CHILLI DRESSING

MAKES: ½ CUP   PREP TIME: 5 MINUTES

Combine 2 tablespoons **sweet chilli sauce**, 3 tablespoons **lemon** or **lime** juice and 2 tablespoons **extra virgin olive oil**. Will keep in the fridge for a week.

TAHINI DRESSING

MAKES: ½ CUP   PREP TIME: 5 MINUTES

Combine 4 tablespoons natural unsweetened **yoghurt**, 2 teaspoons **tahini**, 1 teaspoon liquid **honey**, juice of ½ **lemon** and ½ **clove garlic**, minced. Mix well.

TOMATO + AVOCADO SALSA

MAKES: 2 CUPS   PREP TIME: 10 MINUTES

Mix together 3 diced **tomatoes**, 1 diced ripe **avocado**, ½ small **red onion**, finely diced, ½ cup chopped **coriander** and 2 tablespoons **lime** or **lemon** juice. Season to taste with **salt**.

TOMATO + BASIL SALAD

PREP TIME: 5 MINUTES

Per serving: Toss 1 large (or 2 smaller) **tomatoes**, cut into wedges, with a small handful of **basil** leaves, ½ teaspoon each **extra virgin olive oil** and **balsamic vinegar**.

TANDOORI PASTE

MAKES: ½ CUP   PREP TIME: 5 MINUTES

Mix together 1 tablespoon **ground cumin**, 2 teaspoons **ground coriander**, 1 tablespoon **smoked paprika**, 1 teaspoon **ground turmeric**, ½–1 teaspoon **ground chilli**, 1 teaspoon minced/grated **fresh ginger**, 2 cloves **garlic**, minced, 2 tablespoons **tomato paste**, 1 teaspoon **salt** and 2 tablespoons **natural yoghurt**.

ESSENTIALS

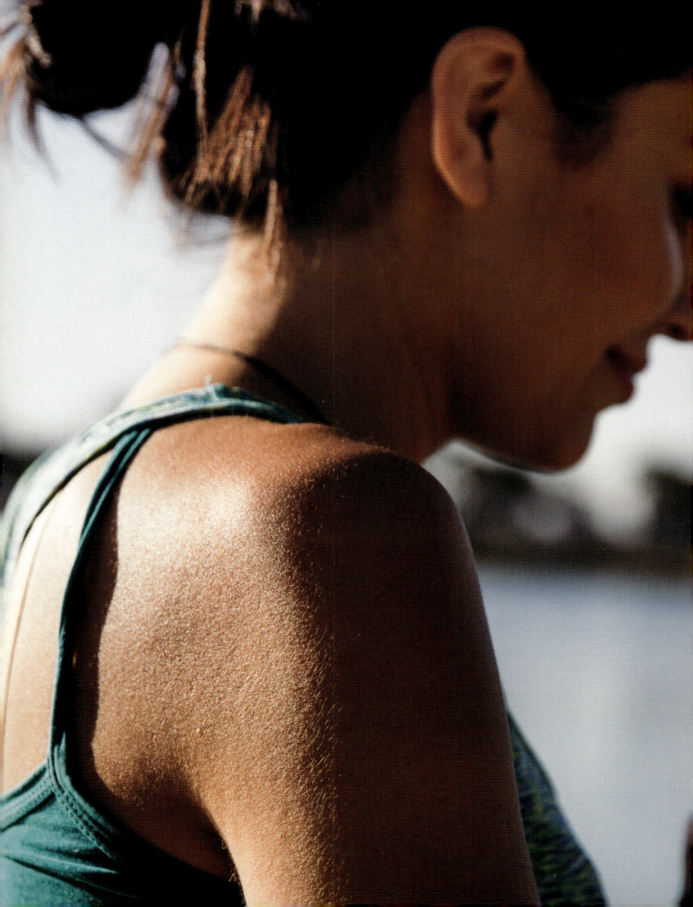

TIME TO GET MOVING

- Exercise is just as important as what you eat, so be sure to make time in your schedule for at least 30 minutes of activity every day. This doesn't have to be all in one go, though — you can break this up into two bouts of 15 minutes or more if that suits you better.

- Use these three levels of exercise programmes to keep stepping up the intensity. Once you get to a certain level of fitness you'll find your body adjusts, so you need to keep pushing the pace.

- Combining a mix of cardio and resistance training gets the best results. Many of us shy away from the weights section at the gym, but we've put together some simple exercises using only your bodyweight (no special equipment or a gym membership needed!) which are easy to master.

- Track your progress by using a notebook, calendar or your smartphone — there are heaps of great apps available for free.

- Most of all, have fun! Exercising shouldn't be a slog or something you dread. Buddy up, join a class, try something you've never done before, and enjoy it. Being active can be something you look forward to every day and it should fit in with your lifestyle.

LET'S GET STARTED
BY MICHAEL McCORMACK

Hey everyone, it's Nadia's friend Michael McCormack here. I've been incredibly passionate about health, fitness and sport for as long as I can remember. I studied Physical Education at Otago University, specialising in Exercise Prescription, and for the last 10 years my wife and I have been working as certified personal trainers both in New Zealand and internationally with all types of clients. Under Nadia's guidance we've designed three levels of exercise programmes — Kick-start, Next Level and Maestro — so that regardless of your fitness level you can get stuck in, see results and enjoy all the benefits of being active.

What's great about these programmes is that you don't need any special equipment or a gym membership — all you need is the right attitude! My aim is to make exercise as practical, convenient and fun as possible. Being active can be something that you look forward to each day and it should fit in with your lifestyle (not the other way around).

Our bodies can adapt very quickly to the lifestyles we live. If you do nothing, your body slows down, you lose muscle tone and you may gain weight. Fortunately, fast adaptation to exercise means that by being active every day you feel results within just one week.

The secret of getting ahead is getting started. Motivation is what gets you started, but habit is what will keep you going. Research shows that it takes at least 21 consecutive days of doing something for it to become a habit — so push through the first four weeks of the programme and it will become second nature. When the going gets tough during a session, I often remind clients that 'if it doesn't challenge you, it won't change you!'.

A lack of time is one of the barriers I hear about all the time, but this programme helps to conquer that. The sequences are short and sweet, and you can do these exercises anywhere, with or without equipment. If the weather is bad, I've provided indoor alternatives to the exercises. So, really, there are no excuses!

It's a good idea to check in with your doctor before starting your new exercise regime — as well as making sure you don't have any medical conditions that might need to be taken into account, it's also a great opportunity to get some baseline measurements before you start.

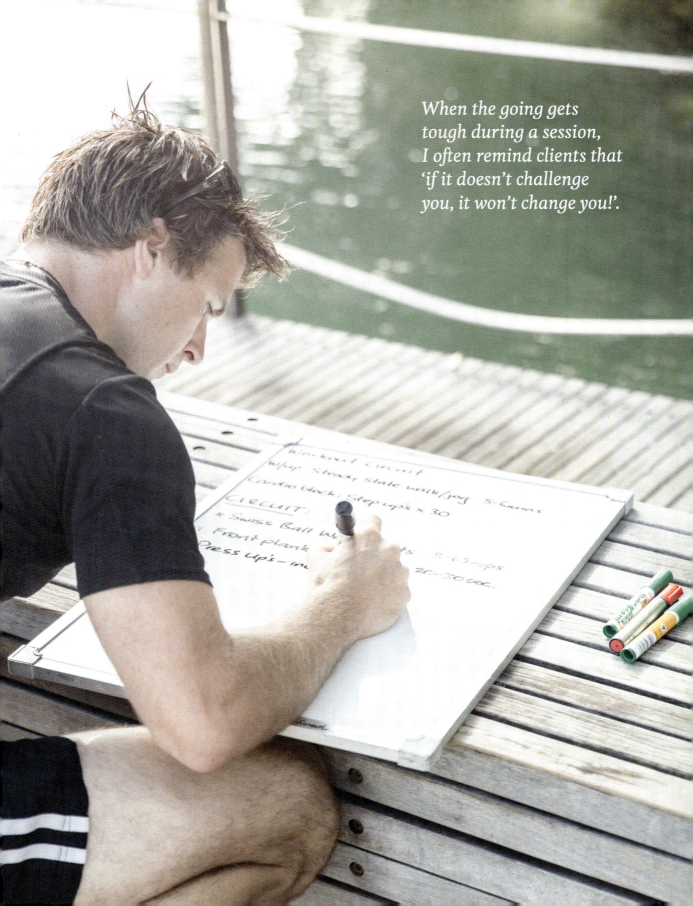

When the going gets tough during a session, I often remind clients that 'if it doesn't challenge you, it won't change you!'.

SET SOME GOALS

To help keep you on track, set yourself both short-term (e.g. fortnightly) and long-term (e.g. 3-6 months) goals. Having short-term goals will help keep you on the right track as you check off each small target with satisfaction. Every 1-2 weeks the goal post should shift closer towards your ultimate goal. Remember, the best goals are habit- and performance-related — focus on achieving these and losing body fat will be a natural outcome. Goals need to be specific, measurable, achievable, realistic and have a timeframe attached (S-M-A-R-T). For example, a short-term goal could be: 'By the end of two weeks (timeframe), I will be able to perform 20 sit-ups on the Swiss ball (measurable), without needing to have a rest (specific)'. For most people this goal is also achievable and realistic. Without a goal, it can be easy to lose sight of what you want to achieve and become complacent. This is what can derail you: being content with where you are now rather than where you want to be. So celebrate achieving your short-term goals and push on from there. It can take around four weeks for you to see your body changing, so don't be discouraged in the early days!

FOLLOWING THE PROGRAMME

Start on the programme level you feel most comfortable with (Kick-start or Next Level for most people), and follow it for six weeks before stepping up to the next programme. You can progress weekly, too, by increasing the number of repetitions for each exercise and shortening the rest periods in between exercises. You could even include a few extra exercises from the next programme up.

You don't need any special equipment; however, a Swiss ball is advised, and also a training diary (a little notebook is fine) and a timing device such as your watch, interval timer or even your phone. If you exercise at the park, gym or elsewhere and don't have this book on hand during your bodyweight resistance sessions, it's a great idea to write down the exercises for that session in your training diary or take a photo of the session plan and exercise demonstrations with your phone to glance at during your workout.

PUSHING THE TEMPO — USING RPE

During the six weeks on each programme the intensity of the sessions will gradually increase. To measure the intensity of the exercise you are doing, you can use a simple scale called RPE (rate of perceived exertion). Perceived exertion is how hard you feel your body is working. It works on a scale of 1 to 10: an RPE of 10 is maximum intensity (e.g. running for your life!), and an RPE of 3 may be equivalent to a casual walk around the block. Keep an eye out for the RPE in the session plans.

Work your way through the weekly sessions as best you can, but if you need more rest than is suggested, take it. Work within your own threshold and not someone else's.

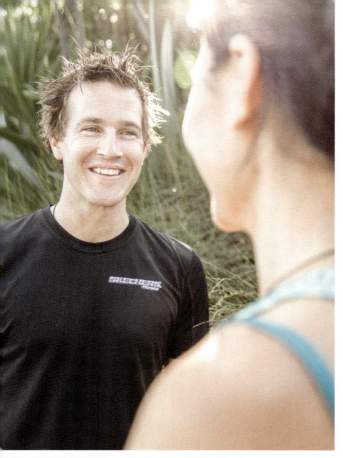
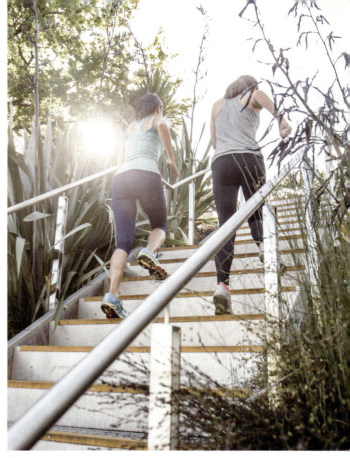
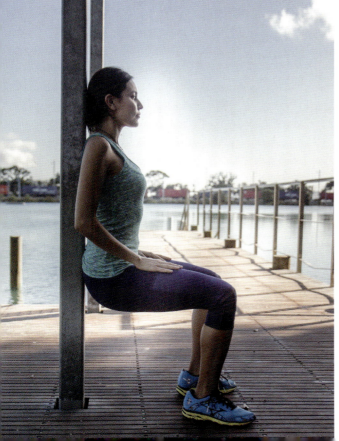
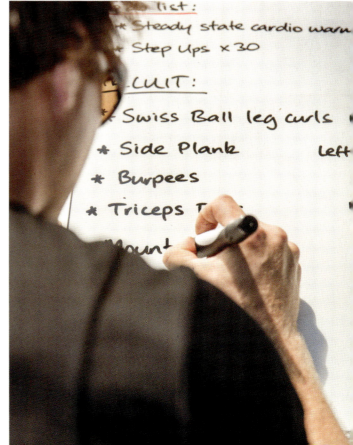

HOW DOES IT ALL FIT TOGETHER?

The programmes offer plenty of variety with a mix of cardio (general fitness) and resistance training (muscle development) working on the upper body, lower body and the core, as well as exercises to help you strengthen weak or inactive muscles. A typical week will include all of the following activities. You can mix up the days to suit your schedule, but make sure you do them all to maximise your results.

Day 1	Charge the Block + Quick-fire
Day 2	Cardio + bodyweight resistance
Day 3	Interval training
Day 4	Flexi-time
Day 5	Cardio + bodyweight resistance
Day 6	Interval training
Day 7	Rest day

WARMING UP

It's a good idea to do a quick warm up before starting each exercise session. You can go for a walk, jog, run up and down stairs or do some skipping. The important thing is to get warm and increase your heart rate. About 5 minutes of warming up is normally enough. Don't eat a large meal within one hour of your session. A piece of fruit beforehand is generally best, along with some water.

CHARGE THE BLOCK + QUICK-FIRE
1 session per week

Find a block near your house or workplace that would take around 30 minutes to walk, bike or run if you were going at a moderate to hard intensity (about 6 on the RPE scale). Once a week you will 'Charge the Block': a race around the block against the clock. This is a simple way of seeing how much your cardio fitness is improving every week. The goal is to take less time to get round the block each week. Make sure you record the time on your calendar or exercise diary each time. When you get back from your Charge the Block all hot and sweaty you will move straight on to 'Quick-fire'.

Quick-fire is a 4-minute bout of four high-energy exercises. Complete 60 seconds of each exercise with a short rest in between to get your breath back. Once you have completed 60 seconds of each exercise you are done.

Stretch after the session for 5–10 minutes. The whole session should take no more than 40 minutes. As the weeks go by, you should be able to do more and more repetitions of each exercise within the 60 seconds.

If it's raining or you prefer to use a gym or you have cardio equipment at home, you can use a treadmill for your power walk or run (around 3–4km), a rower (around 3km) or a bike (around 10km). Each week aim to beat your time from the week before. If you are using an exercise machine, remember to record what setting, incline or level you use and keep it the same going forward so it is consistent each week.

When you progress to the Maestro programme, increase the difficulty of the block challenge by adding more distance or, even better, add in some hills or stairs. If you are using cardio equipment, increase the incline, resistance or cadence (RPM).

CARDIO + BODYWEIGHT RESISTANCE
2 sessions per week

Try to stick to the suggested exercises in each programme; however, you are able to chop and change exercises between the different programme levels if you want to. You might find the corresponding exercise in another programme level a better fit for you, particularly if you have injuries or need to reduce impact on your joints. You should be able to power your way through these sessions in less than 45 minutes. If you aren't sweating by the end of the session, you are either a fitness machine, not working hard enough or could be dehydrated. Sweating during exercise is a good sign!

The cardio + bodyweight resistance sessions run as follows:

Complete the suggested amount of **cardio** (at a moderate intensity) e.g. jogging, skipping, brisk walking.

Complete the suggested number of repetitions (e.g. 10–12 reps) for the first **upper-body exercise**, take a short rest and then move on to the next upper-body exercise.

Repeat this process for the **lower-body exercises**, then move on to the **core exercises**.

When you have completed one set of each exercise, start from the beginning again (excluding the cardio) — you must do three sets of each exercise in total.

When you have finished, enjoy a well-deserved stretch.

How can I challenge myself even more?

Increase the depth (range of motion) of the bodyweight exercises, e.g. getting your chest to the ground in push-ups.

Do the bodyweight exercises more slowly — thus increasing the load on the muscles.

Increase the number of repetitions for each bodyweight exercise — including the weekly Quick-fire set.

Perform exercises such as burpees or the mountain climber faster.

Increase your speed and intensity during the cardio session before you start the bodyweight exercises.

Add an incline (i.e. a hill or some stairs) to your Charge the Block walk, run or bike, or increase the resistance, cadence or RPM on cardio equipment.

Reduce the time you rest between the bodyweight exercises.

Use a lightly weighted backpack during the session (e.g. place tin cans or packets of rice inside it).

As I mentioned before, be sure to challenge yourself. If it's too easy, increase the repetitions or have a look at the exercise progression ideas in the Fit Tips (see pages 307-09). If the repetition range seems too large, do as many as you can and just focus on doing the exercises with good technique.

Resistance training coupled with high-intensity cardio can produce a much better metabolic response than just cardio exercise by itself. After a high-intensity resistance and cardio session your metabolism can remain elevated for up to 18 hours! It is worth working that little bit harder for, as you will burn more calories while you recover.

If an exercise incorporates using one side of the body, make sure you do the same on the other side. If you are doing stationary lunges, for example, and the target repetition range is 10-12, you would do 10-12 reps on the left leg and then 10-12 reps on the right leg.

INTERVAL TRAINING
2 sessions per week

Interval training involves short bursts of high-intensity exercise such as running, skipping or bike sprints, with periods of low-intensity recovery, such as walking, in between. It will lift your heart rate and get you sweating. A watch or phone (there are free interval timer apps available) can make timing super easy. If you live in a residential area, you can even use the distance between power poles as a measure of time or distance. It doesn't need to be exact.

Interval training sessions are high intensity, so the sessions are generally shorter, which should motivate you to keep your effort levels high throughout the session. Ensure you do a 5-minute warm up before starting the session. During the high-intensity phase you should be working near your maximum (an RPE of 9). The recovery phase (an RPE of around 2-3) should allow you to almost get your breath back before starting the next cardio burst. This high-intensity interval training (HIIT) is very effective at boosting your cardio fitness and torching body fat!

FLEXI-TIME
1 session per week

This session is a time to do some activities you enjoy, and that are good for the body and the mind. Try a Pilates or yoga class, do some stretching, play a sport, take part in a dance class or go for a swim.

REST DAY

Take the day off, have a sleep-in and enjoy some down-time. If you are on the Kick-start programme I would suggest you lace up your shoes and go for a short walk. This will keep up the momentum of being active.

KICK-START PROGRAMME

See over the page for exercise descriptions

REPETITION GUIDELINES FOR KICK-START
Make sure you rest for no longer than 60 seconds between exercises.

WEEK 1
8-10 repetitions per exercise per set

WEEK 2
10-12 repetitions per exercise per set

WEEK 3
12-15 repetitions per exercise per set

WEEK 4-6
15-20 repetitions per exercise per set

DAY ONE

20-25 minutes of Charge the Block + Quick-fire

Squats, push-ups, hip bridges and burpees — 60 seconds each

DAY TWO

15 minutes of cardio + bodyweight resistance exercises (see above for repetition guidelines)

UPPER-BODY EXERCISES X 3 SETS
Kneeling push-ups and superman

LOWER-BODY EXERCISES X 3 SETS
Squats and hip bridge

CORE X 3 SETS
Front plank (on your knees or toes)
Aim for a minimum of 30 seconds

DAY THREE

20 minutes of interval training

30 seconds of high-intensity exercise (RPE 9), e.g. running, skipping, running up stairs, followed by 60 seconds of recovery exercise (RPE 3)

DAY FOUR

Flexi-time

45 minutes of your choice of recreational exercise, e.g. swimming, Pilates, yoga, tennis or a walk

DAY FIVE

15 minutes of cardio + bodyweight resistance exercises

UPPER-BODY EXERCISES X 3 SETS
Triceps dips with bent knees and superman

LOWER-BODY EXERCISES X 3 SETS
Wall sit (20–40 seconds) and step-ups

CORE X 3 SETS
Crunches. Aim to do a minimum of 15

DAY SIX

20 minutes of interval training

30 seconds of high-intensity exercise (RPE 9), e.g. running, skipping, running up stairs, followed by 60 seconds of recovery exercise (RPE 3)

DAY SEVEN

Rest day

KICK-START EXERCISE LIBRARY

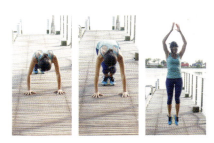

BURPEE

Begin in a standing position. Drop towards the ground into a crouch, jump your feet back into a push-up position, jump your feet back in towards your chest into a crouch, then jump into the air with your arms overhead. For a low-impact option, instead of bouncing your feet backwards when you land, you can walk them back and then forward and finish in a standing position without a jump.

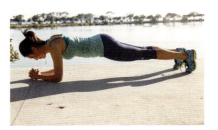

FRONT PLANK

Balance on your elbows and your toes in a face down (prone) position. Engage your core (abdominal) muscles and hold this position keeping your back straight. Balance on your knees for a low-impact option. Don't let your lower back sag down too low.

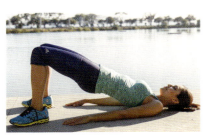

HIP BRIDGE

Lie on your back with your knees bent and feet flat on the ground and hands by your sides. Push through your heels into the floor and raise your hips up to the roof, squeezing your butt. Hold at the top for 2 seconds and slowly lower your hips to the ground and repeat. Try not to touch the ground with your butt between reps.

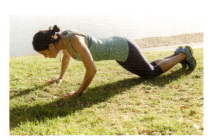

KNEELING PUSH-UP

Same as full-body push-up except that you keep your knees on the ground. Make sure to keep your back straight and that your butt doesn't stick up in the air!

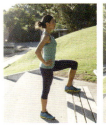
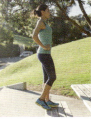

STEP-UPS

Start by stepping onto the bench with your left foot. Bring your right foot up and lift the right knee so it is in line with your hip then lower your right foot down to tap the floor. Keep going on this leg and repeat for the suggested number of reps on each leg. You can use a step, bench, chair or box for this exercise.

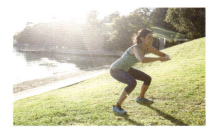

SQUAT

Start in an upright standing position, feet shoulder-width apart. Sit down into a squat, leaning slightly forward with your upper body. Keeping your chest and eyes up, push your butt back and slowly sit down bending your knees, like you are sitting down on an imaginary chair.

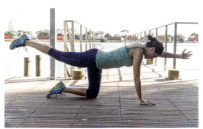

SUPERMAN (OPPOSITE ARM/LEG RAISE)

Start on your hands and knees. Your hands should be flat on the ground directly under your shoulders. Your knees will be directly below your hips, feet resting on the floor. From this position, engage your core (abdominals) and lift and extend one arm straight out the front while extending the opposite leg at the same time out the back, so the arm and the leg are both parallel with the ground. Make sure that your palm faces inwards and your thumb is up towards the roof. Slowly bring the leg and arm back to the starting position. Repeat with the other arm and leg for the set number of repetitions each side.

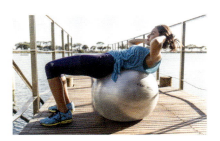

SWISS BALL CRUNCHES/STANDARD CRUNCHES

Lie on your back with the Swiss ball in the lower/middle part of your back. Space your feet shoulder-width apart on the ground and place your fingertips behind your ears. Keeping your chin tucked into your chest, use your abdominals to do a small 'crunch' and slowly return to the start position.

TIP *If the Swiss ball is moving back and forward, you need to tighten your abdominals and keep your hips more stable, or position the ball closer to your butt. You should also feel a good stretch in your upper abdominals when you return to the start position.*

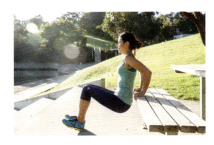

TRICEPS DIPS WITH BENT KNEES

Sit yourself on a bench, chair or step with your hands placed shoulder-width apart. Your fingers will be facing forwards and elbows pointing backwards with a slight bend in them. Extend your legs out in front of you with a slight bend in the knee. Slowly lower your hips off the bench and down towards the ground until there is a 90 degree bend at the elbow. Pause and then push yourself back to the top.

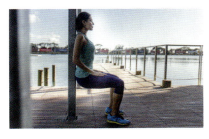

WALL SIT

Start with your back against a wall (or pole) with your feet shoulder-width apart and about two feet from the wall. Adjust your feet if you need to, so that your knees are directly above your ankles. Slowly slide your back down the wall until your thighs are parallel to the ground. Keep your back flat against the wall and your head up. Hold the position for 20 to 60 seconds and increase the length of time as you get stronger.

NEXT LEVEL PROGRAMME

See over the page for exercise descriptions

REPETITION GUIDELINES FOR NEXT LEVEL

Make sure you rest for no longer than 45 seconds between exercises.

WEEK 1
8–10 repetitions per exercise per set

WEEK 2
10–12 repetitions per exercise per set

WEEK 3
12–15 repetitions per exercise per set

WEEK 4–6
15–20 repetitions per exercise per set

DAY ONE

20–25 minutes of Charge the Block + Quick-fire

Squats, crunches, push-ups and alternating lunges — 60 seconds each

DAY TWO

15–20 minutes of cardio + bodyweight resistance exercises (see above for repetition guidelines)

UPPER-BODY EXERCISES X 3 SETS
Full-body push-ups and triceps dips with straight legs

LOWER-BODY EXERCISES X 3 SETS
Alternating lunges and single-leg hip bridge

CORE X 3 SETS
Front plank on toes. Aim for at least 60 seconds

DAY THREE

20–25 minutes of interval training

30 seconds of high-intensity exercise (RPE 9), e.g. running, skipping, running up stairs, followed by 30 seconds of recovery exercise (RPE 3–4)

DAY FOUR

Flexi-time

45 minutes of your choice of recreational exercise, e.g. swimming, Pilates, yoga, tennis or a walk

DAY FIVE

20 minutes of cardio + bodyweight resistance exercises

UPPER-BODY EXERCISES X 3 SETS
Mountain climber and triceps push-ups

LOWER-BODY EXERCISES X 3 SETS
Swiss ball jack-knife and sumo squats

CORE X 3 SETS
Side plank (both sides). Aim for 30 seconds each side

DAY SIX

20-25 minutes of interval training

30 seconds of high-intensity exercise (RPE 9), e.g. running, skipping, running up stairs, followed by 30 seconds of recovery exercise (RPE 3-4)

DAY SEVEN

Rest day

NEXT LEVEL EXERCISE LIBRARY

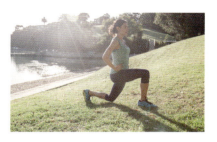

ALTERNATING LUNGES

From a standing position, take a big step forward, while dropping your back knee towards the ground. Your front knee should be bent at a 90 degree angle, so that your thigh is paralled to the ground. Push down through your front foot when you get to the bottom of the movement to push you back up to the starting position. Alternate between legs.

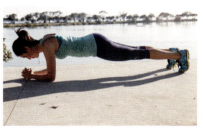

FRONT PLANK

Balance on your elbows and your toes in a face down (prone) position. Engage your core (abdominal) muscles and hold this position keeping your back straight, Balance on your knees for a low-impact option. Don't let your lower back sag down too low.

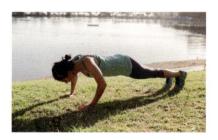

FULL-BODY PUSH-UP

Start in a plank position (face down) with your arms straight and your palms flat on the ground. Engage your abdominals and lower your body until your chest is 15 centimetres from the floor. Make sure your chest, hips and butt all keep in a line and don't drop. Push yourself back up to the starting position.

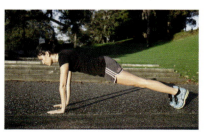

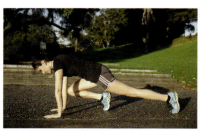

MOUNTAIN CLIMBER

Assume a push-up position so your hands are directly under your chest and shoulder-width apart with straight arms. Your body should form a straight line from your shoulders to your ankles. Lift your right foot off the floor and slowly raise your knee as close to your chest as you can. Return to the starting position and repeat with your left leg. Continue alternating your feet for the desired number of reps or time.

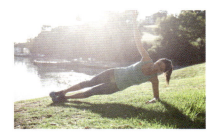

SIDE PLANK

Lie on your side, in a straight line from head to toe, resting your upper-body weight on your forearm. Your elbow should be directly under your shoulder. With your abdominals contracted, lift your hip off the floor. Keep your hips square and your neck in line with your spine as you hold the position for as long as possible. Change sides and repeat.

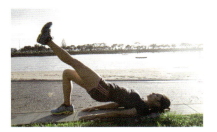

SINGLE-LEG HIP BRIDGE

This is the same as a hip bridge (see page 292) but using only one leg. Keep your foot in line with your hip.

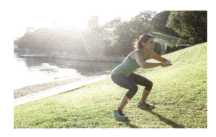

SQUAT

Start in an upright standing position, feet shoulder-width apart. Sit down into a squat, leaning slightly forward with your upper body. Keeping your chest and eyes up, push your butt back and slowly sit down bending your knees, like you are sitting down on an imaginary chair.

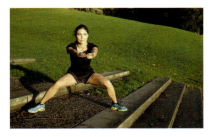

SUMO SQUAT (WIDE SQUAT)

Stand upright with your feet wider than shoulder-width apart, both feet turned out to about 45 degrees. Keeping your chest and head up, lower yourself into a squat, keeping your knees in line with your toes. Come down as far as you can, then push through your heels and come back up to the starting position (don't lock out your knees).

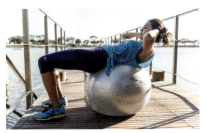

SWISS BALL CRUNCHES/STANDARD CRUNCHES

Lie on your back with the Swiss ball in the lower/middle part of your back. Space your feet shoulder-width apart on the ground and place your fingertips behind your ears. Keeping your chin tucked into your chest, use your abdominals to do a small 'crunch' and slowly return to the start position.

TIP *If the Swiss ball is moving back and forward, you need to tighten your abdominals and keep your hips more stable, or position the ball closer to your butt. You should also feel a good stretch in your upper abdominals when you return to the start position.*

Continued . . .

297

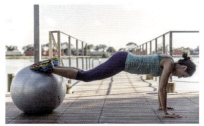

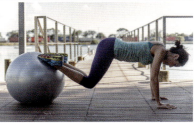

SWISS BALL JACK-KNIFE

Assume a push-up position and place your feet on top of the Swiss ball so your legs are straight and you are hovering above the ground, with shoulders, hips and ankles in line. With your feet on the Swiss ball, pull in your knees to your chest. Pause and then reverse the movement. Repeat.

TIP Get in an 'all fours' position on the floor to start and wriggle your feet up onto the Swiss ball one by one, then lift yourself up to get into the start position.

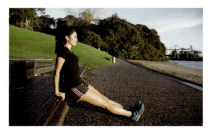

TRICEPS DIPS WITH STRAIGHT LEGS

This is the same as the triceps dip with bent knees (see page 293) except that your legs are extended straight out (knees locked).

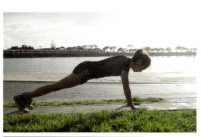

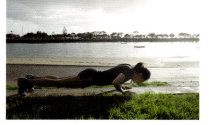

TRICEPS PUSH-UPS (KNEELING OR FULL-BODY)

Hands are positioned close together on the ground underneath the chest. Keep your elbows tucked into your sides to better isolate the triceps. If you need to, balance on your knees intead of your toes.

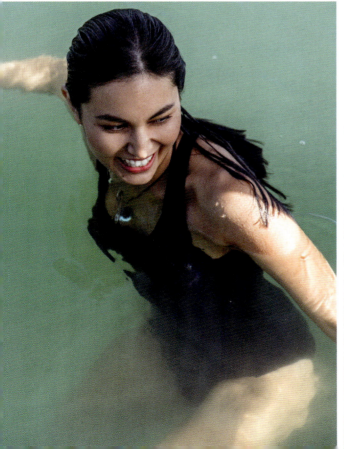
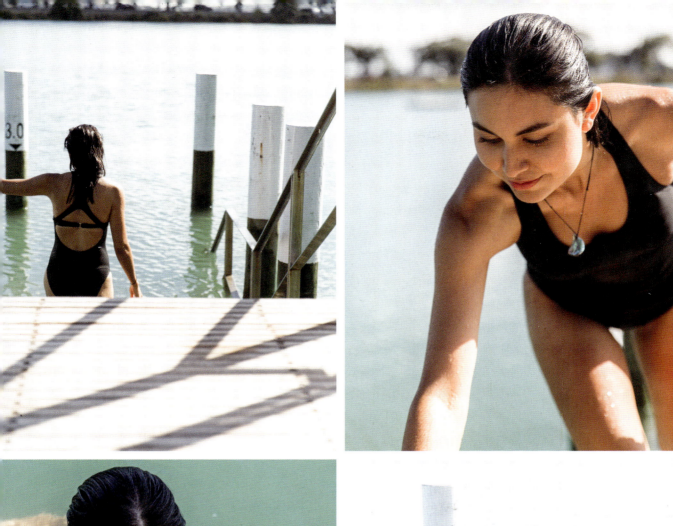
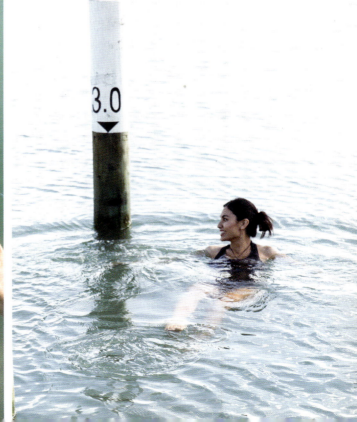

MAESTRO PROGRAMME

See over the page for exercise descriptions

REPETITION GUIDELINES FOR MAESTRO
Complete as many reps as you can for each exercise, focusing on your technique. Make sure you rest for no longer than 45 seconds between exercises.

DAY ONE

25 minutes of Charge the Block + Quick-fire

Squat jumps, burpees and planks — 2 minutes each

DAY TWO

20 minutes of cardio + bodyweight resistance exercises

UPPER-BODY EXERCISES X 3 SETS
Triceps push-ups and Swiss ball jack-knife

LOWER-BODY EXERCISES X 3 SETS
Pulsing sumo squat, burpees and jumping lunges

CORE X 3 SETS
Swiss ball crunches

DAY THREE

25 minutes of interval training

60 seconds of high-intensity exercise (RPE 9), e.g. running, skipping, running up stairs, followed by 30 seconds of recovery exercise (RPE 4)

DAY FOUR

Flexi-time

45 minutes of your choice of recreational exercise, e.g. swimming, Pilates, yoga, tennis, or even just a walk

DAY FIVE

20 minutes of cardio + bodyweight resistance exercises

UPPER-BODY EXERCISES X 3 SETS
Diamond push-ups, Swiss ball plank and mountain climber

LOWER-BODY EXERCISES X 3 SETS
Walking lunges, Swiss ball jack-knife and squat jumps

CORE X 3 SETS
Side plank on both sides
Aim for 45+ seconds each side

DAY SIX

25 minutes of interval training

60 seconds of high-intensity exercise (RPE 9), e.g. running, skipping, running up stairs, followed by 30 seconds of recovery exercise (RPE 4)

DAY SEVEN

Rest day

SO WHAT HAPPENS NEXT?

If you can master the Maestro level it doesn't stop there! Keep setting new goals and look to progress further. You could get a personal trainer to design a personalised programme for you or get some friends together with a personal trainer for a group training session.

You could train towards a triathlon or half marathon to keep the momentum going, or you could just go through the programme again, cutting down on the rest times, adding more repetitions or using extra resistance (see the progression principles in the Fit Tips (see page 307). Your fitness levels will have improved, but there are always ways to challenge yourself even more. Keep your long-term goal in mind and keep moving forwards.

MAESTRO EXERCISE LIBRARY

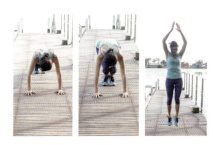

BURPEE

Begin in a standing position, drop towards the ground into a crouch, jump your feet back into a push-up position, jump your feet back in towards your chest into a crouch, then jump into the air with your arms overhead. For a low-impact option, instead of bouncing your feet backwards when you land, you can walk them back and then forward and finish in a standing position without a jump.

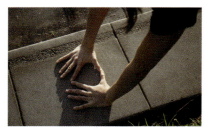

DIAMOND PUSH-UP

Get into a kneeling push-up position with your shoulders directly above your wrists. Now place your hands close together so your thumbs and index fingers form a triangle or diamond shape on the ground. Perform push-ups with your hands in this position.

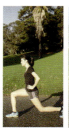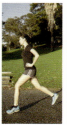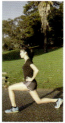

JUMPING LUNGE

Begin in a normal lunge position (see page 296) then jump, moving your back leg to the front and the front leg to the back, into a lunge position again. Repeat.

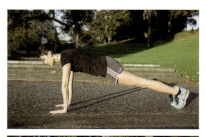

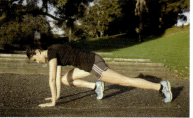

MOUNTAIN CLIMBER

Assume a push-up position so your hands are directly under your chest and shoulder-width apart with straight arms. Your body should form a straight line from your shoulders to your ankles. Lift your right foot off the floor and slowly raise your knee as close to your chest as you can. Return to the starting position and repeat with your left leg. Continue alternating your feet for the desired number of reps or time.

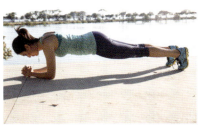

FRONT PLANK

Balance on your elbows and your toes in a face down (prone) position. Engage your core (abdominal) muscles and hold this position keeping your back straight, Balance on your knees for a low-impact option. Don't let your lower back sag down too low.

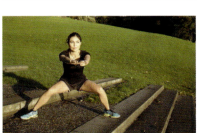

PULSING SUMO SQUAT

Go deep into the squat position with your feet wide apart. Pulse up and down in the deepest position possible.

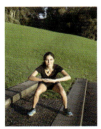

SIDE PLANK

Lie on your side, in a straight line from head to toe, resting your upper-body weight on your forearm. Your elbow should be directly under your shoulder. With your abdominals contracted, lift your hip off the floor. Keep your hips square and your neck in line with your spine as you hold the position for as long as possible. Change sides and repeat.

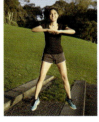

SQUAT JUMP

The starting position is the same for a normal squat, feet slightly wider than shoulder-width apart, chest and head up. From this position, drop down quickly into a deep squat. When you get to the bottom of the squat, power back up explosively into a jump so your feet leave the ground. Land softly in a squat position.

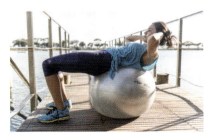

SWISS BALL CRUNCHES/STANDARD CRUNCHES

Lie on your back with the Swiss ball in the lower/middle part of your back. Space your feet shoulder-width apart on the ground and place your fingertips behind your ears. Keeping your chin tucked into your chest, use your abdominals to do a small 'crunch' and slowly return to the start position.

TIP *If the Swiss ball is moving back and forward, you need to tighten your abdominals and keep your hips more stable, or position the ball closer to your butt. You should also feel a good stretch in your upper abdominals when you return to the start position.*

Continued . . .

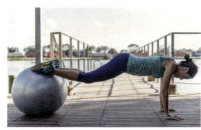

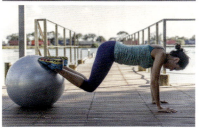

SWISS BALL JACK-KNIFE

Assume a push-up position and place your feet on top of the Swiss ball so your legs are straight and you are hovering above the ground: shoulders, hips and ankles in line. With your feet on the Swiss ball, pull in your knees to your chest. Pause and then reverse the movement. Repeat again.

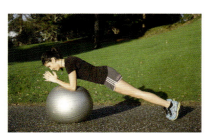

SWISS BALL PLANK

Start in a kneeling position on the floor with your elbows resting on top of the Swiss ball. Now lift your body up so you are in a standard plank position but on the Swiss ball. Your toes will be touching the ground and your elbows will be directly below your shoulders on the Swiss ball. Hold this position for as long as you can, keeping your back flat and abdominals engaged. Don't slouch over the ball.

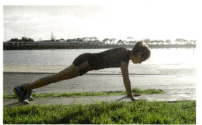

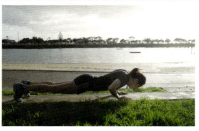

TRICEPS PUSH-UPS (KNEELING OR FULL-BODY)

Hands are positioned close together on the ground underneath the chest. Keep your elbows tucked into your sides to better isolate the triceps.

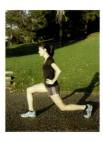
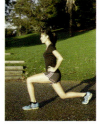

WALKING LUNGES

Step forward with the leading leg into a lunge position. Land on the heel, then the forefoot. Lower your body by flexing the knee and hip of the front leg until the knee of rear leg is almost in contact with floor. Stand on the forward leg with the assistance of rear leg. Lunge forward with opposite leg. Keep lunging forwards, alternating legs.

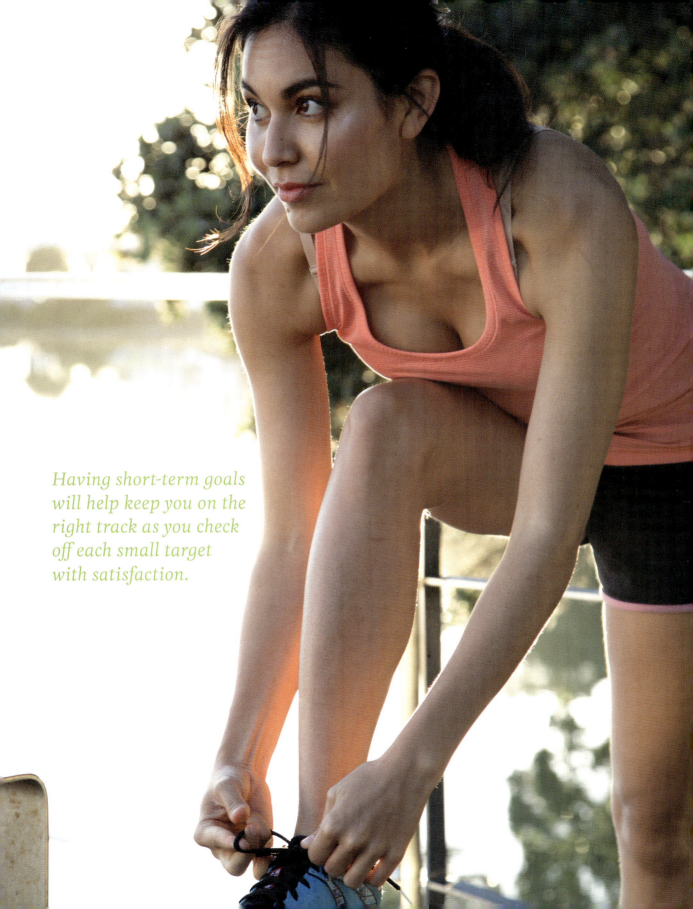

Having short-term goals will help keep you on the right track as you check off each small target with satisfaction.

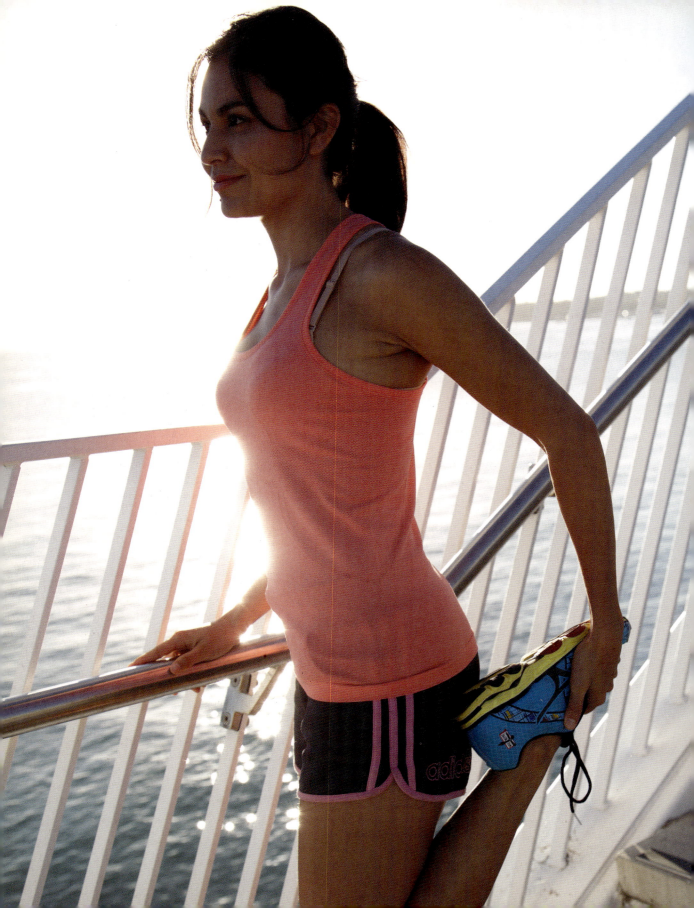

FIT TIPS

Here are a few tips to help you along the way

TRACK YOUR EFFORTS

Write down in a notebook or training diary what you get through each day. Some exercise is always better than none! So even if you only complete 80% of the session, that's okay. Record where you get up to and try to get further next time. You will reach your goals much faster than someone who isn't using a recording system. If you have a smartphone, MyFitnessPal is a free and easy-to-use health and fitness app that can help you along the way; you can even connect with your mates and keep each other accountable.

BODY COMPOSITION

If you want to tone up, focus on body-fat reduction rather than looking at your weight on the scales. With this programme you will lose fat and gain muscle, so the number on the scales may not change every week. However, your body will feel firmer and you will feel more energised.

PROGRESSION PRINCIPLES: FITT

If you stop seeing results, you have reached a plateau and you must change something. To get back on track, identify which one (or two) things might be causing your plateau and make an action plan to change it. The body needs progressive 'overload' to achieve long-term development.

Frequency: One or two workouts a week will improve your health, but will not make much difference to your shape. That's why I suggest at least five bouts of activity a week, to get you looking amazing and turn you into a fat-burning machine.

Intensity (measured by RPE): You will burn some calories when you are working out and then you keep burning calories when you are recovering. The intensity of your workout will determine how long your metabolism remains elevated and how much body fat you will lose. Intensity can be increased by the amount of resistance, speed, tempo (speed of the muscle contraction), distance or time.

Time: Increase the length of your sessions. You may even like to try changing the time of day you exercise, e.g. first thing in the morning to kick-start the fat-burning process all day long.

Type: Your body will only change if it feels it has to, which is why this programme is designed to change the exercise you do each day: cardio, resistance, interval, core and rest. When your body is forced to adapt it gets stronger and develops more lean muscle tissue.

COMMIT TO THE PLAN

Schedule exercise into your day with a variety of before and after work hours (yes, that probably means getting up an hour earlier a couple of times a week — but trust me, you'll feel great afterwards and for the rest of the day!). Identify your barriers to being active and generate a plan that will break them down. Use a big calendar and keep it in a busy place of the house. Every day you don't work out, mark it with a big red 'X', and when you complete a session give yourself a big green tick. If you miss a couple of days in a row, the red marks will be a great visual reminder that it's time to refocus and get going again.

BUDDY UP

Why? For motivation, accountability, companionship, new ideas, competition and fun. Find a friend to do this programme with, try new exercise classes in your area for your Flexi-time or enter an upcoming event. Some of my clients have even paid for another client's entry fee into an event so they have to do it with them — simply brilliant!

CORE OF STEEL

For a healthy back and a toned abdomen, core work is essential. The plank is one of the best exercises to give you a strong core and, in conjunction with an excellent nutrition plan, a flat waistline. People often talk about 'activating the core'. In reality, it is very difficult to isolate one particular deep core muscle at a time. However, stiffening all of the abdominal wall muscles together with your back muscles when performing an exercise will create more spine stability.

REST

Your muscles repair and grow when you rest. If your body is constantly fatigued from long hours at work or stress, you won't get the results you are after. Get into a good bedtime routine and get at least seven hours' sleep a night. People who get enough sleep make better choices with their nutrition and are more successful in their fitness journey.

MUSCLE SORENESS

The muscle soreness that may come with doing new exercises should be expected when you are working your muscles hard and they can sometimes last up to 2–3 days after a session. Dr David J. Szymanski, an expert in exercise physiology, explains that delayed onset muscle soreness (DOMS) 'is normally associated with something negative, but it's actually a physiologically positive reaction'. Muscle tissue is repairing, recruiting more muscle fibres and getting stronger so it is better prepared for those challenging exercises in the coming weeks. There is credibility to the old saying 'No pain, no gain'.

HYDRATE

Cells, especially fat-burning muscle cells, function best when hydrated. Buy a large water bottle (1L or 1.25L) and aim to drink two by the end of the day. Because you are going to be more active, you will need more water than usual. A common mistake is to confuse hunger with thirst. If you think you are hungry, have a full glass of water instead.

BALANCED TRAINING

This programme aims to help you train all your muscles in a balanced fashion. This helps prevent injury, and is why each session includes exercises for upper and lower body and your core. Don't skip the exercises that you find challenging — chances are this is an area of weakness that you need to strengthen most.

STRETCHING GUIDELINES

Some people like to stretch before exercise, and that is fine, but make sure that your stretches are dynamic rather than static. Dynamic stretches involve moving the muscles through a comfortable range of motion a number of times, e.g. swinging your leg back and forth. Dynamic stretching will help to maintain an elevated heart rate after the warm up and prepare your body for action. Static stretching (holding a stretch for 15–30 seconds) should only be done at the end of the session when your muscles are warm.

CREATE CUES

Create an environment at home and in your workplace that provides constant cues to be more active, more often. Put a poster on the kitchen food cupboard of an image and a quote from someone who inspires you, or make it your cellphone background image (how many times do you unlock your phone each day?). Take a Swiss ball to work or leave it in the lounge where it is always visible.

'SNACTIVITY'

Try taking the stairs instead of the lift, or get up to change the TV channel. Try to incorporate incidental activity wherever you can during your day — it all adds up!

FEEL THE BEAT

Create a high-energy playlist of tunes you like on your iPod, and remember to change it up from time to time to stay motivated. Even some upbeat music playing in the car on the way home can help with picking your energy up for a workout in the evening.

COMMUTE

If you have the opportunity to be active on your commute to work, take it! Some ideas include cycling or walking to work, getting off the bus a stop earlier, or parking your car a 10-minute walk from the office.

POSTURE

Take a Swiss ball to work to use as a chair — it will help your posture and strengthen your core. You may even convince your workmates to get one too! Another tip for better posture: whenever you are in your car, take a moment to pull your shoulder blades together and into the seat. Hold the contraction for 10 seconds and repeat five times.

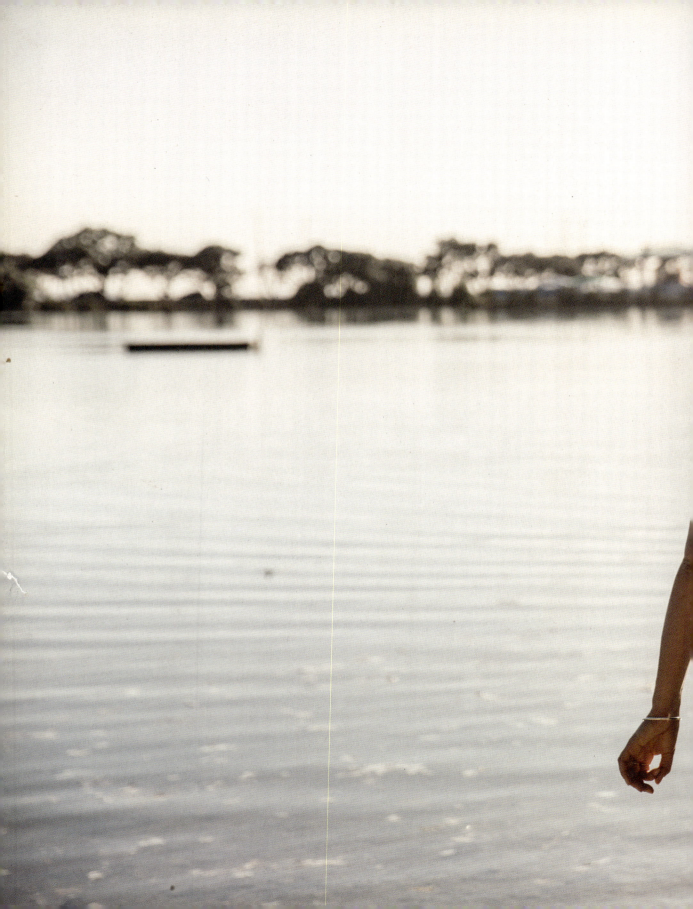

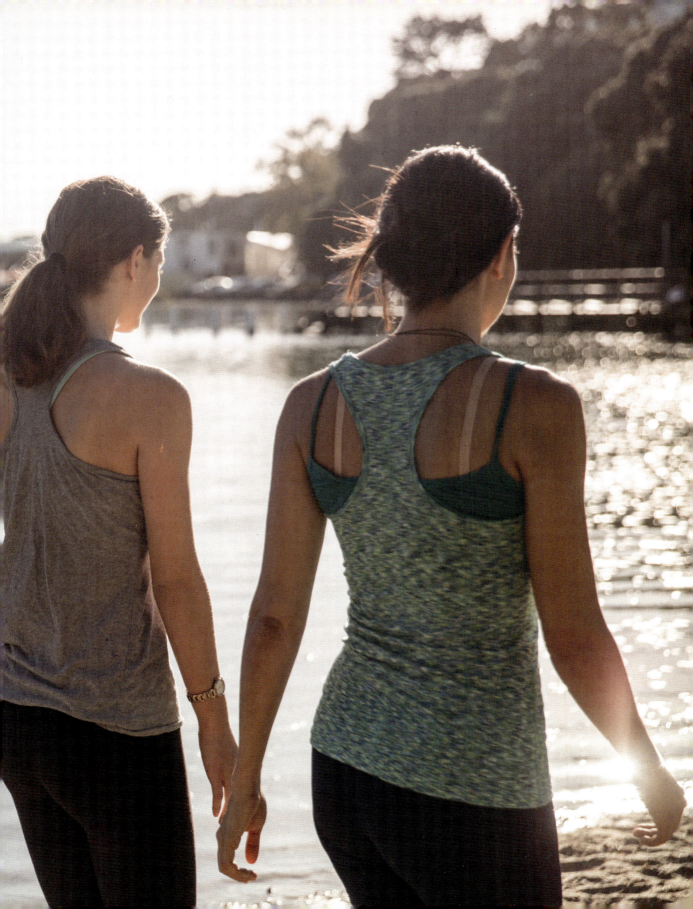

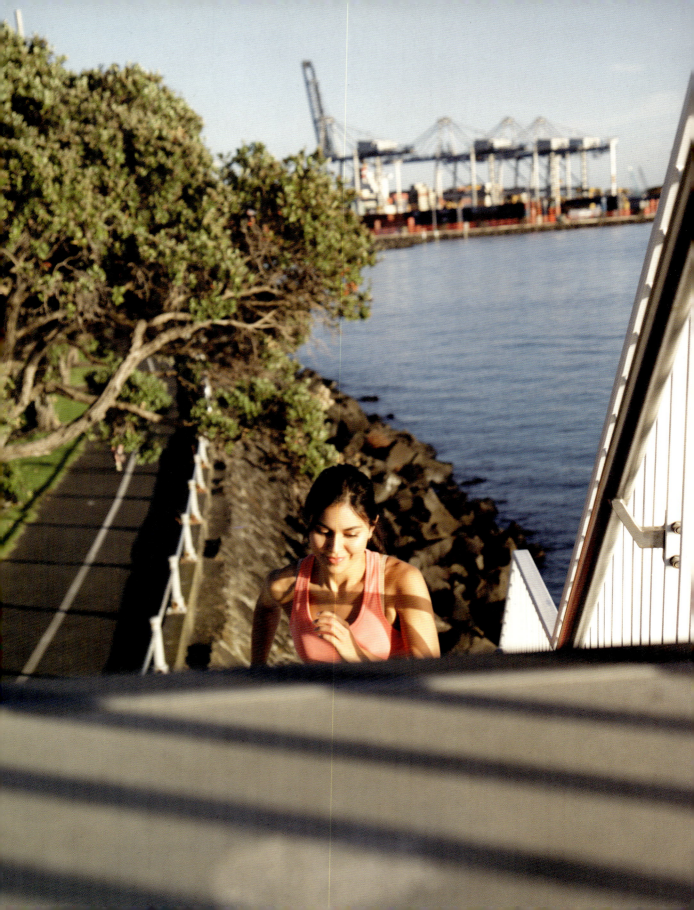

THANK YOU!

Creating this book has been quite a process, and one I couldn't have done without a bunch of awesome, talented and supportive people — family, friends and colleagues — who deserve much more thanks than what I can fit in this paragraph.

Big thanks to Michael McCormack (aka 'Coach Dingo') for creating the exercise programmes and the great exercise tips. I guess I should say thanks, too, for making me run up that hill one more time just when I thought I was going to die!

Thank you Tam West for the beautiful photography, and Factory Ceramics and Taylor Road Homewares for their gorgeous props. Thank you to the team at Strategy Design for their clever design and patience; as well as the Penguin Random House team of Debra Millar, Anna Bowbyes and Carla Sy for getting this book across the line — thanks guys.

Thank you Andreas Eggman, Kay Glendining and my sister Jasmin Lim for helping out with recipe testing — you guys rock, and I really appreciate all your efforts. Extra thanks to Jaz for the nutrition analyses, your patience and being such an awesome sibling. Thanks Nicola Legat for starting off this book, and Jane Collins for the last-minute food styling. Thank you also to the My Food Bag team in both New Zealand and Australia for being such a great bunch of foodies.

Thank you, Mum, for everything. Same goes for my husband, Carlos — my best friend and the best hubby in the world!

Finally, thank you to my fans! It really makes my day meeting you at an event, or chatting on Facebook or Instagram. You have given me amazing support — I'm one lucky cook!

RECIPE INDEX

A
aïoli 208
almond
  honey milk jellies 229
  instant cinnamon, apple + almond bircher bowl 34
  tamarillo, berry, vanilla + almond milk smoothie 33
apples
  apple + sesame slaw 179
  apple, blackberry + date nut crumble 240
  apple, maple + sultana porridge 56
  apple, pear + sultana filo baskets 223
  blackberry + apple porridge 56
  green colada smoothie 32
  instant cinnamon, apple + almond bircher bowl 34
  oaty apple + sultana muffins 257
  raspberry, apple, avocado + yoghurt smoothie 33
apricot cauliflower 'couscous' 182
artichoke, eggplant, mushroom, courgette pizza 127
Asian steak tacos with bok choy slaw 155
asparagus + scorched tomatoes 139
avocados
  avocado, haloumi + grape quinoa salad 102
  avocado, tomato + marmite topping 64
  avocado, tomato, olive + basil Ryvita 267
  guacamole 106
  instant chocolate avocado mousse 247
  Mexican chicken + avocado sandwich 96
  prawn, avocado + mango glass noodle salad 213
  raspberry, apple, avocado + yoghurt smoothie 33
  tomato + avocado salsa 278

B
baba ganoush, roasted red capsicum + sprouts topping 64
bacon
  bacon, pea + egg breakfast fried rice 48
  creamy spiced parsnip soup with crispy bacon 72
  lamb, crushed minted peas, scorched tomatoes, asparagus + bacon 139
  the works 43
baked Cajun tortilla chips with beans + guacamole 106
baked custard 242
baked samosas with pineapple salsa + kasundi 130
baking *see also* confectionery; desserts; muffins
  chocolate berry fudge brownies 238
  chocolate chickpea cookies 266
  coconana bread 66
  cranberry, pistachio + lemon bliss balls 261
  date + cashew caramel chocolate slice 251
  fig + orange bliss balls 261
  garlic naan 190
  home-made biscotti 264
  lemon coconut slice 244
  oat, date + coconut cookies 265
  prune, cocoa + coconut bliss balls 261
balls *see* baking
bananas
  banana + chia porridge 56
  banana coconut caramel smoothie 33
  banana, nut butter, maple + chia seeds topping 64
  chocolate oat smoothie 33
  coconana bread 66
  creamy cashew, banana + cinnamon smoothie 33
  everyday banana pancakes 50
  grilled cinnamon bananas with maple caramelised pecans + yoghurt 226
  hummingbird muffins 256
barley
  braised parsnips, carrots + barley 136
  kale + barley tabouleh 171
  Mexican shredded beef, tomato + barley soup 142
basic hummus 270
basil
  basil, lemon + sundried tomato hummus 270
  creamy basil dressing 118
  tomato + basil salad 279
beans *see also* chickpeas
  bean, corn + kale chilli tacos 122
  chocolate berry fudge brownies 238
  mozzarella quesadillas 78
  prawn, edamame + quinoa stir-fry 100
  Spanish meatballs, beans + cauliflower parsley mash 152
beef
  Asian steak tacos with bok choy slaw 155
  beef tostadas with charred corn salsa 159
  black pepper steak + mushroom pie 146
  broth 145
  ginger hoisin beef, capsicum + peanut noodles 85
  Japanese beef noodle salad 150
  Korean beef + vegetable bowl 149
  Mexican shredded beef, tomato + barley soup 142
  rare beef noodle soup (pho bo) 145
  Spanish meatballs, beans + cauliflower parsley mash 152
  steak, chargrilled capsicum, parmesan + rocket sandwich 97
  steak, smoky kumara fries + salsa verde 141
  vege-packed spaghetti Bolognese 156
beetroot
  apple + berry smoothie 32
  quick beetroot relish 278
berries *see also* particular berries
  berry + cinnamon cream yoghurt mille-feuille 249
  berry yoghurt ice-blocks 260
  chocolate berry fudge brownies 238
  green colada smoothie 32
biscuits *see* baking
bitter chocolate 'ice cream' coated in chocolate + hazelnuts 237
black olive hummus 270
black pepper steak + mushroom pie 146
blackberries
  apple, blackberry + date nut crumble 240
  blackberry + apple porridge 54
bliss balls 261
bok choy slaw 155
braised parsnips, carrots + barley 137
breads *see* baking
breakfast dishes 28–66
breakfast fruit parfaits 55
brie, hummus, caramelised onions + pesto drizzle sandwich 96
broccoli creamy smoked

salmon, leek pasta 200
broccolini, sesame 194
broth 145
burgers, naked burgers 164
buttered lemon cauliflower 'rice' 168
butternut *see also* pumpkin tahini dip 273

C

capsicums
  baba ganoush, roasted red capsicum + sprouts topping 64
  ginger hoisin beef, capsicum + peanut noodles 85
  steak, chargrilled capsicum, parmesan + rocket sandwich 97
caramelised chilli sauce 128
caramelised onions 276
carrots
  braised parsnips, carrots + barley 136
  carrot cake porridge 56
  hummingbird muffins 256
  Moroccan carrot dip 271
cashews
  creamy cashew, banana + cinnamon smoothie 33
  date + cashew caramel chocolate slice 251
  eggplant, tofu + caramelised chilli stir-fry with cashew nuts 128
  Vietnamese chicken, cashew nut + herb noodles 84
cauliflower
  apricot cauliflower 'couscous' 182
  buttered lemon cauliflower 'rice' 168
  cauliflower 'rice' 211
  cauliflower 'couscous' 133
  cauliflower parsley mash 152
  cauliflower-crust pizza with margarita topping 112
charred corn salsa 159
cheese *see also* particular cheeses
  grilled cheese, ham, red onion + pineapple topping 65
  onion + cheese sauce 207
chermoula
  chermoula chicken, pumpkin + cherry tomato bake with coriander + mint yoghurt 184
  chermoula paste 276
  grilled fish with warm chickpea salad 198
cherry + coconut granola 40
chia
  banana + chia porridge 56
  banana, nut butter, maple +

chia seeds topping 64
chia pudding with fruit salsa 232
chicken
  chermoula chicken, pumpkin + cherry tomato bake with coriander + mint yoghurt 184
  chicken + mint salad rolls with peanut dipping sauce 166
  chicken + pineapple curry garlic naan wrap 190
  chicken quinoa tabouleh with yoghurt dressing 99
  chicken + spinach tikka masala with buttered lemon cauliflower 'rice' 168
  chicken, silverbeet, lemon + parsley macaroni soup 172
  harissa chicken steaks with kale + barley tabouleh 171
  lemongrass chicken skewers with mango salad 193
  Mexican chicken + avocado sandwich 96
  oriental poached chicken noodle bowl 181
  paprika chicken with apricot cauliflower 'couscous' 182
  spicy Jamaican jerk chicken, mango salsa + kumara fries 174
  tandoori chicken skewers with lemon, coconut & almond pilaf 176
  teriyaki chicken + crunchy bok choy, apple + sesame slaw 179
  Thai chicken mince salad (laab gai) 188
  Thai roast chicken, pumpkin + spinach bake 187
  Vietnamese chicken, cashew nut + herb noodles 84
chickpea lunch boxes 90–91
chickpeas
  chocolate chickpea cookies 266
  curried chickpea + egg salad 91
  Moroccan chickpea soup (harira) 76
  Moroccan chickpeas 90
  one-pan turkish eggs + chickpeas in smoky tomato sauce 36
  spiced chickpea salad with dates + feta 91
  warm chickpea salad 198
chillies
  eggplant, tofu + caramelised chilli stir-fry with cashew nuts 128
  sweet chilli dressing 279
  tomato jalapeño jam 78
chipotle yoghurt 159
chive yoghurt 78
chocolate
  bitter chocolate 'ice cream' coated in chocolate + hazelnuts 237
  chocolate berry fudge brownies 238
  chocolate chickpea cookies 266
  chocolate oat smoothie 33
  date + cashew caramel chocolate slice 251
  hazelnut coating 237
  instant chocolate avocado mousse 247
  prune, cocoa + coconut bliss balls 261
  topping 251
chorizo, Spanish meatballs 152
chutney *see* sauces
cinnamon, apple + almond bircher bowl, instant 34
coconut
  banana coconut caramel smoothie 33
  cherry + coconut granola 40
  coconana bread 66
  coconut, chilli + coriander steamed fish with soba noodles 202
  green colada smoothie 32
  lemon coconut slice 244
  oat, date + coconut cookies 265
  prune, cocoa + coconut bliss balls 261
confectionery *see also* baking; desserts
  salted caramel fudge 231
coriander + mint yoghurt 184
corn
  bean, corn + kale chilli tacos 122
  charred corn salsa 159
courgettes
  courgette ribbon salad 118
  eggplant, mushroom, courgette + artichoke pizza 127
  cranberry, pistachio + lemon bliss balls 261
cream cheese
  creamy spinach + herb dip 270
  smoked salmon, cream cheese, cucumber + chives topping 64
  sundried tomato + cream cheese-stuffed mushrooms 118
creamed leftover rice 52
creamy basil dressing 118
creamy cashew, banana + cinnamon smoothie 32
creamy mint, mango + kiwifruit smoothie 32

creamy smoked salmon, leek + broccoli pasta 200
creamy spiced parsnip soup with crispy bacon 72
creamy spinach + herb dip 270
cucumber + chives topping 64
curried chickpea + egg salad 91
curried scrambled eggs with tomato + coriander 53
curries
  chicken + pineapple curry garlic naan wrap 190
  chicken + spinach tikka masala 168
  curried chickpea + egg salad 91
  curried potato + spinach hash 71
  lentil + vegetable curry 115

D

dates
  apple, blackberry + date nut crumble 240
  banana coconut caramel smoothie 33
  chocolate chickpea cookies 266
  date + cashew caramel chocolate slice 251
  date nut crumble topping 240
  oat, date + coconut cookies 265
  salted caramel fudge 231
  spiced chickpea salad with dates + feta 91
desserts *see also* baking; confectionery; pancakes; pies
  apple, blackberry + date nut crumble 240
  baked custard 242
  berry + cinnamon cream yoghurt mille-feuille 249
  bitter chocolate 'ice cream' coated in chocolate + hazelnuts 237
  chia pudding with fruit salsa 232
  grilled cinnamon bananas with maple caramelised pecans + yoghurt 226
  honey milk jellies 229
  instant chocolate avocado mousse 247
  lemongrass, ginger + honey poached pears 224
  melon with mint + tamarind, chilli + ginger syrup 218
  pineapple, kiwifruit + passionfruit salad with vanilla syrup + basil 221
  strawberry, basil + lime sorbet 236
dill yoghurt 133

RECIPE INDEX

315

dinner dishes 110–214
dipping sauces *see* sauces
dips 270–273 *see also* sauces
  basic hummus 270
  basil, lemon + sundried tomato hummus 270
  black olive hummus 270
  butternut tahini dip 273
  creamy spinach + herb dip 270
  Moroccan carrot dip 271
  smoky eggplant + chilli dip 272
dressings *see also* salads; sauces
  creamy basil dressing 118
  for apple sesame slaw 179
  for Thai chicken mince salad (laab gai) 188
  for grape quinoa salad 102
  for green mango salad 193
  for Japanese beef noodle salad 150
  ginger hoisin dressing 85
  miso dressing 86
  nuoc cham dressing 160
  sweet chilli dressing 87, 279
  tahini dressing 279
  Vietnamese dressing 84
  yoghurt dressing 99
drinks *see* smoothies

E
edamame, prawn + quinoa stir-fry 100
eggplant
  eggplant, mushroom, courgette + artichoke pizza 127
  eggplant, tofu + caramelised chilli stir-fry with cashew nuts 128
  lentil ragu + eggplant 'lasagne' 121
  roast eggplant, tomato, feta + lime quinoa salad 105
  smoky eggplant + chilli dip 272
eggs
  bacon, pea + egg breakfast fried rice 48
  baked custard 242
  curried chickpea + egg salad 91
  curried potato + spinach hash with smoked fish 71
  curried scrambled eggs with tomato + coriander 53
  egg + spinach topping 65
  French tuna, egg + caper pan bagnat 97
  kale + prosciutto scrambled eggs 53
  Lebanese breakfast wrap with hummus, tomato, spinach + feta 61
  lentil + parmesan mushroom melts with a fried egg 109
  one-pan turkish eggs + chickpeas in smoky tomato sauce 36
  pumpkin, kale + feta frittata 81
  smoked salmon + chives scrambled eggs 52
  spinach + parmesan scrambled eggs 52
  Swedish breakfast smörgås 47
  vegetarian pad thai 124
everyday banana pancakes 50

F
feta
  cauliflower 'couscous' 133
  eggplant, mushroom, courgette + artichoke pizza 127
  hummus, tomato + feta topping 65
  one-pan turkish eggs + chickpeas in smoky tomato sauce 36
  pumpkin, kale + feta frittata 81
  roast eggplant, tomato, feta + lime quinoa salad 105
  spiced chickpea salad with dates + feta 91
fig + orange bliss balls 261
fillings *see* toppings
fish *see also* prawns; salmon; tuna
  chermoula grilled fish with warm chickpea salad 198
  coconut, chilli + coriander steamed fish with soba noodles 202
  curried potato + spinach hash with smoked fish 71
  Mediterranean baked fish with herby spinach + potatoes 204
  oven-baked fish with capers, dill + parsley, wedges + aïoli 208
  root veg topped smoked fish + silverbeet pie 207
flounder, whole flounder with ratatouille 197
French tuna, egg + caper pan bagnat 97
fried rice
  bacon, pea + egg breakfast fried rice 48
  sauce 48
fruit *see also* desserts; particular fruits
  fruit salsa 232
  grilled stone fruit + vanilla lemon ricotta 44
  parfaits 57

G
ginger
  ginger hoisin beef, capsicum + peanut noodles 85
  ginger hoisin dressing 85
  lemongrass, ginger + honey poached pears 224
grape + quinoa salad 102
Greek lamb + spinach spiral filo pie 135
green colada smoothie 32
green mango salad 193
grilled cheese, ham, red onion + pineapple topping 65
grilled cinnamon bananas with maple caramelised pecans + yoghurt 226
grilled stone fruit + vanilla lemon ricotta 44
guacamole 106

H
haloumi
  avocado, haloumi + grape quinoa salad 102
  haloumi + tomato kebabs with roast pumpkin quinoa + tahini dressing 116
  maple-roasted pumpkin + onion soup with haloumi, mint and chilli 75
ham, grilled cheese, red onion + pineapple topping 65
harissa
  harissa chicken steaks with kale + barley tabouleh 171
  harissa paste 276
hazelnut chocolate coating 237
herby spinach + potatoes 204
hoisin pork + vege stir-fry 162
home-made biscotti 264
hummingbird muffins 256
hummus
  basic hummus 270
  basil, lemon + sundried tomato hummus 270
  black olive hummus 270
  hummus, caramelised onions, brie + pesto drizzle sandwich 96
  hummus, tomato + feta topping 65
  Lebanese breakfast wrap with hummus, tomato, spinach + feta 61

I
ice cream, ice-blocks & sorbets *see also* desserts
  berry yoghurt ice-blocks 260
  bitter chocolate 'ice cream' coated in chocolate + hazelnuts 237
  strawberry, basil + lime sorbet 236
icings, chocolate 251
instant chocolate avocado mousse 247

J
Japanese beef noodle salad 150
Japanese salad dressing 150
Jamaican jerk paste 276
jazzed-up porridge 54
jazzed-up scrambled eggs 52

K
kale
  bean, corn + kale chilli tacos 122
  chermoula chicken, pumpkin + cherry tomato bake with coriander + mint yoghurt 184
  kale + barley tabouleh 171
  kale chips 274
  kale + prosciutto scrambled eggs 53
  pumpkin, kale + feta frittata 81
kasundi (indian spiced tomato chutney) 279
kebabs *see* skewers
kiwifruit
  creamy mint, mango + kiwifruit smoothie 32
  fruit salsa 232
  pineapple, kiwifruit + passionfruit salad with vanilla syrup + basil 221
kofte, Turkish lamb 133
Korean beef + vegetable bowl 149
kumara
  chips 164
  fries 174
  smoky fries 141

L
laab gai dressing 188
laksa paste 277
lamb
  Greek lamb + spinach spiral filo pie 135
  lamb baharat with braised vegetables, barley, lemon + olives 136
  lamb with Moroccan chickpeas 90
  lamb, crushed minted peas, scorched tomatoes, asparagus + bacon 139
  steak, smoky kumara fries + salsa verde 141
  Turkish lamb kofte + cauliflower 'couscous' 133
leafy green salad 277
Lebanese breakfast wrap with hummus, tomato, spinach + feta 61

leek, creamy smoked salmon + broccoli pasta 200
lemon
  basil, lemon + sundried tomato hummus 270
  coconut slice 244
  cranberry, pistachio + lemon bliss balls 261
lemongrass
  chicken skewers with mango salad 193
  ginger + honey poached pears 224
  lemongrass paste 277
lentils
  lentil + parmesan mushroom melts with a fried egg 109
  lentil + vegetable curry 115
  lentil ragu + eggplant 'lasagne' 121
lime, strawberry + basil sorbet 236
loaves *see* baking
lunch dishes 68–109

M

macadamias, salted caramel fudge 231
mandarin, peach + ginger parfait 55
mango
  creamy mint, mango + kiwifruit smoothie 32
  fruit salsa 232
  green mango salad 193
  mango salsa 174
  prawn, avocado + mango glass noodle salad 213
maple syrup
  apple, maple + sultana porridge 56
  banana, nut butter, maple + chia seeds topping 64
  carrot cake porridge 56
  maple caramelised pecans 226
  maple-roasted pumpkin + onion soup with haloumi, mint and chilli 75
margarita topping 112
marinades *see* pastes and marinades
marmite, avocado + tomato topping 64
Mediterranean baked fish with herby spinach + potatoes 204
melon with mint + tamarind, chilli + ginger syrup 218
Mexican chicken + avocado sandwich 96
Mexican shredded beef, tomato + barley soup 142
mint
  chicken + mint salad rolls with peanut dipping sauce 166
  crushed minted peas 139

coriander + mint yoghurt 184
creamy mint, mango + kiwifruit smoothie 32
melon with mint + tamarind, chilli + ginger syrup 218
strawberry, mint + lime parfait 57
miso dressing 86
Moroccan carrot dip 271
Moroccan chickpea soup (harira) 76
Moroccan chickpeas 90
mozzarella
  cauliflower-crust pizza with margarita topping 112
  eggplant, mushroom, courgette + artichoke pizza 127
  grilled cheese, ham, red onion + pineapple topping 63
  lentil ragu + eggplant 'lasagne' 121
  mozzarella quesadillas 78
muesli
  instant cinnamon, apple + almond bircher bowl 34
muffins *see also* baking
  hummingbird muffins 256
  oaty apple + sultana muffins 257
mushrooms
  black pepper steak + mushroom pie 146
  eggplant, mushroom, courgette + artichoke pizza 127
  Korean beef + vegetable bowl 149
  lentil + parmesan mushroom melts with a fried egg 109
  sundried tomato + cream cheese-stuffed mushrooms 118
  the works 43

N

naan, garlic 190
noodle boxes 84–87
noodles
  coconut, chilli + coriander steamed fish with soba noodles 202
  ginger hoisin beef, capsicum + peanut noodles 85
  Japanese beef noodle salad 150
  oriental poached chicken noodle bowl 181
  prawn laksa 214
  prawn, avocado + mango glass noodle salad 213
  rare beef noodle soup (pho bo) 145

rice noodle salad 160
roast vegetable + miso dressing noodles 86
sweet chilli prawns, snow peas + sesame noodles 87
vegetarian pad thai 124
Vietnamese chicken, cashew nut + herb noodles 84
nuoc cham dressing 161
nuts *see also* particular nuts
  banana, nut butter, maple + chia seeds topping 64

O

oats 56 *see also* porridge
  cherry + coconut granola 40
  chocolate oat smoothie 33
  instant cinnamon, apple + almond bircher bowl 34
  oat, date + coconut cookies 265
  oaty apple + sultana muffins 257
olives
  avocado, tomato, olive + basil Ryvita 267
  black olive hummus 270
one-pan turkish eggs + chickpeas in smoky tomato sauce 36, 39
onions
  caramelised onions 276
  grilled cheese, ham, red onion + pineapple topping 65
  hummus, caramelised onions, brie + pesto drizzle sandwich 96
  maple-roasted pumpkin + onion soup with haloumi, mint and chilli 75
  onion + cheese sauce 207
open sandwiches 96–97 *see also* sandwiches
oriental poached chicken noodle bowl 181
oven-baked fish with capers, dill + parsley, wedges + aïoli 208

P

pad thai sauce 124
pancakes, everyday banana 50
paprika chicken with apricot cauliflower 'couscous' 182
parmesan
  cauliflower-crust pizza with margarita topping 112
  lentil + parmesan mushroom melts with a fried egg 109
  lentil ragu + eggplant 'lasagne' 121
  root veg topped smoked

fish + silverbeet pie 207
spinach + parmesan scrambled eggs 53
steak, chargrilled capsicum, parmesan + rocket sandwich 97
sundried tomato + cream cheese-stuffed mushrooms 118
vege-packed spaghetti Bolognese 156
parsnips
  braised parsnips, carrots + barley 136
  creamy spiced parsnip soup with crispy bacon 72
passionfruit, pineapple + kiwifruit salad with vanilla syrup + basil 221
pasta
  chicken, silverbeet, lemon + parsley macaroni soup 172
  creamy smoked salmon, leek + broccoli pasta 200
  vege-packed spaghetti Bolognese 156
pastes and marinades *see also* sauces
  chermoula paste 276
  harissa paste 276
  Jamaican jerk paste 276
  laksa paste 277
  lemongrass paste 277
  tandoori paste 279
  Thai marinade 187
peaches
  mandarin, peach + ginger parfait 57
peanuts
  ginger hoisin beef, capsicum + peanut noodles 85
  peanut dipping sauce 166
pears
  apple, pear + sultana filo baskets 223
  lemongrass, ginger + honey poached pears 224
  ricotta, pear, honey + walnuts topping 65
peas
  bacon, pea + egg breakfast fried rice 48
  crushed minted peas 139
  sweet chilli prawns, snow peas + sesame noodles 87
pecans, maple caramelised 226
pesto, hummus, caramelised onions, brie + pesto drizzle sandwich 96
pies *see also* desserts
  apple, pear + sultana filo baskets 223
  black pepper steak + mushroom pie 146

RECIPE INDEX

317

Greek lamb + spinach spiral filo pie 135
pineapples
  chicken + pineapple curry garlic naan wrap 190
  green colada smoothie 32
  grilled cheese, ham, red onion + pineapple topping 65
  hummingbird muffins 256
  pineapple + coconut salsa 278
  pineapple, kiwifruit + passionfruit salad with vanilla syrup + basil 221
  pistachio, cranberry + lemon bliss balls 261
pizza
  cauliflower-crust pizza with margarita topping 112
  eggplant, mushroom, courgette + artichoke pizza 127
  sauce 280
poached eggs + smoked fish 71
pork
  hoisin pork + vege stir-fry 162
  Vietnamese pork meatballs with rice noodle salad 160
porridge 56 *see also* oats
potatoes
  cauliflower parsley mash 152
  curried potato + spinach hash with smoked fish 71
  herby spinach + potatoes 204
  wedges + aïoli 208
prawns
  prawn laksa 214
  prawn, avocado + mango glass noodle salad 213
  prawn, edamame + quinoa stir-fry 100
  sweet chilli prawns, snow peas + sesame noodles 87
prune, cocoa + coconut bliss balls 261
pulses *see* barley; chickpeas; lentils
pumpkins
  butternut tahini dip 273
  chermoula chicken, pumpkin + cherry tomato bake with coriander + mint yoghurt 184
  maple-roasted pumpkin + onion soup with haloumi, mint and chilli 75
  pumpkin, kale + feta frittata 81
  roast pumpkin quinoa 116

Thai roast chicken, pumpkin + spinach bake 187

Q
quesadillas 78
quick beetroot relish 278
quinoa
  avocado, haloumi + grape quinoa salad 102
  chicken quinoa tabouleh with yoghurt dressing 99
  prawn, edamame + quinoa stir-fry 100
  quinoa lunch boxes 99-105
  quinoa salad dressing 102
  roast eggplant, tomato, feta + lime quinoa salad 105
  roast pumpkin quinoa 116

R
raita 176
rare beef noodle soup (pho bo) 145
raspberry
  raspberry, apple, avocado + yoghurt smoothie 33
  tamarillo, berry, vanilla + almond milk smoothie 33
ratatouille 197
relishes *see* sauces
rice
  bacon, pea + egg breakfast fried rice 48
  creamed leftover rice 52
rice noodle salad 160
ricotta
  ricotta, pear, honey + walnuts topping 65
  vanilla lemon ricotta 44
roast eggplant, tomato, feta + lime quinoa salad 105
roast pumpkin quinoa 117
roast vegetable + miso dressing noodles 86
rocket, steak, chargrilled capsicum + parmesan sandwich 97

S
salad dressings *see* dressings
salad rolls, chicken + mint with peanut dipping sauce 166
salads *see also* desserts; vegetables
  apple sesame slaw 179
  avocado, haloumi + grape quinoa salad 102
  bok choy slaw 155
  cauliflower 'couscous' 133
  chicken quinoa tabouleh with yoghurt dressing 99
  courgette ribbon salad 118
  curried chickpea + egg salad 91

  green mango salad 193
  Japanese beef noodle salad 150
  leafy green salad 277
  prawn, avocado + mango glass noodle salad 213
  rice noodle salad 160
  roast eggplant, tomato, feta + lime quinoa salad 105
  spiced chickpea salad with dates + feta 91
  Thai chicken mince salad (laab gai) 188
  tomato + basil salad 279
  warm chickpea salad 198
salmon
  creamy smoked salmon, leek + broccoli pasta 200
  smoked salmon cakes 39
  smoked salmon + chives scrambled eggs 52
  smoked salmon, cream cheese, cucumber + chives topping 64
  sticky chilli salmon with beans, asian herbs + cauliflower 'rice' 211
  Swedish breakfast smörgås 47
  teriyaki salmon skewers with sesame broccolini 194
salsa *see* sauces
salsa verde 278
salted caramel fudge 231
samosas, baked samosas with pineapple salsa + kasundi 130
sandwiches *see also* toppings; wraps
  chicken + pineapple curry garlic naan wrap 190
  French tuna, egg + caper pan bagnat 97
  hummus, caramelised onions, brie + pesto drizzle sandwich 96
  Mexican chicken + avocado sandwich 96
  steak, chargrilled capsicum, parmesan + rocket sandwich 97
  Swedish breakfast smörgås 47
sauces *see also* dips; dressings; pastes and marinades
  aïoli 208
  caramelised chilli 128
  charred corn salsa 159
  chipotle yoghurt 159
  coriander + mint yoghurt 184
  dill yoghurt 133
  guacamole 106
  hoisin pork + vege stir-fry 162
  kasundi 277
  mango salsa 174
  onion + cheese sauce 207
  pad thai 124

  peanut dipping sauce 166
  pineapple + coconut salsa 278
  pizza sauce 278
  quick beetroot relish 278
  raita 176
  salsa verde 278
  smoky tomato sauce 36
  sticky chilli sauce 211
  teriyaki 194
  tomato + avocado salsa 279
  tomato jalapeño jam 78
sauces, sweet
  fruit salsa 232
  tamarind, chilli + ginger syrup 218
  vanilla syrup 221
sausages, Spanish meatballs 152
scorched tomatoes + asparagus 139
sesame broccolini 194
silverbeet chicken, lemon + parsley macaroni soup 172
skewers
  haloumi + tomato kebabs with roast pumpkin quinoa + tahini dressing 116
  lemongrass chicken skewers with mango salad 193
  tandoori chicken skewers with lemon, coconut & almond pilaf 176
  teriyaki salmon skewers with sesame broccolini 194
  Turkish lamb kofte 133
slices *see* baking
smoked salmon cakes 39
smoked salmon, cream cheese, cucumber + chives topping 64
smoky eggplant + chilli dip 272
smoky kumara fries 141
smoky tomato sauce 36
smoothies *see also* drinks
  banana coconut caramel 33
  beetroot, apple + berry smoothie 32
  chocolate oat 33
  creamy cashew, banana + cinnamon 32
  creamy mint, mango + kiwifruit smoothie 32
  green colada 32
  raspberry, apple, avocado + yoghurt 33
  tamarillo, berry, vanilla + almond milk 33
snacks 252-274
sorbets *see* ice cream
soups 145
  chicken, silverbeet, lemon + parsley macaroni soup 172
  creamy spiced parsnip

soup with crispy bacon 72
maple-roasted pumpkin + onion soup with haloumi, mint and chilli 75
Mexican shredded beef, tomato + barley soup 142
Moroccan chickpea soup (harira) 76
oriental poached chicken noodle bowl 181
prawn laksa 214
rare beef noodle soup (pho bo) 145
Spanish meatballs, beans + cauliflower parsley mash 152
spiced chickpea salad with dates + feta 91
spicy Jamaican jerk chicken, mango salsa + kumara fries 174
spinach
  chermoula chicken, pumpkin + cherry tomato bake with coriander + mint yoghurt 184
  chicken + spinach tikka masala 168
  creamy spinach + herb dip 270
  curried potato + spinach hash with smoked fish 71
  egg + spinach topping 65
  Greek lamb + spinach spiral filo pie 135
  green colada smoothie 32
  herby spinach + potatoes 204
  spinach + parmesan scrambled eggs 53
  Thai roast chicken, pumpkin + spinach bake 187
steak, chargrilled capsicum, parmesan + rocket sandwich 97
steak, smoky kumara fries + salsa verde 141
sticky chilli salmon with beans, asian herbs + cauliflower 'rice' 211
sticky chilli sauce 211
stir-fry
  bacon, pea + egg breakfast fried rice 48
  eggplant, tofu + caramelised chilli stir-fry with cashew nuts 128
  hoisin pork + vege stir-fry 162
  Korean beef + vegetable bowl 148
  prawn, edamame + quinoa stir-fry 100
  teriyaki chicken with apple sesame slaw 178
  vegetarian pad thai 124
strawberries
  strawberry, basil + lime sorbet 236
  strawberry, mint + lime parfait 57
sultanas
  apple, maple + sultana porridge 56
  apple, pear + sultana filo baskets 223
  oaty apple + sultana muffins 257
sundried tomato + cream cheese-stuffed mushrooms 118
Swedish breakfast smörgås 47
sweet chilli dressing 279
sweet chilli prawns, snow peas + sesame noodles 87
syrups *see* sauces, sweet

T
tacos *see* tortillas
tahini
  butternut tahini dip 273
  dressing 281
tamarillo, berry, vanilla + almond milk smoothie 33
tamarind, chilli + ginger syrup 218
tandoori paste 279
tandoori roast chicken + vegetables with raita 176
teriyaki chicken + crunchy bok choy, apple + sesame slaw 179
teriyaki salmon skewers with sesame broccolini 194
teriyaki sauce 194
Thai chicken mince salad (laab gai) 188
Thai marinade 187
Thai roast chicken, pumpkin + spinach bake 187
the works 43
toast toppings 64–64
tofu, eggplant + caramelised chilli stir-fry with cashew nuts 128
tomatoes
  avocado, tomato + marmite topping 64
  avocado, tomato, olive + basil Ryvita 267
  basil, lemon + sundried tomato hummus 270
  chermoula chicken, pumpkin + cherry tomato bake with coriander + mint yoghurt 184
  haloumi + tomato kebabs with roast pumpkin quinoa + tahini dressing 116
  hummus, tomato + feta topping 65
  margarita topping 112
  Mexican shredded beef, tomato + barley soup 142
  roast eggplant, tomato, feta + lime quinoa salad 105
  scorched tomatoes + asparagus 139
  smoky tomato sauce 36
  sundried tomato + cream cheese-stuffed mushrooms 118
  the works 43
  tomato + avocado salsa 279
  tomato + basil salad 279
  tomato jalapeño jam 78
toppings *see also* sandwiches; wraps
  apple, blackberry + date nut crumble 240
  avocado, tomato + marmite topping 64
  avocado, tomato, olive + basil Ryvita 267
  baba ganoush, roasted red capsicum + sprouts topping 64
  banana, nut butter, maple + chia seeds topping 64
  chocolate 251
  chocolate hazelnut coating 237
  egg + spinach topping 65
  grilled cheese, ham, red onion + pineapple topping 65
  hummus, tomato + feta topping 65
  margarita topping 112
  ricotta, pear, honey + walnuts topping 65
  smoked salmon, cream cheese, cucumber + chives topping 64
  vegetable topping for pie 207
tortillas
  Asian steak tacos with bok choy slaw 155
  baked Cajun tortilla chips with beans + guacamole 106
  bean, corn + kale chilli tacos 122
  beef tostadas with charred corn salsa 159
  mozzarella quesadillas 78
tuna, French tuna, egg + caper pan bagnat 97
Turkish lamb kofte + cauliflower 'couscous' 133

V
vanilla
  vanilla lemon ricotta 44
  vanilla syrup 221
vege-packed spaghetti Bolognese 157
vegetable topping 207
vegetables *see also* salads; particular vegetables
  avocado, haloumi + grape quinoa salad 102
  baked samosas with pineapple salsa + kasundi 130
  Korean beef + vegetable bowl 149
  lentil + vegetable curry 115
  ratatouille 197
  roast vegetable + miso dressing noodles 86
  roasted 176
  vege-packed spaghetti Bolognese 156
  vegetarian pad thai 124
  with raita 176
vegetarian pad thai 124
venison
  black pepper steak + mushroom pie 146
  naked burgers with quick beetroot relish + kumara chips 164
Vietnamese chicken, cashew nut + herb noodles 84
Vietnamese dressing 84
Vietnamese pork meatballs with rice noodle salad 160

W
walnuts
  ricotta, pear, honey + walnuts topping 65
warm chickpea salad 198
wedges 208
whole flounder with ratatouille 197
wraps *see also* sandwiches; toppings
  chicken + pineapple curry garlic naan wrap 190
  Lebanese breakfast wrap with hummus, tomato, spinach + feta 61

Y
yoghurt
  berry + cinnamon cream yoghurt mille-feuille 249
  berry yoghurt ice-blocks 260
  chipotle yoghurt 159
  coriander + mint yoghurt 184
  dill yoghurt 133
  raita 176
  raspberry, apple, avocado + yoghurt smoothie 33
  yoghurt dressing 99

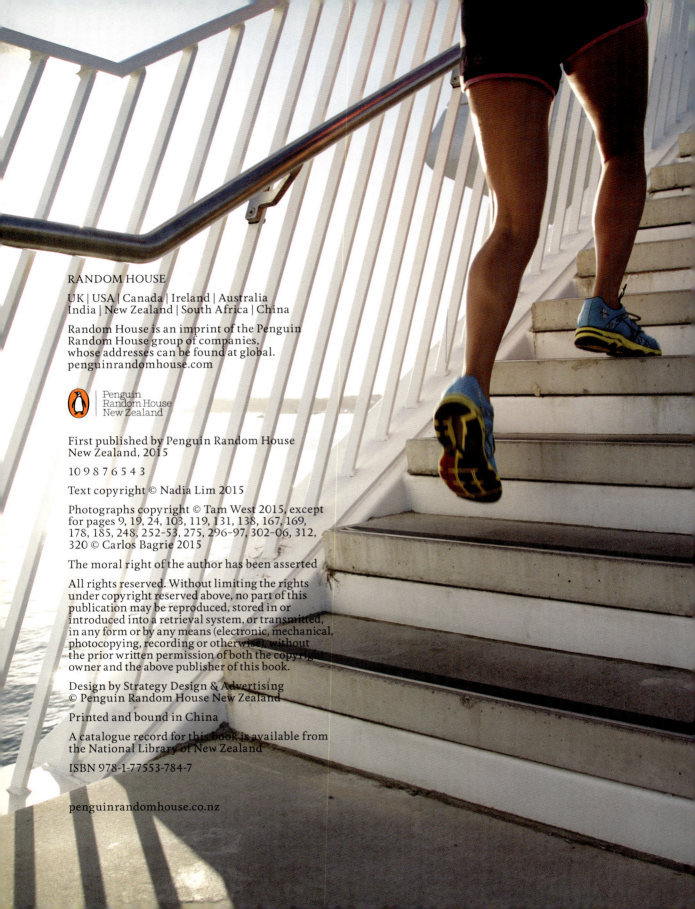

RANDOM HOUSE

UK | USA | Canada | Ireland | Australia
India | New Zealand | South Africa | China

Random House is an imprint of the Penguin Random House group of companies, whose addresses can be found at global.penguinrandomhouse.com

Penguin Random House New Zealand

First published by Penguin Random House New Zealand, 2015

10 9 8 7 6 5 4 3

Text copyright © Nadia Lim 2015

Photographs copyright © Tam West 2015, except for pages 9, 19, 24, 103, 119, 131, 138, 167, 169, 178, 185, 248, 252-53, 275, 296-97, 302-06, 312, 320 © Carlos Bagrie 2015

The moral right of the author has been asserted

All rights reserved. Without limiting the rights under copyright reserved above, no part of this publication may be reproduced, stored in or introduced into a retrieval system, or transmitted, in any form or by any means (electronic, mechanical, photocopying, recording or otherwise), without the prior written permission of both the copyright owner and the above publisher of this book.

Design by Strategy Design & Advertising
© Penguin Random House New Zealand

Printed and bound in China

A catalogue record for this book is available from the National Library of New Zealand

ISBN 978-1-77553-784-7

penguinrandomhouse.co.nz

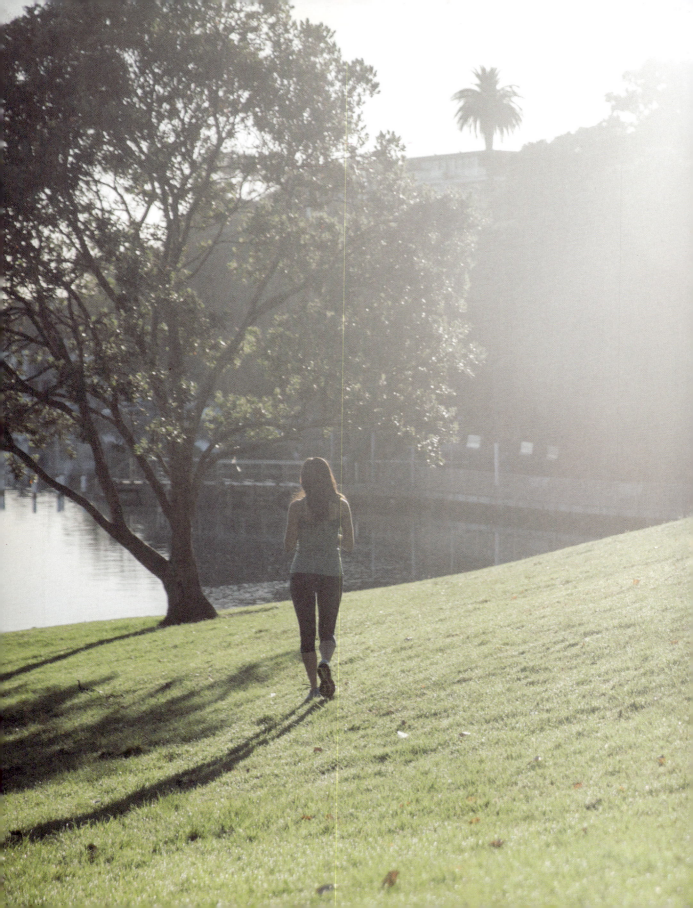